*a clinician's view
of neuromuscular diseases*

The cover illustrations are from photographs taken at the Muscular Dystrophy Association's Summer Camp held in the Center for the Handicapped, Babler State Park, Missouri, 1976.

a clinician's view
of neuromuscular
diseases

Michael H. Brooke, M.D.

*Professor of Neurology and Director, Jerry Lewis Neuromuscular
Research Center*
Washington University
School of Medicine
St. Louis, Missouri

The Williams & Wilkins Company/Baltimore

Library of Congress Cataloging in Publication Data

Brooke, Michael H
  A clinician's view of neuromuscular diseases.

  Includes bibliographies and index.
  1. Neuromuscular diseases. I. Title. [DNLM: 1. Neuromuscular diseases. WE550 B872c]
RC925.B76   616.7'4   76-54356
ISBN 0-683-01063-8

Composed and printed at the
Waverly Press, Inc.
Mt. Royal and Guilford Aves.
Baltimore, Md. 21202, U.S.A.

preface

This book will be prefaced by an apology, although probably not that which many will demand. It is a short work and will disappoint those who expect an encyclopedic compendium. Such tomes are often accompanied by so large a price that they are a luxury not to be afforded by the average physician with a peripheral interest in the subject. This book is aimed at the neurologist, pediatrician, orthopedist, and general practitioner who are aware that a bewildering array of neuromuscular diseases has surfaced in the last few decades unaccompanied by a simple text to describe them.

My own prejudices, carefully nurtured over a period of years, are here displayed for all to see. I have tried to identify such idiosyncrasies when appropriate but I do not apologize for them. They have been garnered during the time spent caring for patients with muscle diseases and I am reluctant to abandon them. A book is after all a personal thing. It is also delicate and the impassive citation of contradictory articles or the recitation of 200 rare but possible complications of a given disease can wilt it. I have chosen to emphasize some aspects of the illnesses and to ignore others. Such selectivity is not without purpose, reflecting the amount of time spent discussing the various topics in my own clinic and the frequency with which certain questions are asked.

My approach to the bibliography may appear capricious. I have often not quoted the original article, and those whose pioneer work is recognized in dozens of other texts may not necessarily find themselves in this one. Whenever possible I have tried to list the most recent references in the hope that the interested reader will consult their bibliographies and begin that backward chase in the literature which will culminate in the discovery of the original sources. In areas which have been subject to much recent research or change I have tried to include a complete list of references. In other areas, where knowledge has progressed not in leaps but in a shuffle, the bibliography is less complete.

Of all these shortcomings I am unrepentant. The substance of my apology is of an entirely different matter. I was raised in a country where style was thought more important than substance; even, harsher critics may say, to the point of supplanting it on occasions. I was determined to write a literate book. Regrettably I failed. I found myself tainted by jargon, cliche, and tautology in a most inexcusable fashion. Inappropriate gerunds jostled with split infinitives. Weakness existed, not in isolation, but had to be "significant" or, even

v

worse, "motor." Tenses mixed more readily than tonic water and the proper use of the comma eluded me, totally. The sentences which failed to contain the word "however" were all prefaced by "although." In short, it had all the characteristics of a standard medical text. Thanks to the unflagging efforts of the copy editor, the damage done to the English language has been healed but my literary style remains moribund.

And so, to our predecessors who felt that men of science were necessarily men of letters, to those whose clinical descriptions sparkled from the early texts so that in the reading of them one glimpsed the patient himself, to those whose letters to the editor made medical journals prior to 1920 so much less dusty than their recent counterparts—my apologies.

                                                                    M.H.B.

acknowledgments

I would like to acknowledge the support of the Muscular Dystrophy Association. Those of us who work in their clinics or attend their summer camps have found that the MDA is more than just a source of research funds. The James H. Woods Foundation was kind enough to provide some much needed support during the writing of this book. I would also like to thank Ms. Candy Palmer in Denver and Mrs. Sally Kraus and Ms. Linda Klippel in St. Louis. Their secretarial help was invaluable but, more remarkably, they tolerated my importuning with great good humor.

contents

1 the symptoms and signs of neuromuscular diseases

Please listen to the patient, he's trying
to tell you what disease he has

THE SYMPTOMS

It often seems that the urgency with which physicians rush their patients off for laboratory studies has its historical equal only in the migration of lemmings or the precipitous rush of the Gadarene swine. I sometimes suspect that students entering medical school are issued with a pamphlet entitled "How To Employ Your Time Usefully While the Patient Is Giving His History." It unnerves me when a physician misses the classical history of myasthenia because he is busy filling out requests for laboratory tests which will cost the patient a month's wages. Perhaps these feelings are unwarranted, but the exercise of diagnosing a patient's illness from his own words is a rewarding one and worth a few comments.

The way in which the history is obtained from a patient with neuromuscular disease is no whit different from the method used in any other illness. The symptoms may be different but the principles are identical. As each symptom is given, it should be pursued with a dogged tenacity until all the details are known. Thus, inquiry is made into the duration of the symptom, whether it is constant or intermittent, exacerbating or relieving factors, whether or not there are associated symptoms (such as pain), the effect of medications, and whether the symptom is progressing or diminishing.

In general, the symptoms of neuromuscular illnesses are those of weakness. However, the English language is on occasion an inexact form of communication. The statement that certain muscles are "weak" should not be accepted at face value. Indeed, patients often use the words "weak," "numb," and "tired" interchangeably. Some patients with a dense sensory loss complain that their legs are "weak." Equally, people with a marked motor disturbance may use the word "numb" for this loss of power. Any patient who complains of weakness must be pressed to describe the fashion in which the weakness affects him and what tasks he finds difficult.

1

It should be possible after obtaining the history of a patient with neuromuscular disease to predict with some accuracy which muscle groups are weak. When muscle strength is lost, the resulting symptoms depend more upon the muscle groups involved than upon the type of disease that causes the weakness. A patient who has a peripheral neuropathy may have the same difficulty with hand movement as one whose weakness is due to a distal myopathy. Thus, from the patient's own description of his disease one will be able to say where the weakness is, but perhaps not what the disease is.

Much of what follows is self-evident, but the frequency with which these complaints occur in patients with neuromuscular disease and the infrequency with which hysterical patients manifest these symptoms make it worthwhile to catalog them.

Head and Neck

When the muscles of the head and neck are weak, clear cut difficulties occur. Weakness of the upper eyelids may be perceived by the patient, who may complain that they are drooping. On the other hand, this is not always the case and one patient with a moderate degree of ptosis presented with the complaint that her head was falling backwards. In an attempt to peer from under her ptotic lids she would hold her chin tilted upwards, the very image of the proverbial haughty dowager.

Weakness of the extraocular muscles is noted initially as blurring of vision and ultimately as diplopia. Since diplopia is not infrequently seen as an hysterical complaint, it is wise to ask whether the patient has discovered any maneuvers which improve the double vision. Those with diplopia due to extraocular weakness will usually state that if they cover one eye the diplopia disappears. By and large, this fact is unknown to the hysteric and although there are many causes of monocular diplopia, from lesions of the occipital lobe to abnormalities of the retina and cornea, the history of monocular diplopia must be regarded with some suspicion.

Weakness of the masseter and temporalis muscles is noted as a difficulty in chewing. Although the chewing of any food may be impaired, it is usually steak or other meat which causes the first symptoms. Occasionally the jaw weakness may be so severe as to give rise to the complaint that the jaw sags and the mouth opens uncontrollably.

Weakness of the facial muscles produces several characteristic difficulties. When severe, the face is expressionless, the mouth is unsmiling, and, when the patient sleeps, his eyes are open, only the whites showing between the unclosed lids. In a moderate degree of facial weakness the smile may have the appearance of a rather unpleasant snarl which is embarrassing to the patient. Ordinarily in smiling and laughing the orbicularis oris keeps the lips inverted in the nature of a purse string. In facial weakness the lips are allowed to evert. This snarling appearance may be so disturbing that the mouth is reflexly hidden behind the hand whenever the patient laughs. Other tasks that are impeded by facial weakness are whistling, drinking through a straw, and blowing up a balloon. All of these functions may be impaired in patients who have no idea that their face is at all weak. Patients presenting in middle age with facioscapulohumeral dystrophy who state that their disease began two or three years ago often admit on direct questioning that they have never been able to whistle with the lips pursed. This is not regarded by the patient as an abnormality, but as more of an idiosyncrasy.

It is not easy to get a clear history of speech abnormality from most patients. The abnormalities of speech are quite characteristic when one hears the patient talk, but it is often difficult to distinguish a spastic dysarthria from that due to palatal weakness on the basis of the history. Difficulty with swallowing, however, is usually well described. Patients with palatal weakness and weakness of the pharynx due to lower motor neuron disease or to a myopathy frequently complain of choking. They have more difficulty swallowing liquids than solids, although both may present a problem, and they may suffer the regurgitation of fluids through the nose; the last symptom is less likely to occur with bilateral upper motor neuron disease (pseudobulbar palsy). With upper motor neuron lesions, there is a difficulty with the initiation of swallowing and often liquids will be aspirated into the trachea producing a coughing and choking spell.

Dysphagia is frequent enough in the hysteric and the symptoms are so similar in different patients that the term "globus hystericus" has been given to it. This symptom is usually associated with solid food; the patient has the sensation of a large ball of food which sticks in the back of the throat and will not go down or will descend part way to be lodged behind the larynx. This hysterical ball may last for hours and may be painful; nasal reflux and aspiration are not hallmarks of hysteria.

Other abnormalities of swallowing are produced by disturbance of esophageal function. The causes are varied and range from diseases of the esophagus such as scleroderma to compression by malignant lymph nodes. The patient often complains of a sensation of food sticking retrosternally. Unfortunately, the hysteric may complain of the same thing and it is difficult to distinguish this clinically.

Weakness of the neck muscles again produces difficulty in a characteristic situation. This is most striking when the patient is riding in a car or a bus. With sharp acceleration or braking, the strength of the neck muscles is not sufficient to counteract the inertia of the head and the head will snap uncontrollably backwards and forwards. This can be very disconcerting, and most patients with significant neck weakness give this history upon questioning. Neck weakness may give rise to problems in more bucolic situations, as illustrated by a man with weakness of the posterior muscles of the neck who was tending his rosebushes. As he bent forward from the waist to pluck one of the blossoms, his head fell onto his chest and he was unable to lift it again.

Limbs and Trunk

Weakness of the muscles of the limbs and trunk gives roughly four sets of symptoms: those associated with weakness of the shoulders, of the hands and forearms, of the hips and thighs, and of the lower legs.

Weakness of the shoulders is first noticed in performing tasks with the arms above the head: the housewife has difficulty lifting plates down from a high shelf; a carpenter complains that hammering nails into a beam which is over his head is becoming impossible. A more severe degree of difficulty may give problems with much simpler tasks. Thus, a man may have to use both hands to hold his razor while shaving or a patient may not be able to comb her hair without resting her elbows on a table and bringing her head down to a lower level. Patients may also complain that they have to "throw" their arms in order to get their hands onto a shelf at shoulder height. This throwing motion is a truncal movement which results in the arm being flung upwards; the hand then catches the desired spot and pulls the arm up onto the shelf.

Weakness of the muscles of the hands and forearms gives rise to difficulty opening the screw cap tops on jars or opening door handles, particularly of the door knob type. Additionally, car door handles may present a problem. Occasionally very specific disabilities may occur with hand weakness. One lady's chief complaint was that she could not reach behind her back and undo her brassiere. Her abnormality was a median nerve palsy with weakness of the abductors of the thumb and of the opponens muscle.

Most are familiar with the symptoms associated with hip weakness. With mild hip weakness the patient runs poorly and in an ungainly fashion. He is unable to jump and, as the weakness becomes more severe, he cannot easily get up from a sitting position on the floor and may have difficulty climbing stairs or arising from a chair. In arising from the floor patients will mention that they have to pull themselves up on a nearby chair or use their hands to support their knees. They may suddenly grow to dislike a favorite arm chair because it is low enough to present difficulties in arising from it. In trying to stand they have to push themselves up with their hands on the arms of the chair. Often they will prefer to sit on a kitchen chair and then, eventually, a high stool to allow them to stand up using the minimum amount of muscle effort. Climbing stairs always presents a problem to the patient with hip and thigh weakness. Patients with hip weakness will find it necessary to hang onto the banister to pull themselves up the stairs or to support the thigh with one hand while ascending. Interestingly, patients with thigh weakness have more difficulty coming down stairs than they do going up. As one foot descends to the lower step, the opposite quadriceps must take up the strain of the bent knee and support the entire body weight until the foot rests on the lower step. In those with quadriceps weakness there is a tendency for the knee to give way and collapse causing the patient to fall the rest of the way down the stairs. This quadriceps weakness also may cause the patient to fall if he is jostled in a crowd.

It is important to distinguish the symptoms listed above from those which are seen in hysterical weakness. I try to avoid the use of leading questions while taking a history and, if a patient complains of weakness and does not spontaneously volunteer the information with regard to stairs and chairs, I will ask whether he has any difficulty with common objects around the house. If this does not elicit the history above, I will ask about difficulty with chairs or with stairs. The patient with real weakness immediately seizes upon this and provides the appropriate complaint. The patient with imagined weakness is still not clear as to the direction of the inquiry. Finally, when pressed to give specific details of their difficulty in getting out of a chair, patients with hysterical weakness will often say that they are just too tired and they cannot get out of the chair. When asked about climbing stairs they usually admit to climbing two or three, after which effort they must rest. Seldom do they experience the difficulties listed in the previous paragraphs.

Weakness of the calf muscles and the anterior tibial group of muscles leads to problems while walking. Weakness of the evertors of the foot and the dorsiflexors of the foot causes the patient to lift his knee high in the air, and the gait may have a noticeable slapping quality. When the weakness is not so severe, the patient may complain only that he sprains his ankles very easily and that he finds it difficult to walk over a pebbled surface or a cobblestone street. This is due to the fact that if he steps on a pebble with the medial side of the foot, the foot is inverted and the weight of the body acts to accentuate this inversion. The evertor muscles are too weak to correct the movement; the foot is twisted and the ankle sprained. One of my patients, when asked about walking over rough or uneven surfaces, told me that he thought he would trip over a cigarette paper if it was in his path. Patients with such anterior tibial and peroneal weakness also catch their toes on curbs as they step over them. This may cause them to trip and fall. One interesting aspect of anterior tibial weakness is the problem which occurs in standing up from a sitting position. In order to stand up from a chair, the feet have to be dorsiflexed. If a patient is sitting in a chair with the knees at 90 degrees and the feet firmly on the floor, the initial movement in getting out of the chair is a dorsiflexion of the feet. If you wish to prove this for yourself, sit in a chair with your hands over the anterior tibial muscles and feel them contract as you start to arise from the chair.

Weakness of the muscles of the calf will result in a loss of the "spring" to the step, which assumes a "flat footed" character, and, of course, the patient has difficulty standing on his toes.

THE SIGNS

The physical examination of patients with neuromuscular disease often perplexes those who are unfamiliar with these illnesses. Such perplexity is unnecessary since the examination is basically very simple. There are four aspects to it: inspection, palpation, examination of reflexes, and evaluation of muscle strength. It is also convenient to take the various parts of the body in sequence. The head and neck, the shoulders, the arms, the torso, the hips, and the legs are all examined separately. If one does this conscientiously, it is difficult to miss significant findings.

Inspection

Inspection of the muscles reveals the presence or absence of wasting as well as the occurrence of any spontaneous movements such as fasciculations or myokymia. Weakness of muscles also alters a patient's resting posture in some quite characteristic fashions. These postural alterations are often far more helpful in determining the extent of weakness than is the more formal evaluation of strength.

Examination of the muscles of the head and neck may reveal ptosis (Figures 1.1 and 1.2). With ptosis of moderate degree the affected lid or lids will be obviously droopy and part of the iris will be covered. Ptosis may be so severe that the lid covers the pupil, making vision impossible in any direction other than downward. The patient must then retroflex the neck in order to see straight ahead. In a mild ptosis, the lower border of the affected eyelid

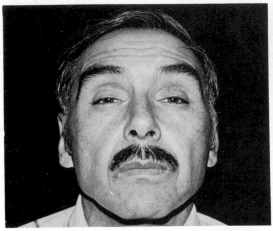 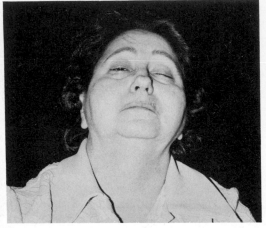

Figure 1.1 (*left*). Ptosis. Notice the compensatory elevation of eyebrows with consequent wrinkling of the forehead. Oculopharyngeal dystrophy.

Figure 1.2 (*right*). Ptosis. The head is retroflexed, allowing the patient to see from under her ptotic lids. This lady also has compensatory elevation of the eyebrows; she is keeping her left eye closed because of the diplopia from which she suffers. Myasthenia gravis.

may actually be at the same level with regard to the iris as the normal side. This is due to an elevation of the eyebrow, which hoists the ptotic lid upward. Such compensatory elevation of the eyebrow may be suspected when there is an increase in the number of forehead creases on the abnormal side. In such a case, when the forehead is smoothed out by the examiner's hand and the eyebrows are at the same level, the ptosis will become apparent. Hysterical ptosis is one of the easiest diagnoses to make from inspection. Because of the fact that one cannot voluntarily close the upper eyelid without raising the lower lid at the same time, the patient with an hysterical ptosis always has a contraction of the lower lid. In other extraocular weaknesses the axes of the eyes may no longer be parallel and esotropia or exotropia may be noted.

Wasting of the temporalis muscles gives a hollowing of the temples and when it is associated with masseter atrophy imparts a cadaveric appearance. Severe weakness of the masseter muscles, such as is seen occasionally in myasthenia gravis, causes the jaw to open spontaneously. The patient counteracts this by supporting the jaw with one hand. The sight of a patient with his arm adducted and elbow flexed, propping the jaw on a table formed by the knuckles of his hand, is a characteristic and unmistakable one.

A large part of our communication with others is expedited by the play of emotion over our facial muscles. It is not surprising that weakness of these muscles is easily perceived. Although mild facial weakness may not be noticeable at rest, when the patient smiles or laughs the normally pleasant expression may be converted to a snarl. Spontaneous eye closure is frequently incomplete and when the patient blinks, the lids move slowly and without fully closing the eyes (Figure 1.3). Sometimes facial weakness may be detected by having the patient open his mouth. During this maneuver the normal activity of the facial muscles causes an elevation of the upper lip. If

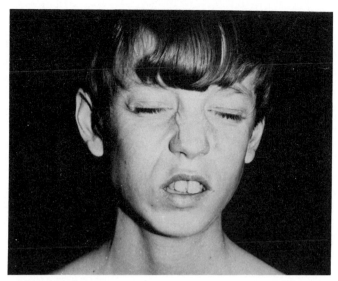

Figure 1.3. Facial weakness. Attempted eye closure does not result in complete occlusion of the palpebral fissure. The eyelashes are still visible and not 'buried' within the tightly closed lids. Inflammatory myopathy with IgA deficiency.

there is facial weakness, particularly unilateral facial weakness, the elevation of the upper lip is lacking. This results in a flattening of the upper border of the "cupid's bow," that area of the upper lip to which lipstick is applied. Severe weakness wipes the face clean of all expression: the skin is smooth and unwrinkled, and the mouth with its downturned corners lends an unusually mournful cast to an immobile mask.

Although one of the characteristic signs of facial weakness is the "bouche de tapir" — the tapir's mouth — in which the lips are protruded in unconscious mimicry of the animal, my experience has been that facial weakness is more easily noticed when viewed full face, because the lips have a flat, two-dimensional appearance. Instead of showing the normal curve, they look like two opposed rectangles. There is a classical neurological dogma that if the muscles of the forehead are spared the weakness affecting the rest of the face the lesion is of the upper motor neuron. Oddly, in neuromuscular diseases there are many exceptions to this rule.

Weakness of the palate may be difficult to see, although on occasion it hangs limp and unmoving. It is usually noted while listening to the patient talk. Although this section is devoted to inspection of the patient, it seems a convenient place to discuss abnormalities of speech. In lower motor neuron lesions involving the palate, the voice has an echoing, nasal quality, rather like that associated with a cleft palate. The vowels become hollow and the consonants, particularly such guttural sounds as the hard "G" and "C," are difficult to pronounce. Facial weakness will, of course, also give rise to speech abnormalities, but in this case the difficulty lies in the plosive sounds such as "P" and "B." Two other abnormalities of speech, although not due to palatal weakness, should be easily recognized. Spastic speech, that associated with pseudobulbar palsy (bilateral upper motor neuron lesions), has a forced quality. The voice sounds strained and monotonous. One perceives a sense of great effort on the part of the patient as he attempts to force words out through a reluctant musculature. On the other hand, speech associated with cerebellar difficulties is quite different. Here the speech is broken up and disjointed, sometimes described as "scanning." When the patient is asked to say test phrases, such as "liquid electricity" or "methodist episcopal," not only are the syllables disjointed, but the emphasis occurs on the wrong ones. Indeed, the whole manner of speech is as irregular and ataxic as is the violent intention tremor associated with lesions of the cerebellum. Laryngeal weakness may be noticed as a hoarseness of the voice with a rasping, brassy quality. A useful test of laryngeal function is to listen for the glottal stop. Ordinarily, when one coughs there is a small click at the beginning. This click is the same sound that is produced when the phrase "sofa and chair" is pronounced correctly. It occurs between the word "sofa" and the word "and." It may disappear in those of us with slovenly speech habits, in which case an "R" is substituted, as in "sofa-r-and chair." In laryngeal weakness, when the patient is asked to cough the initial glottal stop may be lost, the cough then resembling that of a dog in which the glottal stop is frequently not present.

Wasting of the sternocleidomastoids and of the trapezius is fairly easily noticed. When wasting of the sternocleidomastoids and the anterior neck muscles becomes marked, there is an odd appearance to the clavicles, which jut out in front of the wasted muscles (Figure 1.4). Wasting of the tongue is often hard to see but when present the tongue may become characteristically wrinkled or scalloped, especially at the lateral border.

Wasting of the muscles around the shoulders is easily seen (Figures 1.5 and 1.6). The bony prominences become more noticeable. Posteriorly, the spine of the scapula juts out, no longer hidden by the suprapinatus above and the infraspinatus below. The deltoid may be wasted, and a marked "step" is

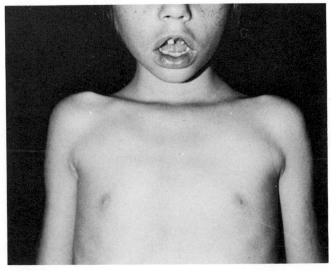

Figure 1.4. Neck and shoulder weakness. The clavicles form a "step" at the base of the neck. Infantile facioscapulohumeral dystrophy.

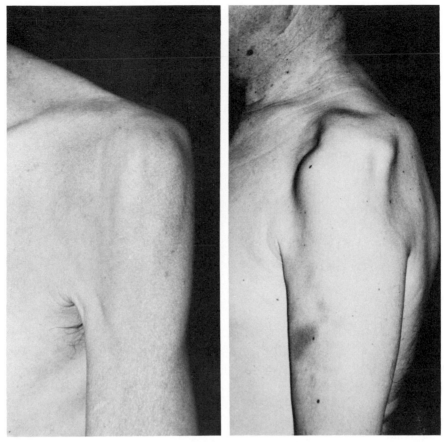

Figure 1.5 (*left*). Mild deltoid atrophy. Notice the stranded appearance of the underlying muscle, giving the appearance of ridges and hollows as one looks at the skin in oblique light. Motor neuron disease.

Figure 1.6 (*right*). Severe shoulder girdle atrophy. Motor neuron disease.

formed at the point of the shoulder. Seen from the front there may be a quite characteristic sign. As the shoulders become weak, the scapulae tend to slide laterally and upwards on the thorax as the muscle tone is no longer sufficient to brace them backwards. When this happens, the points of the shoulders tend to fold anteriorly, rather as if one were folding over the corner of a piece of paper in a dog-ear fashion. Since there is often associated pectoral muscle wasting, a crease is formed which runs diagonally from the axilla towards the neck (Figure 1.7). Winging of the scapula, in which the lower medial corner or sometimes the entire medial border of the scapula just backwards, may also be noticed (Figure 1.8). In slender people it may be difficult to determine whether or not this winging is of pathological significance. Many physicians employ the technique of having the patient push against the wall in order to determine whether or not the winging is real. I have found the following maneuver more reliable: The patient is asked to raise his arms outstretched in front of him until they are horizontal. He is then told to bring the arms slowly down again until the hands are at his side. In patients with winging of the

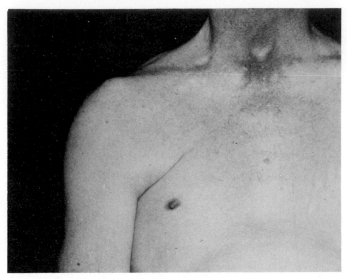

Figure 1.7. Shoulder weakness. The deep crease running from the axilla obliquely toward the neck is an indication of shoulder weakness with underlying pectoral atrophy. Limb girdle dystrophy.

scapula this downward movement always exacerbates the winging, and very often during the maneuver the medial inferior corner of the scapula pops backwards with a sudden rotary movement (Figure 1.9). Another sign of shoulder weakness which is extremely useful is the "trapezius hump." This is a prominence in the mid portion of the belly of the trapezius which is easily seen from in front (Figures 1.10 and 1.11). In patients with mild weakness, it is probably due to the activity of this muscle in trying to provide some support in fixation of the scapula. In more severe weakness the scapula itself rides up over the shoulder and is visible from in front (Figure 1.8). The trapezius hump is especially prominent during abduction of the arms, but may also be noticeable at rest. A secondary effect of shoulder weakness is on the position of the hands. In the normal standing posture the hands are held with the thumbs facing forwards. Weakness of the shoulder, with the attendant displacement of the scapula, causes the arm to turn so that the back of the hand now faces forwards (Figure 1.12). This is an extremely sensitive sign of shoulder weakness.

Inspection of the arms and hands is relatively straightforward. One looks for wasting in the biceps, triceps, and forearm muscles. As a practical tip, it is easier to look for wasting of the forearm muscles when the patient holds the arms forward with the elbows flexed, putting the forearms in a vertical position, a posture similar to that used in boxing at the turn of the century. The bellies of the muscles on the medial and lateral side of the forearms may then be compared and any wasting detected.

In examining the muscles of the hands the signs of flattening of the thenar and hypothenar eminence and of "guttering" of the interossei muscles are well known. One maneuver which is useful in patients who are suspected of having wasting of the first dorsal interosseous is to ask them to adduct the

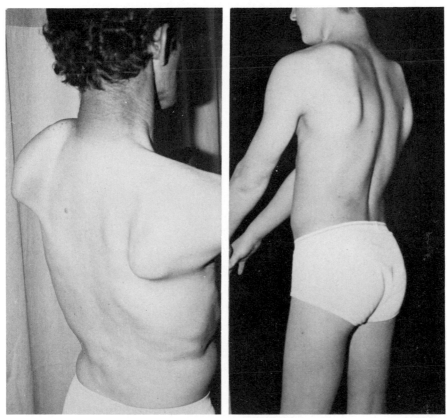

Figure 1.8 (*left*). Scapular winging. The patient cannot hold his arms out in front of him, and an attempt to do this results in the scapulae riding upwards and laterally over the back of the thorax. Facioscapulohumeral dystrophy.

Figure 1.9 (*right*). Mild scapular winging. When the patient is asked to hold his arms out in front of him and then to bring them slowly down again, as in this picture, the inferior medial corners of the scapulae pop back with a sudden movement. Limb girdle dystrophy.

thumb to the first finger. Normally this results in a prominent belly of the first dorsal interosseous muscle. In patients with wasting, the belly does not develop and palpation of the muscle reveals it to be rather flabby (Figure 1.13). Weakness of the muscles of the hand causes characteristic changes in the posture of the hand. Ordinarily a hand's normal posture is with the fingers semiflexed at all joints and the thumb held in a plane at right angles to the fingers (so that the thumbnail faces forwards when the hands are held by the side). In weakness of muscles of the thenar eminence the thumb rotates so that it lies in the same plane as the fingers—the so-called simian or ape-like hand. An additional abnormality is associated with weakness of the other small muscles of the hand. The fingers are held loosely, neither adducted nor abducted, and the fingers, although remaining flexed at the interphalangeal joints, become extended at the metacarpophalangeal joints producing the "claw" hand (Figure 1.14).

Inspection of the thorax and abdomen is less likely to be helpful in muscle

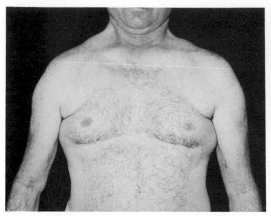 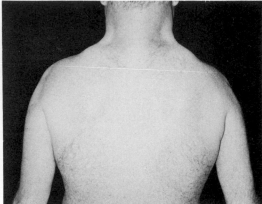

Figures 1.10 and 1.11. Shoulder weakness. Diagonal creases running from the axilla to the neck are visible. The clavicles slope downwards, and the "trapezius hump" is visible midway between the shoulder and the neck (1.10, *left*). This is also seen from the back, and some webbing of the lateral aspects of the neck is noted (1.11, *right*). Scapuloperoneal dystrophy.

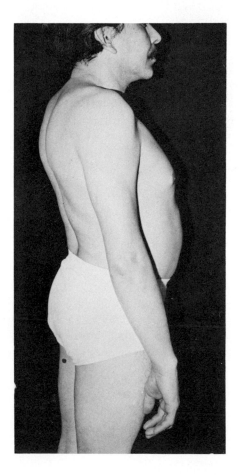

Figure 1.12. Shoulder weakness. Weakness of the shoulders allows the arms to rotate internally, and the backs of the hands face forward. This is an abnormal posture. In addition, this patient has a slight lumbar lordosis. Limb girdle dystrophy.

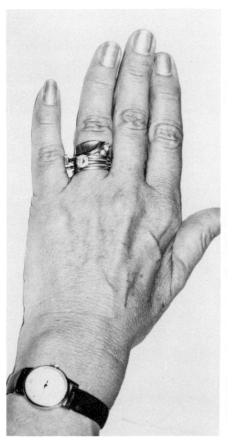 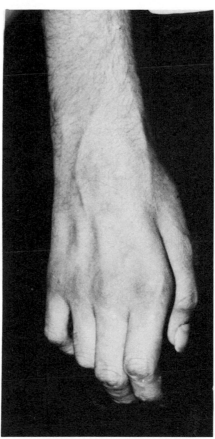

Figure 1.13 (*left*). Wasting of the hand. Notice the hollowing between the first two fingers and between the first finger and the thumb. Even the apposition of the thumb to the first finger has failed to produce any palpable muscle mass. Motor neuron disease.

Figure 1.14 (*right*). The posture of the paralyzed or claw hand. The fingers are held semiflexed, and there is some extension at the metacarpophalangeal joint. Motor neuron disease.

illnesses. Wasting of the intercostal and paraspinal muscles accentuates the bony prominences of ribs and vertebrae. Laxity of the abdominal muscles may cause sagging and folding of the skin when the patient stands, but, in general, these signs are more often associated with the chronically ill patient than one selectively affected by neuromuscular disease. About the most useful sign is the lumbar lordosis with its accompanying protuberant belly that is seen in cases with proximal hip and lumbar weakness. This is discussed in further detail below.

The quadriceps femoris, above all other muscles in the body, are most susceptible to wasting, and it is the vastus lateralis and medialis that bear the brunt of this wasting. The diagnosis of disuse atrophy should always be made with some reluctance, since focal atrophy of muscle groups is generally due to disease of the neuromuscular system rather than disuse, but it is remarkable how rapidly the quadriceps will waste following even a brief period of bedrest or as a result of pain in the hip or knee. Quadriceps wasting can be noticed more easily if the patient is asked to tense the thigh by making the knee stiff or fixing the kneecap. When this is done, the bellies of the normal medial and lateral vasti are prominent just above the knee. A wasted thigh is not only slender but also tapers perceptibly towards the knee.

When the muscles of the anterior tibial and peroneal groups are lost, the tibia assumes a "knife-edge" configuration owing to the prominence of its anterior border. A groove is seen immediately lateral to this knife-edge border. Sometimes a similar groove is seen in normal people of slight build, but if the patient is asked to dorsiflex the foot a distinction between the normal and abnormal can be made. Normally during such dorsiflexion the bulge of the anterior tibial muscle obliterates this groove. In abnormal wasting the muscle belly is not prominent and the groove persists. Loss of the gastrocnemii causes the medial and lateral bellies of this muscle to change from their normally rounded configuration to a tapering and flabby appearance. It is also useful to inspect the size of the extensor digitorum brevis. Both myopathies and neuropathies may cause a foot drop, but if the cause be due to a disease of the peripheral nerve, the extensor digitorum brevis is usually reduced in size. In a foot drop caused by a myopathy, such as in the scapuloperoneal syndrome, the extensor digitorum brevis is often hypertrophied, perhaps because this small muscle is used in a futile attempt to dorsiflex the feet by pulling up on the toes.

Finally, all the muscle groups should be examined to look for the presence or absence of fasciculations or other involuntary movements. One of the many unanswered questions in neuromuscular disease is how to differentiate benign fasciculations from those of pathological significance. Some have maintained that the benign fasciculation is a brief, repetitive twitch of the same group of muscle fibers occurring over a period of two to three minutes, whereas pathological fasciculations appear in many muscle groups in a random fashion. Watching a patient with diffuse fasciculations is reminiscent of watching the surface of a pond in summer when the fish are rising: the ripples arise here and there with no seeming pattern. Unfortunately, there is no hard and fast differentiation of benign from pathological fasciculations. It has been our experience that perfectly normal people without any neuromuscular disease have periods of time when fasciculations may be quite intense and diffuse. Isolated fasciculations may last for many days in a patient who fails to develop any sign of neuromuscular disease when followed over many years. Fasciculations are exacerbated by many factors, such as fatigue, both physical and mental, cigarette smoking, and the consumption of coffee or other caffeine-containing drinks. There is perhaps one clue to the fact that a fasciculation is of pathological significance, and this is related to the size of the fasciculation. A fasciculation is an involuntary discharge of one motor unit resulting in the contraction of all the muscle fibers supplied by a single nerve cell. When denervation occurs, the several hundred muscle fibers supplied by a particular nerve may become devoid of their nerve supply. Ordinarily they atrophy, but reinnervation from a neighboring nerve cell may occur. This results in the accumulation of additional muscle fibers within the newly formed motor unit. By a constant process of denervation and reinnervation, motor units may come to contain several thousand muscle fibers rather than a few hundred. If such a large motor unit is the site of a fasciculation, a large part of the muscle may be involved in a single fasciculation so that the twitch extends across a good portion of the muscle belly. This has a clinical correlation with the large fasciculations seen in denervating disease. Thus, the presence of a sizable fasciculation may be some indication of pathology. Unfortunately, this is less useful in practice, since by the time denervation and reinnervation are extensive and the fasciculations are large the disease is clinically apparent by other criteria.

A fasciculation is a brief twitch of a small portion of the muscle and should be distinguished from the phenomenon of myokymia. Some confusion has arisen in the literature, and on occasion the distinction is obscured. Myokymia is a repetitive train of action potentials causing a brief tetanic contraction of the muscle fibers of a motor unit. Because of the repetitive nature of the discharge, the visible contraction is much longer in its time course. The twitch-like character of a fasciculation is different from the more sinuous movement of myokymia. Moreover, myokymia seldom involves one nerve fiber alone. The same abnormality affects many motor units, and their contraction and relaxation gives an undulating character to the whole muscle which resembles the movement seen in a field of wheat as the wind blows across it. Myokymia is also more apt to move the joint across which the muscle acts than are fasciculations.

Palpation

After the muscles have been examined, additional information may be obtained by palpating the muscle and by percussing it. There is really no way to describe the texture of normal muscle except to say that it has a certain resilience; it is equally difficult to describe the abnormal. However, the physician who learns to tell the difference between a flabby, atrophic, denervated muscle and the peculiar rubbery consistency of muscle in Duchenne's dystrophy will find that palpation is a useful means of examination. One of the most characteristic signs is the feeling of the gastrocnemius muscle of a patient with the pseudohypertrophic form of muscular dystrophy (Duchenne's). The children's stores often carry toys fashioned after spiders, snakes, or monsters of various kinds. They are made of a plastic which has a jelly-like consistency and shakes and trembles in an all too life-like fashion, and they are usually an iridescent green or other inexcusable color. The muscle of a patient with Duchenne's dystrophy has almost exactly the same kind of feel as the substance out of which these toys are made.

A patient may experience pain while the muscle is being palpated, and this may also be helpful in the diagnosis. Sometimes fine nodules are felt beneath the skin or in the substance of the muscle in patients with inflammatory myopathies.

The evaluation of a patient's tone is more important in children than it is in adults. Even the concept of tone is a difficult one to explain. It means different things to physiologists, pediatricians, and neurologists. The word is used here to indicate the degree of resistance to movement that a limb has when the patient is relaxed. When the arm is picked up and the elbow flexed or the forearm gently shaken, the movements which occur at the elbow and the wrist are damped slightly by the normal tone in the muscles. The joints move freely and readily enough but a minimal amount of resistance can be perceived, even though it does not hamper the movement. In a patient who is hypotonic, the limb has all the resilience of overcooked spaghetti. It is impossible to describe this in words, and only the examiner's experience with patients with various degrees of tone will enable him to make an accurate assessment.

In children, the degree of head lag and the position of the body in ventral suspension are examined in addition to passive movement of the limbs. To evaluate head lag, the baby is placed on his back and his shoulders are raised by pulling his arms. Even the newborn child will make some attempt to flex his neck and bring the head up with the shoulders. Head lag is a phenomenon in which the head droops passively backwards and no attempt is made to raise it (Figure 1.15). The degree of tone may also be evaluated by holding the child under the trunk and lifting him clear of the surface in the supine position. In hypotonic conditions the body will assume the posture of an inverted U, whereas in a normal child, shortly after birth, the back will be relatively straight and the arms and legs flexed.

Very often in hypotonic children the joints are hyperextensible; for example, the fingers may be bent backwards to touch the forearms or the feet dorsiflexed so that the toes can be made to touch the shins. Although the term hypotonic is sometimes used for such joints, it is better to name them hyperextensible or hypermobile.

Increased tone in neuromuscular disease is usually associated with contractures of the muscles. A contracture is a shortening which occurs in the muscle in the absence of any voluntary activity or any electrical signs of muscle activity. It is most often associated with a fibrotic shortened muscle. The muscles around any joint may be involved; they usually shorten into the

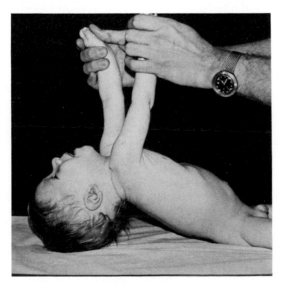

Figure 1.15. Abnormal "head lag." The baby is being pulled upwards by the arms, and the head lolls backwards without control. Infantile spinal muscular atrophy.

position which the patient adopts at rest. Thus, a patient confined to a wheelchair will have flexion contractures of the hips, knees, and elbows.

Percussion of the muscle may reveal the presence of myotonia, myoedema, or other abnormal direct percussion responses. Percussion myotonia is a sustained and uncontrollable contraction, associated with a delay in relaxation, produced by a sharp blow. It is characteristically sought in the thenar eminence, percussion of which causes an abrupt abduction of the thumb. The patient then struggles to get his hand back into the normal relaxed position. However, myotonia should also be looked for in muscles other than those of the hand. Percussion of the forearm over the extensor muscles of the fingers may result in the abrupt extension of the fingers followed by a slow downward drift as the myotonia relaxes. Another way of detecting myotonia is to slant a light obliquely across the belly of a muscle such as the deltoid. Percussion will then cause the contraction of a strip of the muscle, producing a depression which will be shadowed by the oblique light. This method is useful in eliciting myotonia of the tongue and muscles acting across large joints.

Myoedema is a phenomenon seen in hypothyroidism and in other metabolic abnormalities. Percussion of the muscle produces an initial depression which spreads outwards across the muscle rather like the ripples on a pond when a stone is thrown into the water. The initial depression then mounds upwards, giving the appearance of a small hillock where the muscle was percussed. The hillock may last for many seconds to minutes. Some have used the term myoedema for actual swelling of the muscle, as in a patient with a tender, painful muscle during an acute attack of polymyositis or of rhabdomyolysis. I think these two usages should be carefully differentiated and, at least in this book, myoedema will be used to indicate the percussion response.

Normal muscle will also contract upon percussion, particularly over the thenar eminence and the muscles of the forearm. However, the normal response is a brief contraction which immediately relaxes. It is usually not very marked, and the joint moves little if at all. Occasionally this percussion response may become quite brisk without having the characteristic delayed relaxation phase of myotonia. It is particularly seen in denervating illnesses and also in electrolyte imbalance in which the direct response to muscle percussion is augmented.

Reflexes

Examination of the deep tendon reflexes is an important part of the muscle examination. The reflexes which are evaluated are those of any standard neurological examination and include the biceps, triceps, supinator, knee, and ankle jerks together with the superficial reflexes of the abdomen and the plantar responses. With regard to the deep tendon reflexes, I have never really understood the sytem of grading which is used by many. I refer to the +, ++, +++, etc. system. I would like to believe that there are others equally baffled by this system, and I would, therefore, make a plea that reflexes be described as either absent, diminished, normal, or hyperactive. If it is necessary to add the comment that there is associated clonus, then so be it. At least this has the advantage of clarity when others subsequently read the patient's chart. In judging whether a reflex is hyperactive, attention is paid to the spread of the reflex to neighboring muscle groups and, most importantly, to the degree of "snap" in the muscle contraction. Ordinarily, when a tendon is tapped, the initial contraction of the muscle has a rather smooth quality before relaxing. If a tension recording were taken from the muscle, the familiar curve would be seen. In a hyperactive reflex, the initial upsweep of such a curve is very steep. This gives the appearance of a distinct snap to the muscle contraction. The tendon jerk becomes more jerky than usual, so to speak.

Muscle Strength

The evaluation of muscle strength is at the heart of the examination of the neuromuscular system. For the detailed evaluation of individual muscles, the classical monograph "Aids to the Investigation of Peripheral Nerve Injuries" by the Medical Research Council is enthusiastically recommended.[1] The grading system used therein is most useful. Strength is evaluated in the following categories: 0, no movement of the muscle; 1, flicker or trace of contraction; 2, active movement when gravity is eliminated; 3, active movement against gravity; 4, active movement against gravity and resistance; and 5, normal power. This elegant system of grading has been corrupted by at least a generation of neurologists. All of us insist on grading muscle as 4+, 3−, and so on. The disadvantage inherent in the system is that once a muscle becomes weak (i.e. grade 4) there is a wide variation in the degree of strength until a muscle loses the ability to move the joint against any resistance and becomes grade 3. This dilemma is a difficult one, and attempts to quantitate muscle strength exactly, by the use of dynamometers and so forth, have not yet produced a more reliable method. This led to the adoption of a system of functional muscle testing, a heresy which will be explained later.

It is time consuming to examine every muscle in the body, and most of us develop a shortened method. I think that an acceptable compromise is to examine the strength at each joint with all the movements possible at that joint. Thus, neck flexion, extension, and rotation are examined. Abduction, adduction, extension, and flexion of the shoulder, extension and flexion of the elbow are tested, and so on with all the joints of the body. This may not be pleasing to the purists, but it does have the advantage of enabling the examiner to see more than two patients in an afternoon.

It is important here to discuss another aspect of the evaluation of strength. It has been a frequent experience to see a patient whose weakness has been described as severe, only to find that his trouble is more psychological than muscular. Organic weakness gives very characteristic signs. The examiner can overcome the patient's best efforts to resist him, and the resistance which the muscle displays is uniform throughout the range of movement. Thus, if one is testing the abductors of the shoulders in a patient who is slightly weak, the patient is instructed to "make wings," the arms are held up horizontally, and pressure on the elbow allows the examiner to push the patient's arms downwards towards his side. The resistance that the examiner feels is the same at the beginning of this movement as it is when the patient's elbows have been forced down to 45 degrees. This is quite different from hysterical weakness, in which there is a sudden "giving way" phenomenon. In the same situation of testing shoulder abduction, it may initially be quite difficult to depress the patient's elbow but then the muscle suddenly collapses and the arm falls down to the side. In fact a repetitive "catch and give" phenomenon may occur, resulting in a feeling rather like cog wheel rigidity in which small contractions are succeeded by periods of relaxation. This is never due to muscle weakness; however, if the patient has pain in the joint being tested, the same result may be obtained. Thus, when the phenomenon of "sudden give" is detected in examining a muscle, the patient should be asked whether the joint or the muscle hurts. If such pain is present, it is impossible to get an accurate assessment of muscular strength. This last point cannot be stressed too strongly.

If a patient is suspected of having hysterical weakness, he should be observed closely to see whether, when he is unaware of scrutiny, he makes movements with the limb, which he denies being able to perform upon command; a patient who is totally unable to step onto a small stool may do so readily when he uses the stool to climb onto the examining couch. Another sign of value in the testing of a patient with suspected hysteria is to palpate the antagonist muscles while testing muscle strength. Thus, if one feels contraction of the triceps while the biceps is being examined, one may surmise that all is not well. Since this paragraph is degenerating into the nature of random thoughts, I will add one further which is of value. The presence of biceps weakness carries with it a useful clinical sign. The biceps strength is obviously tested with the wrists supinated. Patients with biceps weakness invariably use one of two tricks to try and overcome the examiner. The first is to rotate the forearm midway between pronation and supination, in which position the added help of the brachioradialis comes into play. The other maneuver is to pull the elbow backwards. This is so like the movement used by a bartender in pulling up a pint of beer that it has been called "the bartender's sign."

If heresy is to be preached it might as well be florid heresy. That which follows will, I am sure, provoke disagreement. I have found that the formal examination of muscle strength in the fashion mentioned above has not been as useful as the functional evaluation of a patient's abilities. The whole concept of functional muscle testing is to determine in what way the patient's functional abilities such as stepping onto a stool, climbing, getting up from a chair, and so on are disturbed. It is remarkable how the way in which a patient walks and does certain tasks will allow a quite accurate deduction of the muscle groups that are weak. An evaluation of the functional disability of the patient also provides more accurate testing of the progression or improvement of an illness. A patient may be able to arise from the floor only with difficulty and with the support of both hands when first seen, but some months later may get up with transient hand support on one knee. Formal testing of muscle strength in both these situations may reveal only grade 4 muscles. Thus the improvement cannot really be gauged from formal strength testing. I think we all find it difficult to put down in words how strong a muscle is, and functional testing is an attempt to make the evaluation more accurate.

Gait

Functional evaluation begins with an examination of the gait. Consider what happens to the gait if the patient has progressive weakness of the hip muscles. In normal walking, as the heel hits the ground and the weight of the body is transferred to that leg, the strain is taken up by those muscles which abduct the leg on the hip. Obviously, this does not cause an abduction of the leg while walking but, rather, prevents the pelvis from tilting sharply so that the opposite hip is dropped. This function of the hip abductors is best thought of as a shock absorbing mechanism which smooths out the shock transmitted from the leg to the pelvis. In minimal hip weakness, this action is lost. The patient's heel frequently hits the ground with a quite audible thud and the pelvis tilts abruptly to the opposite side. When the trouble is bilateral, as it usually is, this produces a heavy footed gait and a mild waddle. As the hip weakness becomes worse, other muscle groups are involved, particularly those of the hip and back extensors. This spreading weakness adds another characteristic to the walk. One normally stands with the back straight, and the body's weight acts through the center of gravity in a line which lies anterior to the hip joints. Thus, without the help of any muscle tone, the body would jack-knife forward at the hips. The hip and back extensors prevent such a collapse. When these muscles become weak, the patient develops a compensatory posture. The shoulders are thrown backwards and a lumbar lordosis becomes apparent. This enables the body's weight to be thrown on a line behind the hip joints, further accentuating the backward lean. The body cannot collapse from this position, since it is supported as much by bony and ligamentous structures as it is by muscle. The walk in such circumstances has the previous waddling characteristic, superimposed on which is a lumbar lordosis and an associated protrusion of the abdomen. The attitude in which the patient waddles gently down the street, arms thrown back and belly thrust forward, has been termed the aldermanic posture, a term which will become obsolete as the literature of Dickens gives way to video tapes of Westerns.

Weakness of the quadriceps muscles gives rise to a phenomenon called "back-kneeing" (Figure 1.16). During normal walking, the quadriceps act to stabilize the knee joint. There used to be a schoolboy trick, and I doubt that the practice has disappeared, in which one approached the victim from behind and tapped sharply on the backs of the knees. In the unwary, this resulted in a sudden collapse of the knees causing the victim some momentary panic before the quadriceps took up the strain. It is exactly this collapse of the knee joint that the patient with quadriceps weakness fears most. To protect himself, he will lock the knee backwards in a position of hyperextension. He does this while standing and also with each step that he takes. As his heel hits the ground the knee is thrust backwards; the joint is stabilized mechanically by this thrust.

At first one might think that shoulder weakness would give little abnormality in the way a patient walks. However, abnormal posture of the shoulder is easily noticed during walking. The scapulae are allowed to slide forward and laterally when the muscle tone is no longer sufficient to keep them braced backwards. This causes the shoulders to hunch and allows the arms to rotate so that the backs of the hands are facing forward. As the patient walks, a curious floppiness of the arms is added to this hunched appearance. The floppiness is due to the lack of stabilization of the upper arm by normal muscle tone. With each step the arm swings passively to and fro, a pendulum suspended from the shoulder.

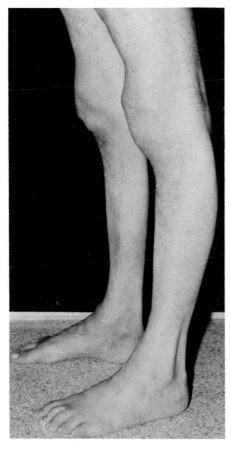

Figure 1.16. "Back-kneeing." In an attempt to stabilize the knee joint, it is thrust backwards and locked in a hyper-extended position. Limb girdle dystrophy.

Distal weakness of the legs causes another characteristic abnormality of gait. Weakness of the peroneal and anterior tibial groups hinders dorsiflexion of the foot. Walking is not easy for a patient with this problem; as the heel is lifted off the ground, the foot hangs limply from the ankle. The patient is in danger of tripping over any object which catches his toes, a danger which can be avoided only by lifting the knee high in the air. The patient is now faced with another problem. If he brings his foot downwards in a normal fashion, the toe will hit first and, because of weakness of eversion, he may well sprain his ankle as the foot collapses under him. Somehow or other he has to dorsiflex the foot, and since he cannot do this under muscular control he uses a short flinging movement of the lower leg in order to throw the toes upwards. He must get the foot quickly down on the ground following this, lest it passively falls back into plantar flexion. This quick throw and rapid descent produce the foot slapping gait. The sight of the high stepping walk with the foot being slapped onto the ground producing a noise like a clapperboard is almost unmistakable. Perhaps the word "almost" should be emphasized, because there is another gait that is superficially similar. Patients with loss of position sense in the feet also raise the legs high and stamp the feet on the ground, since they are not quite sure where the feet are nor yet where the ground is. They like to make firm contact with the foot, not only so that the forcible shock of the foot hitting the ground will force proprioceptive impulses through a somewhat jaded nervous system, but also so that they may hear the comforting sound of foot upon path. This results in a stamping gait as the patient goes on his uncertain way. The essential difference between these two kinds of walk is that in the stamping gait of a patient with position sense loss the foot is dorsiflexed when the knee is high, whereas in the steppage gait of a patient with anterior tibial or peroneal weakness the foot dangles limply from the leg. In weakness of the muscles of the posterior aspect of the calf, the spring to the step is lost and the patient may walk with a shuffle. It should be stressed that a significant amount of gastrocnemius weakness may be present without any detectable abnormality of gait.

In patients with weakness of the muscles of both anterior and posterior compartments of the leg, the ankle joint is unstable in quiet standing and the patient may shift his weight uneasily from foot to foot.

Perhaps brief mention should be made of the hysterical abnormalities of gait. These are always difficult to evaluate and the patient's disturbance is usually a bizarre one. All varieties are seen, from the patient whose every step is a slow and cautious exploration into unknown territory to those whose wild and acrobatic movements seem to bring them to the brink of disaster. It is interesting that if the physician can forbear from holding out a helping hand when the patient seems imminently on the point of collapsing to the floor, the hysteric will miraculously regain his balance and proceed unsteadily to some new predicament.

There are, of course, other abnormalities which may be seen when a patient walks. It is beyond the scope of this book to describe the walk in upper motor neuron illnesses, the gait of a patient with Parkinsonism, or the gait of those with cerebellar disorders. Each has its own characteristics and these are well described in the standard neurological texts.

Observation of a patient while he is carrying out some simple tasks is an important part of the examination. The activities which are most useful to watch are arising from a sitting position on the floor, arising from a chair, stepping onto a chair, stepping onto a foot stool, walking on the heels, hopping on the toes, and raising the arms above the head. Weakness of muscles produces definite alterations in the way these tasks are carried out. The fact that it is easier to get the cooperation of young patients with this series of tests than in attempting a more formal evaluation of strength is an added advantage.

Arising from the Floor

Ordinarily, a patient can arise from a sitting position on the floor swiftly and easily. He flexes his legs, drawing the feet under him; one hand may be transiently placed on the floor to provide an added push; he then adopts a squatting position. From this position he stands, keeping the trunk erect, simply by straightening his legs. Children usually dispense with any hand support and bounce to their feet before one really has time to analyze the movement. With the development of hip weakness, there is a rather systematic deterioration in this performance (Figures 1.17 to 1.27). Starting from the same position, sitting on the floor with legs outstretched, the patient with proximal hip weakness will start by making a quarter turn of the trunk,

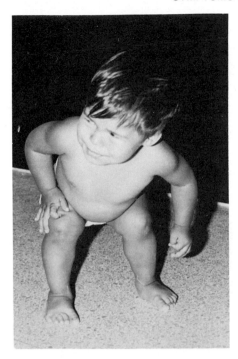

Figure 1.17. Mild hip weakness. In arising from the floor, this child placed his right hand transiently on his knee but required no other assistance. Duchenne's dystrophy.

usually to the weaker side. The hand towards which he is turning is then placed on the floor, and simultaneously the knees are drawn up under the body. The whole weight is then shifted, so that the patient is resting either on hands and knees or on one hand and one knee. In the next movement the patient straightens his knees raising his hips in the air. Colloquially, I know this as the "butt first" maneuver; the patient forms an arch with the buttocks at the apex. It is much easier for a patient to stand upright by straightening at the hips from this position than to arise from a squatting position. When the weakness is mild, a patient may arise readily from the floor when asked to do so; only the fact that he hoists his hips in the air before the rest of his body reveals his loss of strength. When the weakness of the hips is severe, the patient adopts the butt first posture more laboriously and, indeed, the arch that the body forms is precariously balanced. The feet are wide spread and the hands firmly planted on the ground. One hand is then placed upon the thigh, leaving the body supported on both feet and one hand. This is the "tripod sign," so called because of the three point base upon which the patient rests. A firm thrust of the hand on the thigh is sufficient to brace the trunk upwards and to allow some patients to stand. In others, both hands must be placed on the thighs to support the weight of the trunk. When viewed from the side, the body forms the shape of a capital A on its side with the apex being the hips and the cross bar the arms. The trunk is then inched laboriously upwards by the hands walking up the thighs. This entire maneuver is often known as Gower's sign. Because the hand support on the thighs is crucial to the performance of this movement it should be noted that variations exist. Some patients, particularly children with mild weakness, bend the arm and rest the elbow on the thigh when assuming the upright position. In others with

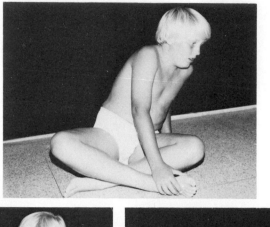

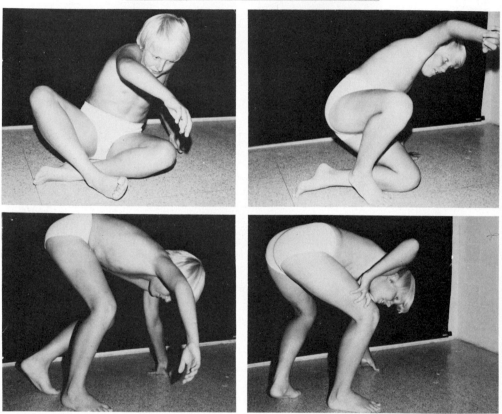

Figures 1.18 through 1.22. This series of photographs illustrates the various components which are analyzed in watching a patient arise from the floor. With a moderate degree of weakness such as this patient has, the first movement is a quarter turn of the body toward the weak side (1.18, *top*). Supporting himself with one hand on the floor, he rolls over, bringing his knees and feet under him (1.19 and 1.20, *center left and right*). The hips are then raised in the air while maintaining the support with one hand, the "butt first" maneuver (1.21, *lower left*). Finally, one hand is placed on the thigh to provide the additional support needed in straightening the body from this position (1.22, *lower right*). Non-progressive congenital myopathy, undiagnosed.

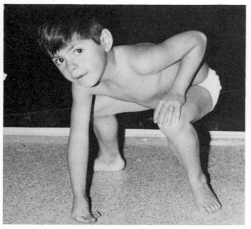
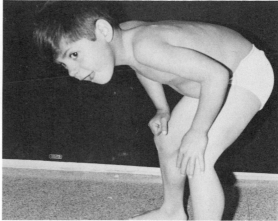

Figures 1.23 and 1.24. This patient arises from the floor with unilateral hand support on the floor but then requires bilateral hand support on the thighs in order to attain the upright position. Duchenne's muscular dystrophy.

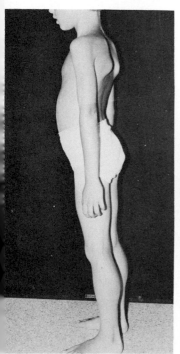
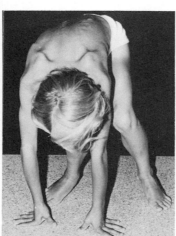
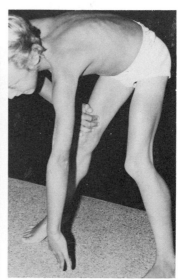

Figures 1.25 through 1.27. In this child, the degree of weakness is sufficient to produce a moderate degree of lumbar lordosis. The shoulder weakness is also apparent in the way in which the scapulae jut backwards (1.25, *left*). When he tries to arise from the floor (1.26, *center*), he needs bilateral hand support on the floor in the "butt first" maneuver. He then transfers his hand to his thigh (1.27, *right*), and stands by using bilateral hand support on the thighs. Duchenne's muscular dystrophy.

very mild weakness the hand may touch the thigh only transiently in a rather fluid movement as the patient stands. Some patients adopt a maneuver which is slightly different from the Gower's maneuver. They find it easier to arise from a sitting position by first placing both hands slightly behind them flat upon the floor. This is termed "backhanding" (Figures 1.28 to 1.30). The knees are then drawn up, and the initial few inches of movement are obtained by a push from both arms. The patient then arises from a squatting position in the usual fashion. This initial bilateral arm push is another indication of mild hip weakness.

In analyzing the various ways in which patients arise from the floor, each component movement should be noted. These are as follows: hand support on the floor, either unilateral or bilateral; the turning movement of the trunk; the butt first maneuver; and hand support on the thighs, either unilateral or bilateral, transient or labored. If all these aspects are observed during a

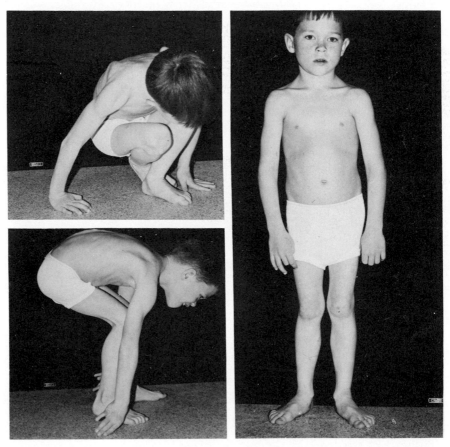

Figures 1.28 through 1.30. This patient adopts a slightly different maneuver in standing. He places his hands behind him on the floor (1.28, *upper left*), and then pushes upwards to assume the upright position (1.29, *lower left*). This is colloquially known as the "back-hand" maneuver. This child also had some distal weakness, and in quiet standing (1.30, *right*) it is seen that he has bilateral flat feet. In Figure 1.28, the scapular winging should be noted as he thrusts upwards off the floor. Juvenile spinal muscular atrophy.

course of an illness, there will be an easily noticed change in performance. This change may well occur at a time when formal testing of muscle strength does not show any difference.

Arising from a Chair

The patient is asked to sit in a chair and then to stand up. Most standard kitchen chairs are about 18 inches high. Ordinarily, this movement is performed without any assistance from the hands. Various changes are produced by different degrees of hip weakness. In early hip weakness the patient may need to put one hand on his knee or on the side of the chair and push briefly with this hand during the movement. As the weakness becomes more severe, it may be necessary to use both hands for support. Finally, not only must both hands be placed on the chair for support, but the patient then uses both hands to "climb up his thighs" in the typical fashion described above (Gower's maneuver). The patient may also begin the task by rocking the trunk backwards and forwards in order to gain the momentum to enable him to stand.

Stepping onto a Chair

Stepping up onto a chair between 18 and 20 inches high is a difficult task and, unless the patient feels secure in doing it, the examiner should not insist. Anyone who can do this movement quickly, without hand support and without pulling himself up on neighboring objects, has fairly good muscle strength. Early weakness of the hips results in a slight "pause" during the step. The patient places one foot on the chair and seems to gather himself for the effort. This hesitation is one of the earliest signs of hip weakness. The patient bends the knee of the leg which is still standing on the ground and then thrusts himself upwards. He now has to transfer his weight to the foot which is on the chair; in patients with some hip weakness, this is very often a moment of difficulty. Patients who are unable to do the task will fall back to stand on the other leg. Other patients may start to fall backwards momentarily but then catch themselves and are able to pull themselves up onto the chair. This results in a sag of the hip in mid movement, known as the "hip dip." Both the hesitation and the hip dip are indications of proximal weakness.

Stepping onto a Stool

I use a stool about 8 inches high for evaluating the stepping power of patients who are unable to step up onto a chair. This movement is usually an easy one and should be within the capabilities of even the elderly or the debilitated patient. Abnormalities in this movement associated with mild hip weakness are very similar to those described when the patient steps onto a chair. There may be a slight hesitation at the beginning of the movement. The hip dip presents often as a wobble in mid movement, almost as if the leg is about to give way. In addition, patients who have hip weakness may attempt to "throw" themselves up onto the foot stool. It is as if the whole body takes part in the movement upwards in a "throwing" motion, in which the shoulders seem to take as great a part as the hips. When the weakness becomes more severe, the patient may place one hand upon his knee in order to straighten the knee out and brace the trunk upwards, rather in the fashion that he does when arising from the floor (Figure 1.31). As the loss of strength progresses, the patient may have to use both hands, one on the knee and one on a nearby support, to pull himself up onto the stool. The movement is evaluated for both legs individually and is graded as to whether there is hesitation, a hip dip, an upward throw, and unilateral or bilateral hand support.

Walking on the Heels

Normally one can walk on the heel of either foot with the foot dorsiflexed, with no alteration in the posture of the trunk. Weakness of the anterior tibial muscles impedes this movement. It may be severe enough that the toes cannot be lifted from the ground at all. But in mild weakness the patient uses an alteration in his posture to enable him to do this. The knees are held stiffly and the hips are thrust backwards while slightly flexed, so that the trunk counterbalances the change in the weight distribution. This new posture results in the legs' slanting backwards when viewed from the side and gives the weakened anterior tibial muscles additional help in pulling the toes off the ground. Persons with normal strength never need to use this additional backward thrust of the hips to dorsiflex the feet.

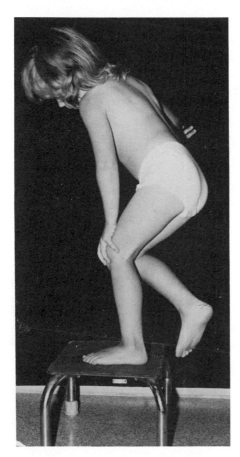

Figure 1.31. In stepping onto a stool a patient with a moderate degree of hip weakness uses the support of the hand on the knee to complete the task. Dermatomyositis.

Hopping on the Toes

The patient is asked to hop on the toes of one foot and then the other. Some patients whose walk is almost normal are not able to do this at all. This is one of the few sensitive tests to bring out weakness of the plantar flexors of the feet. The test should be interpreted with caution in those with severe thigh and hip weakness since the performance may be hampered by the patient's real fear of the leg collapsing at the knee. In such cases the patient can be asked simply to walk on his toes.

Raising the Arms above the Head

Ordinarily there is no difficulty in holding the arms straight and abducting them from the sides to bring them up above the head until the hands touch. When viewed from in front, the hands follow the circumference of a circle from the sides of the body to the mid line above the head. Patients with shoulder weakness adopt several tricks to try and overcome their difficulty. One of the earliest is a tendency to flex the elbows during the maneuver. A moment's reflection on the nature of levers and fulcrums will reveal that if the elbow is flexed the shoulder muscles have less work to do in supporting an arm abducted to 90 degrees. The second abnormality that may occur is the use of the trapezius and other accessory muscles during the movement. This results in a shoulder shrug as the movement is attempted. The last abnormality, which is seen in severe weakness, is found when a patient is unable to get the arms above the head unless he clasps his hands in front of him and pulls. I am not sure what the mechanism is, but this makes it easier for the patient to get his hands above his head.

The preceding series of tests can be done quite quickly and will give much useful information with regard to proximal weakness of the hips and shoulders and distal weakness of the legs. It is also obvious that these maneuvers will not give information with regard to the strength in the hands, forearms, and upper arms. This means that formal examination of the biceps and triceps, of the forearm extensors and flexors, and of the small muscles of the hands must be carried out.

CLINICAL DIFFERENCES BETWEEN MYOPATHIES AND DENERVATION

One of the most hallowed tenets of physicians interested in neuromuscular disease has been that disease caused by denervation is quite different from that caused by primary illnesses of the muscles. What was at one time a clear cut difference is now becoming a little blurred. Many times the distinction will be irrelevant because the actual diagnosis will be so apparent; a patient may be said to have facioscapulohumeral dystrophy or myasthenia gravis without even considering whether the disease is myopathic or neurogenic. At other times the cause of the weakness may be puzzling and it may then be useful to attempt the diagnosis of myopathy or neuropathy. The presence or absence of weakness is of no help, since both denervating diseases and myopathies cause weakness. It has been said that wasting is more associated with the denervating conditions than with myopathies. This is by no means always true, particularly in the chronic dystrophies. However, if the degree of weakness is out of proportion to the severity of the wasting, the disease is more likely to be due to a myopathic process. An illustration of this is seen in Duchenne's dystrophy, in which the muscles are bulky although the weakness may be quite pronounced. If, on the other hand, the wasting is severe and particularly if the muscle has a rather stranded appearance, as though it were broken up into individual bundles which can be seen through the skin, the disease is more likely to be a denervating one. Changes in the deep tendon reflexes tend to occur earlier in the myopathic conditions than they do in denervation. Again, the bulky muscle which is weak and in which the deep tendon reflex is absent is more likely to reflect a myopathy.

The presence of fasciculations, particularly when numerous, may indicate a denervating disease. Fasciculations occurring in the absence of weakness do not mean denervating disease, but if there is obvious weakness and wasting and fasciculations are pronounced, it is more nearly certain that denervation underlies the process. In addition, the more pronounced the fasciculation the more likely it is that the disease is of the anterior horn cell or of the proximal part of the nerve. Contractures may occur in either process but are more likely to occur early in the myopathies. This is particularly true of young children.

However when all is said and done, there are so many exceptions to the rules given above that one can only make a cautious interpretation. It is, indeed, much easier to arrive directly at the diagnosis after the physical examination and history than to become embroiled in the argument as to whether a disease is myopathic or neurogenic.

Most of the diseases in which weakness occurs are due to abnormalities of the anterior horn cell, peripheral nerve, neuromuscular junction, or the muscle itself. Upper motor neuron lesions will also cause paralysis, but the physical findings in this situation are so different that it rarely gives rise to confusion. It is true that in cerebral hypotonia in young children, diffuse diseases of the central nervous system may present with floppiness, but weakness is generally not a prominent part of this picture. At any rate, it is useful in considering the differential diagnosis of muscle diseases to consider the neuromuscular unit in this sequential fashion. The diseases to be described will also be listed in this order and will commence with illnesses which are known to involve the anterior horn cell.

BIBLIOGRAPHY

1. Medical Research Council. Aids to the investigation of peripheral nerve injuries. Her Majesty's Stationery Office, London, 1943.

FUNCTIONAL EVALUATION AND GRADING SYSTEM FOR NEUROMUSCULAR PATIENTS

The following forms are used in evaluating patients with neuromuscular disease.

In the first part (Chart 1.1), a detailed analysis is made of the way in which patients perform certain tasks, such as walking or stepping onto a footstool. This analysis is derived from descriptions given above.

In the second part (Chart 1.2), an attempt is made to grade the severity of

Chart 1.1.   Functional Evaluation—Muscle Patients

Date _____

Name_____

Diagnosis_____

Gait
1. Normal
2. Not possible
3. Loss of "shock absorbers"   Mild   Moderate   Severe
4. Compensatory lordosis   Mild   Moderate   Severe
5. "Back knee"   Mild   Moderate   Severe
6. Foot drop   Mild   Moderate   Severe
   Time to walk 30 feet

Stepping onto a Footstool

Right foot   Left foot

_____   Normal   _____
_____   Not possible   _____
_____   Hesitation   _____
_____   "Hip dip"   _____
_____   Throw   _____

             Hand support
_____   Unilateral   _____
_____   Bilateral   _____
_____   Transient   _____
_____   Sustained   _____

Arising from Floor
1. Normal
2. Not possible
3. Initial turn   0°   90°   180°
4. "Butt first" maneuver   Yes   No
5. Hand support
   1. Floor   Left   Right   Both
   2. Thigh
      A.   Left   Right   Both
      B.   Transient Sustained Repetitive
   3. "Back hand" support
6. Time

Arising from Chair
1. Normal
2. Not possible
3. Hand support
   1. Chair   Left   Right   Both
   2. Thigh
      A.   Left   Right   Both
      B.   Transient Sustained Repetitive
4. Time

Chart 1.1 — *Continued*

Stepping onto a Chair

Right foot		Left foot
_____	Normal	_____
_____	Not possible	_____
_____	Hesitation	_____
_____	"Hip dip"	_____
_____	Throw	_____
	Hand support	
_____	Unilateral	_____
_____	Bilateral	_____
_____	Transient	_____
_____	Sustained	_____

Chart 1.2. Grading System — Muscle Patients

Date _____

Name_____

Diagnosis_____

Hips and Legs

1 Walks and climbs stairs without assistance.
2 Walks and climbs stairs with aid of railing.
3 Walks and climbs stairs slowly with aid of railing (over 25 seconds for 8 standard steps or over 3 seconds for a single step).
4 Walks unassisted and rises from chair but cannot climb stairs.
5 Walks unassisted but cannot rise from a chair or climb stairs.
6 Walks only with assistance or walks independently with long leg braces.
7 Walks in long leg braces but requires assistance for balance.
8 Stands in long leg braces but unable to walk even with assistance.
9 Is in wheelchair.
10 Confined to bed.

Arms and Shoulders

1 Starting with the arms at the sides, the patient can abduct the arms in full circle until they touch above the head. Can place a weight of 2-kg or more on a shelf above eye level.
2 Can raise arms above head as previously but cannot place a 2-kg weight on a shelf.
3 Can raise arms above head only by flexing the elbow (i.e. shortening the circumference of the movement) or using accessory muscles.
4 Cannot raise hands above head but can raise 8 oz. glass of water to mouth.
5 Can raise hands to mouth but cannot raise 8 oz. glass of water to mouth.
6 Cannot raise hands to mouth but can use hands to hold pen or pick up pennies from table.
7 Cannot raise hands to mouth and has no useful function of hands.

Bulbar Function

1 Normal speech and swallowing.
2 Speech and/or swallowing is abnormal but presents no practical difficulty.
3 Speech is occasionally difficult to understand and/or the swallowing difficulty causes occasional choking (on a daily basis).

4   Speech can be understood by close friends or relatives but it is difficult for casual acquaintances to understand and/or swallowing difficulty is always present and prolongs mealtimes.

5   Speech is impossible to understand even by close friends or swallowing is impossible.

Composite Grade ＿ ＿ ＿

Chart 1.3.   Pulmonary Evaluation – Muscle Patients

Date＿＿＿＿＿＿＿＿

Name＿＿＿＿＿＿＿＿＿＿＿＿＿＿＿＿＿＿＿＿＿＿＿＿＿＿

Diagnosis＿＿＿＿＿＿＿＿＿＿＿＿＿＿＿＿＿＿＿＿＿＿＿＿

Forced vital capacity	＿＿L
% predicted vital capacity	＿＿
Peak flow	＿＿L/second
% FEV* 0.5 seconds	＿＿
% FEV 1 second	＿＿
% FEV 3 seconds	＿＿
Resting ventilation (L/minute)	＿＿L
Maximum voluntary ventilation (L/minute)	＿＿L

---

the patient's illness. The grading basically follows the outline suggested by Vignos et al.,[1] but has been modified and expanded. The method which these authors proposed was of particular use in Duchenne's muscular dystrophy and focused mainly on hip weakness. In any neuromuscular disease it is the hip weakness that produces the maximum disability; therefore, this emphasis has been retained. In order to give some weight to disability of the arms and of the bulbar musculature we adopted a modification. Patients are rated using a three digit number. The first digit is determined by hip and leg function. The second digit refers to the shoulder and arm function, and the third to bulbar function. This makes the method applicable to other diseases although the first digit still gives the most useful evaluation of the overall severity of the disease. Thus a patient with Duchenne's dystrophy who is confined to a wheelchair, can feed himself, cannot raise his hands fully above his head, but has no difficulty swallowing or talking would be graded 941. A patient with motor neuron disease, on the other hand, who is able to walk relatively normally but cannot use his arms and has severe difficulty with bulbar musculature might be graded 164.

Pulmonary evaluation is also carried out, as illustrated in Chart 1.3.

BIBLIOGRAPHY

1. Vignos, P. J., Spencer, G. E., and Archibald, K. C. Management of Progressive Muscular Dystrophy in Childhood. JAMA *184:*89–96, 1963.

2

diseases of the motor neurons

ACUTE INFANTILE SPINAL MUSCULAR ATROPHY (ACUTE WERDNIG-HOFFMANN DISEASE, SPINAL MUSCULAR ATROPHY TYPE 1)

Clinical Aspects

This illness is a degenerative disease of the anterior horn cells and of the motor nuclei of some cranial nerves, generally inherited as an autosomal recessive gene. The majority of patients with acute infantile spinal muscular atrophy present a rather stereotyped picture. The child's mother may notice during the last months of pregnancy that the normal abrupt kicking movements of the healthy fetus are enfeebled or disappear entirely. When questioned about this change in fetal movements, as many as a third of the mothers acknowledge the symptom,[1] although it is seldom volunteered. In more than half of the patients, abnormality is noticed at birth or within the first few days. The baby may be extremely limp, and the infant's lusty cry is supplanted by a plaintive mewling. Respiratory distress is apparent early, and the generalized weakness is often severe enough to prevent the child from moving arms or legs. Weakness of bulbar muscles may make each feeding time an arduous procedure lasting an hour or more.

In other cases the infant is normal for the first few weeks of life and then a generalized weakness of limbs, trunk, and bulbar muscles ensues. The child's parents often have difficulty in deciding the exact time of the first symptoms and it is only when one of the motor milestones, such as lifting the head, is missed that the effects of the illness are noted. Rarely, the weakness seems to appear with surprising suddenness and may be thought by the parents to be related to an injury, infection, or immunization. Whatever the mode of onset, the symptoms of acute spinal muscular atrophy are manifest by the age of 3 to 6 months. Early in the disease the child's posture is typical: he lies spread-eagled with the thighs splayed apart, flat upon the surface of the examining table. The knees are flexed in the characteristic "frog-leg" position (Figure 2.1). The arms assume a similar posture of abduction with the elbow flexed. The child's arms are usually externally rotated so that the forearms rest on the examining table beside his head. On occasions the arms may be internally rotated, bringing the forearms down parallel to the trunk. There may be small flickering movements of the feet and hands at rest. The chest is thin, with the ribs easily visible, and is often flattened as if the thorax were unable to support its own weight. Paradoxical movement of the thorax occurs so that during inspiration the descent of the diaphragm causes further flattening of

34

the thorax; the rise and fall of the abdominal muscles are the major movements to be seen (Figure 2.2). Almost uniformly, such children have an alert and lively expression. The eyes turn quickly to the examiner even though the head cannot. The muscles of facial expression are only mildly weak; one does not see in spinal muscular atrophy the paralysis of the face which is so common in infantile myotonic dystrophy and infantile facioscapulohumeral muscular dystrophy. The mild amount of facial weakness and wasting may give the expression an elfin look. The children are quick to smile and become the favorites of nurses and doctors alike. The extraocular muscles are not affected. The muscles involved in feeding may be severely affected, and feeding difficulties are often the initial complaint. Pooling of saliva in the nasopharynx together with the diminished respiratory movements results in a faint and continuous bubbling sound. Fasciculations of the tongue are seen in about half of the patients. They occur as discrete, tiny indentations which appear to be close to the surface of the tongue, and should not be confused

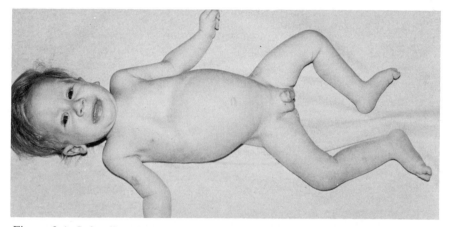

Figure 2.1. Infantile spinal muscular atrophy. This hypotonic child lies motionless with legs in the characteristic "frog leg" position.

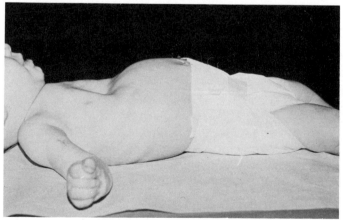

Figure 2.2. Infantile spinal muscular atrophy. The same child as in the previous photograph. Pectus excavatum is to be noted. The protuberant abdomen is associated with respiratory movement; most of the respiratory effort is abdominal.

with the slightly tremulous movement of the tongue at rest which is seen in a normal infant. Fasciculations of the limb muscles are seldom seen, perhaps because of the covering of subcutaneous fat. In those children who can move their limbs there may be an associated fine tremor, but it is not as marked in the acute form of spinal muscular atrophy as it is in some of the more chronic forms. A sensory examination, when it can be evaluated, is quite normal. Loss of the deep tendon reflexes is the rule.

It is sometimes said that the proximal muscles are more involved than the distal ones and that the legs are more involved than the arms. In evaluating the degree of weakness it should be realized that it takes less effort to move fingers and toes than to move arms or legs, and this may give the impression that the proximal muscles are more affected. In our clinic we have been struck by the rather generalized and symmetrical weakness in acute infantile spinal muscular atrophy. Children with the typical acute form of the illness are usually dead by 2 years of age and almost certainly are dead by 3 years of age. This should imply that the disease is progressive, but the progress of an illness in a patient who has lost almost all muscle function is difficult to evaluate. Respiratory difficulties do seem to be progressively worse, whether because of increasing weakness or because of the effects of repeated respiratory infections is difficult to say. The terminal event is usually a pneumonia with respiratory failure. In patients whose disease has lasted for some months contractures may develop in the muscles; this sign is not often found early in the illness. Congenital deformities such as a hip dislocation and contractures at birth are uncommon and occur in less than 10 per cent of patients.[2] This may on occasion serve to distinguish acute spinal muscular atrophy from some of the other causes of severe hypotonia, such as congenital fiber type disproportion.

The disease is genetically determined and is almost always inherited as an autosomal recessive. Suggestions have been made that there are modifying factors to the expression of this autosomal gene,[3, 4] but by and large, genetic counseling may be given on the basis of an autosomal recessive inheritance. The risk to any future children born to parents of a child with acute spinal muscular atrophy will stand at one in four. The frequency of the carrier state in an English population is about 1 in 80[3] and is probably of the same order in the American population. The risk of having an affected child will be about 1 in 400 for any unaffected sibling of a patient with spinal muscular atrophy if the carrier state of the sibling's spouse is not known. The incidence of the illness is about 1 in 15,000 to 1 in 25,000 live births.[3, 5]

A complete discussion of genetic counseling must take into consideration the relationship of this illness to the chronic or arrested form of spinal muscular atrophy. It has been suggested that the various spinal muscular atrophies form a continuous spectrum from patients with severe infantile disease dying in the first year to those whose disease begins in late childhood and in whom survival until late adult life is commonplace.[6–8] Families have been described in which some members have the acute variety whereas others have more benign disease. Some investigators have put forward convincing arguments that these appearances are deceptive and that acute spinal muscular atrophy is genetically and clinically distinct from the more chronic forms.[5, 9] They have suggested that the acute variety of spinal muscular atrophy has its onset usually before 3 months and certainly before 6 months. Death is considered inevitable by 3 years of age and usually occurs much earlier. If a child has this clinical course a similar prognosis may be given for any future siblings who are affected. Conversely, the chronic form usually commences at about 6 months of age and rarely before 3 months. These patients may live until early adult life or even later. There is a small area of overlap in the two groups. Some affected members of a family with the chronic variety may die before 3 years of age, but this is unusual enough to permit prognostic and genetic counseling on the basis of discrete forms of illness.

Laboratory Studies

The two most useful laboratory studies are electromyography and muscle biopsy. The serum muscle enzymes, such as aldolase and creatine phosphokinase, may be slightly elevated, but in general are normal. Electromyography often shows fibrillations at rest and either a decreased interference pattern or an absence of motor units if the limb is paralyzed. One does not see the bizarre giant polyphasic complexes characteristic of denervation and reinnervation which are found in other illnesses. Muscle biopsy may reveal changes which are diagnostic of the illness and different from those seen in other forms of denervation. Whether this merely represents the age at which the denervation begins or indicates a change specific to the disease is not known. At any rate, there are sheets of round atrophic fibers among which are interspersed clumps of markedly hypertrophied fibers. The majority of these hypertrophic fibers are Type 1 when evaluated with the ATPase reaction (Figure 2.3).

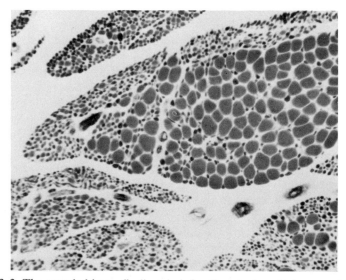

Figure 2.3. The muscle biopsy findings in infantile spinal muscular atrophy are quite characteristic, with large numbers of round, atrophic fibers and clumps of hypertrophic fibers of uniform histochemical type (Type 1). (ATPase reaction pH 9.4)

Treatment

There is no drug therapy for the illness, but physical therapy is important, particularly when done at home by the parents. The limbs must be kept supple and contractures prevented if the child is to remain comfortable. Respiratory toilet and postural drainage together with breathing exercises are important in those children who are old enough to cooperate with such therapy. I think that the philosophy of many people who look after large numbers of children with acute spinal muscular atrophy disease is to avoid any heroic measures should the child develop a pneumonia. The advent of antibiotics does not seem to have altered the life span of children with acute Werdnig-Hoffman's disease.[6] Before genetic counseling is undertaken, a prognosis given, or a particular form of therapy recommended, the diagnosis should be confirmed with all appropriate studies since there are some severe weaknesses of the first year which may spontaneously improve. These will be discussed in later chapters.

CHRONIC INFANTILE SPINAL MUSCULAR ATROPHY (CHRONIC WERDNIG-HOFFMANN DISEASE, SPINAL MUSCULAR ATROPHY TYPE 2, INTERMEDIATE SPINAL MUSCULAR ATROPHY)

Clinical Aspects

The idea that spinal muscular atrophy represents a clinical continuum between its most acute and its most chronic forms has been disputed by those who believe that the acute form is a genetically distinct entity. Whatever the final resolution of this matter, the discussion of chronic infantile spinal muscular atrophy as a separate category serves to emphasize that not all patients pursue a rapid and fatal course. The illness usually begins in the middle of the first year. Its onset may be so insidious that it is difficult for parents to be precise as to the date. As in the acute form, cases have been described which begin abruptly following immunizations, but this is the exception. A physician is often consulted when a major milestone, such as sitting unsupported or rolling over, is delayed or is not attained. Most of the children are able to move the arms and legs and to lift the head from a prone position, and about a third of the patients are able to roll over at some stage in their life. The child may be able to sit independently for a brief period of time and may even learn to stand. Only the minority maintain such independent sitting and standing, and most are confined to life in a wheelchair during the second and third year. Children who do manage to sit unsupported do so by being placed in this position. They either sit with back straightened and chin tucked in, balancing so precariously that it seems as if the faintest breeze will cause them to tumble backwards, or they are hunched over with their spine forming an arc that owes its support more to the strength of ligaments than of muscle (Figures 2.4 to 2.6). Exceptionally, children with this illness may learn to walk with the aid of long leg braces for a few years.

The distribution of weakness in the chronic form is a little different from the acute illness. There may be mild facial weakness, but this is unusual. Fasciculations and wasting of the tongue are seen in at least one half of the patients[1] (Figure 2.7), but children with the chronic form of spinal muscular atrophy seldom have difficulty in chewing and swallowing. Truncal weakness

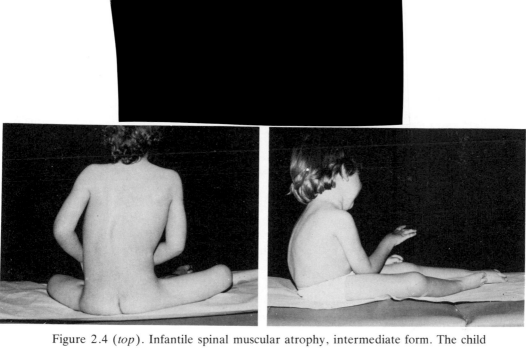

Figure 2.4 (*top*). Infantile spinal muscular atrophy, intermediate form. The child lies in the typical frog leg position. The posture of the weak hands should also be noted.

Figure 2.5 (*lower left*). Infantile spinal muscular atrophy, intermediate form. When this girl sits upright, which she can do unsupported, scoliosis is evident.

Figure 2.6 (*lower right*). Infantile spinal muscular atrophy, intermediate form. A characteristic posture of these patients during unsupported sitting is a rounded kyphosis, which this child exhibits. Notice, once again, the hand posture.

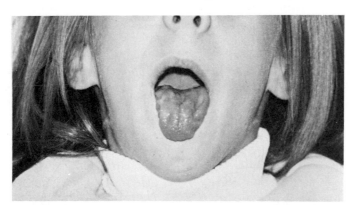

Figure 2.7. Infantile spinal muscular atrophy, intermediate form. The tongue is scalloped and atrophic.

and weakness o   end to be
more severely i   arms were
found to be we   [6, 11] A fine
tremor of the   egarded as
substantiating t   deformities
are inevitably s   e kyphoscoliosis seen in c   nd, indeed,
more frequent   his probably
reflects the sev   than being a
specific change   the hips and
knees are ofte   ts of the arm
and hands are   s in the child
confined to a   es are usually
decreased but

The course of the illness is difficult to evaluate. After the initial progressive weakness the disease may remain static or brief periods of worsening may be interspersed with long periods of stability. The terminal event is respiratory insufficiency which may be provoked as much by the increasing chest deformity as by any progressive weakness of the respiratory muscles, and even the patients who are most severely involved may survive until adult life. Perhaps the wisest course is not to try and predict the time at which death may occur but to plan for possible survival into adult life.

Genetic counseling can be given on the assumption that the illness is inherited as an autosomal recessive. The majority of cases are so inherited, and those which conform to other patterns are rare enough[13] that the possibility can be ignored unless the family history clearly indicates otherwise.

Laboratory Studies

The laboratory studies of most help in the diagnosis are the same as those described under the acute form. The muscle biopsy will show the changes of denervation but may be slightly different from that seen in the acute disease. Although some patients with prolonged life span have biopsies which are identical to acute infantile spinal muscular atrophy (with rounded fibers and the majority of the hypertrophied fibers being Type 1), many of the biopsies show fiber type grouping and large Type 2 fibers. I have not seen the latter change in those children who die of the disease in the first 2 years, and it may be helpful in making the distinction. Again, it is possible that the changes on the biopsy merely represent the severity of the disease rather than reflecting a different etiology. The levels of the serum "muscle" enzymes, such as creatine phosphokinase (CPK), may be either normal or elevated. The degree of elevation may be up to five times normal, but one does not see the astronomical levels of CPK characteristic of Duchenne's muscular dystrophy. There is also a difference in the progression of the serum CPK values. In Duchenne's dystrophy these are highest in the preclinical stage of the disease and drop progressively as the disease becomes more advanced. In spinal muscular atrophy, on the other hand, elevation of the CPK usually occurs as the disease advances and is not noted early in the illness. Electromyography shows the pattern of denervation with occasional signs of reinnervation. Conduction velocities are usually normal. X-rays of the back and limbs are helpful in evaluating the progression of the kyphoscoliosis, the degree of osteoporosis, or the presence of hip dislocations but are not helpful in establishing the diagnosis.

JUVENILE SPINAL MUSCULAR ATROPHY (KUGELBERG-WELANDER DISEASE, SPINAL MUSCULAR ATROPHY TYPE 3)

Clinical Aspects

In the middle 1950's two reports[14, 15] focused attention on an illness beginning in childhood in which proximal weakness was due to denervation. Under the title of juvenile muscular atrophy simulating muscular dystrophy, a clinical entity was outlined with a slow progression, with the life of the patient measured in decades rather than in years. Since then there have been numerous case reports and several review articles.[7, 16–18]

Typically, the disease is first noted between the ages of 5 to 15 years, although it may begin earlier. Cases have been described in which the illness begins in later adult life. As with all the spinal muscular atrophies, it is difficult to decide whether this variability of the age of onset is due to the fact that this is not one disease but a collection of separate and unrecognized illnesses. Nevertheless the great majority of cases seem to occur in childhood or early adolescence. There is some suggestion that the disease may be more severe and perhaps more frequent in the male than in the female, although this too has been disputed.

The disease begins gradually and, although there are sporadic reports of sudden exacerbations associated with acute illnesses such as intercurrent infections, the weakness pursues a slowly progressive course. The muscles around the hips are among the first to be involved and cause difficulty in walking. As the weakness gets worse, the child's walk becomes a waddle and there is an increasing problem with climbing stairs. Later, the weakness is severe enough for the patient to use a Gower's maneuver in arising from the floor. By this time, there is always some associated weakness of the shoulder muscles. This may not be noticed by the patient but is found on physical examination. The calf muscles have been described as pseudohypertrophic in about a fifth of the patients. Whether this really represents pseudohypertrophy or whether the atrophic thigh muscles make the normal gastrocnemius stand out in contrast is unresolved. Toe walking and early contractures of the gastrocnemii are unusual, which helps to differentiate the "pseudohypertrophy" from that seen in Duchenne's muscular dystrophy. Skeletal deformities are not common early in the disease, although the muscular weakness of the hips is associated with a compensatory lordotic posture. The progress of the disease may be slow enough to allow the patient to walk, although with difficulty, ten, twenty, and even thirty years after the start of the illness. Most patients, however, will be using a wheelchair in their mid 30's and some will have a more rapid form of the disease which takes them off their feet by the time they are 20.

Shoulder and arm weakness becomes troublesome in the later stages of the illness. The muscles of the hands and forearms are among the last to be affected and there is sometimes a discrepancy between the flexors of the wrist, which may become quite weak, and the extensors, which retain a fair amount of strength. Although the weakness spreads in the late stages to involve almost all the muscles of the body, the general pattern, in which the legs are more involved than the arms and the proximal muscles are more involved than the distal muscles, holds true for most patients. Weakness of the neck flexors and extensors is also noted, and patients may find some difficulty in lifting the head off the pillow. Rarely, facial weakness, weakness of the tongue, and weakness of the palate are seen. It is seldom noticed by the patient, but friends may comment on the development of nasal speech. Cases have also been described in which ptosis has been found. However, the involvement of the cranial musculature is the exception rather than the rule. As with so many chronic neuromuscular diseases, skeletal deformities, kyphoscoliosis, and contractures of muscles around inactive joints occur in the later stages. There is no intellectual handicap in juvenile spinal muscular atrophy.

The disease is inherited as an autosomal recessive. Other patterns such as autosomal dominant and x-linked recessive inheritance have been described, but they usually occur in cases which are otherwise atypical for juvenile spinal muscular atrophy and give rise to the suspicion that there may be forms of motor neuron disease which are as yet imperfectly characterized.[19]

Fasciculations are found in about half of the patients at some stage. Typically, these are seen around the shoulders and hips and are more noticeable in adolescence and early adult life than later on. Wasting of the involved muscles may be prominent. The deep tendon reflexes are often depressed, particularly at the knees and elbows, although some patients have normal or increased reflexes in spite of quite severe weakness. Extensor plantar responses have been noted in some patients but are extremely rare; no satisfactory explanation has been found for them.

Laboratory Studies

The laboratory studies which are most useful are the serum "muscle" enzymes, the muscle biopsy, and the EMG. Indeed, without these studies, the diagnosis may be impossible. Elevation of the level of serum creatine phosphokinase (CPK) is reported in about half of the patients. In my own experience, abnormally high values were found in over three quarters of the patients. Usually, the values are about doubled, but they may be elevated up to ten times the normal. One rarely sees in juvenile spinal muscular atrophy the very high elevation of CPK which is so common in Duchenne's dystrophy and, as with some of the other denervating diseases, the level of elevation remains steady or even increases with the progress of the disease rather than decreasing as it does in Duchenne's muscular dystrophy. The EMG shows the changes of denervation and reinnervation. Fibrillations, fasciculations, positive denervation potentials, and giant polyphasic potentials may all be found. The muscle biopsy also shows the typical findings of denervation, with a mixture of large and small groups of atrophic fibers and with some markedly hypertrophied fibers. Histochemical studies show type grouping and often a predominance of Type 2 fibers. This is a pattern which is quite different from that of the infantile form of the illness. Whether it is an expression of the age at which the disease begins or whether it is, in fact, a specific change associated with the illness is not known. Much has been written about the presence of "myopathic" changes in the muscles of patients with spinal muscular atrophy, some of which may cloud rather than clarify the issue. There is probably no immutable law which decrees that basophilia, fiber splitting, and internal nuclei must imply a primary disease of the muscle. Their presence in the spinal muscular atrophies merely reflects the variety of changes which muscle undergoes in a chronic disease.

The disease may be mistaken for other illnesses causing slowly progressive proximal weakness. There are, obviously, many of these but the classic confusion has arisen between limb girdle dystrophy and juvenile spinal muscular atrophy. It is almost axiomatic that if you can make the clinical diagnosis of one, the other also remains a possibility. Even the serum CPK cannot clearly separate the two entitites, and EMG and muscle biopsy are necessary to allow an accurate differentiation. In the young patient with juvenile spinal muscular atrophy, the possibility of Duchenne's muscular dystrophy must be considered, and evaluation of serum CPK may be helpful as mentioned.

Treatment

Treatment of the disease is similar to that of the other forms of spinal muscular atrophy. Active assisted exercises should be carried out in order to strengthen the available muscles. Skeletal deformities should be prevented or corrected when they do occur. The use of a heavy back brace to prevent the kyphoscoliosis in patients with spinal muscular atrophy is not possible while the patient is still ambulatory. However, once the patient is confined to a wheelchair, such a back brace is eventually necessary. Very frequently, the patient with an increasing lumbar lordosis is troubled by low back pain. The possibility of degenerative disc disease should not be ignored in a patient complaining of pain and increased weakness.

BIBLIOGRAPHY

1. Pearn, J. H. Fetal movements and Werdnig-Hoffman's disease. J. Neurol. Sci. *18:* 373–379, 1973.
2. Pearn, J. H., and Wilson, J. Acute Werdnig-Hoffman's disease: Acute infantile spinal muscular atrophy. Arch. Dis. Child. *48:* 425–430, 1973.
3. Pearn, J. H. The gene frequency of acute Werdnig-Hoffman's disease (SMA Type I): A total population survey in northeast England. J. Med. Genet. *10:* 260–265, 1973.
4. Zellweger, H., Hanhart, E., and Schneider, H. J. A new genetic variant of the spinal muscular atrophies in infancy. J. Med. Genet. *9:* 401–407, 1972.
5. Pearn, J. H., Carter, C. O., and Wilson, J. The genetic identity of acute spinal muscular atrophy. Brain *96:* 463–470, 1973.
6. Dubowitz, V. Infantile muscular atrophy: A prospective study with particular reference to a slowly progressive variety. Brain *87:* 707–718, 1964.
7. Gardner-Medwin, D., Hudgson, P., and Walton, J. N. Benign spinal muscular atrophy arising in childhood and adolescence. J. Neurol. Sci. *5:* 121–158, 1967.
8. Byers, R. K., and Banker, B. Q. Infantile muscular atrophy. Arch. Neurol. *5:* 140–164, 1961.
9. Fried, K., and Emery, A. E. H. Spinal muscular atrophy, Type II. Clin. Genet. *2:* 203–209, 1971.
10. Munsat, T. L., Woods, R., Fowler, W., and Pearson, C. M. Neurogenic muscular atrophy of infancy with prolonged survival. Brain *92:* 9–24, 1969.
11. Van Wijngaarden, G. K., and Bethlem, J. Benign infantile spinal muscular atrophy: A prospective study. Brain *96:* 163–170, 1973.

12. Moosa, A., and Dubowitz, V. Spinal muscular atrophy in childhood: Two clues to clinical diagnosis. Arch. Dis. Child. *48:* 386–388, 1973.
13. Zellweger, H. and Hanhart, E. The infantile proximal spinal muscular atrophies in Switzerland. Helv. Paediatr. Acta *27:* 355–360, 1972.
14. Kugelberg, E., and Welander, L. Heredofamilial juvenile muscular atrophy simulating muscular dystrophy. Arch. Neurol. Psychiatr. *75:* 500–509, 1956.
15. Wohlfart, G., Fex, J., and Eliasson, S. Hereditary proximal spinal muscular atrophy: A clinical entity simulating progressive muscular dystrophy. Acta Psychiatr. Scand. *30:* 395–406, 1955.
16. Emery, A. E. H. The nosology of the spinal muscular atrophies. J. Med. Genet. *8:* 481–495, 1971.
17. Namba, T., Aberfeld, D. C., and Grob, D. Chronic spinal muscular atrophy. J. Neurol. Sci. *11:* 401–423, 1970.
18. Hausmanowa-Petrusewicz, I., Askanas, W., Badurska, B., Emeryk, B., et al. Infantile and juvenile spinal muscular atrophy. J. Neurol. Sci. *6:* 269–287, 1968.
19. Emery, A. E. H., Davie, A. M., and Smith, C. Spinal muscular atrophy: Resolution of heterogeneity. In: *Recent Advances in Myology*, Edited by W. G. Bradley, D. Gardner-Medwin, and J. N. Walton. Excepta Medica, Amsterdam. 1975, pp. 557–565.

MOTOR NEURON DISEASE (AMYOTROPHIC LATERAL SCLEROSIS)

Clinical Aspects

The symptoms of this illness are associated with degeneration of the motor nerve cells throughout the nervous system. There is a progressive wasting and weakness of those muscles which lose their nerve supply, and signs of spasticity and hyperreflexia betoken the damage to the upper motor neurons. Various clinical varieties have been described, depending on the part of the nervous system which bears the brunt of the disease. There is probably no more terrifying disease in the medical textbooks than the acute form of motor neuron disease. The appalling plight of the patient in whom a rapidly progressive weakness of the arms and legs is associated with an inability to speak or swallow but whose mind remains clear to the end is obvious. One patient commented that having motor neuron disease was being given the privilege of a ringside seat at one's own dissolution. It is a disease that commands the respect of those who witness it, even if only briefly. Hence, more physicians and medical students have entertained the delusion that they are suffering from motor neuron disease than from any other neuromuscular disease. Most of us working in neuromuscular clinics have suspected occasionally that our common benign fasciculations represented the early ravages of this disease.

Because of the ominous prognosis which the disease usually carries, we have tended to ignore a significant percentage of patients with motor neuron disease who have a relatively benign course, with survival up to twenty or thirty years after the onset. In the following paragraphs a subdivision of motor neuron diseases into the more classical varieties of progressive spinal muscular atrophy, progressive bulbar palsy, and amyotrophic lateral sclerosis will not be attempted. Instead, the typical severe form of the illness will be described, followed by an outline of the milder varieties.

Motor neuron disease usually occurs sporadically in the population with a prevalence which has been estimated between 2 and 7 in 100,000 population.[1, 2] The higher figure is probably more accurate. Approximately five per cent of patients have a family history of the illness, although the mode of inheritance is not clear and the other cases may be quite remote from the patient's immediate family. Sometimes an autosomal dominant pattern of inheritance is seen.[3] It is said that males are more affected than females and that the disease most often commences in middle or late life. Statistical evaluation of populations at the Mayo Clinic and elsewhere has suggested that the average age of onset is between 50 and 60 years,[4] but motor neuron disease is really no respecter of age or gender.

The early symptoms reflect a patchy distribution of weakness which is often distal. Frequently the hands become clumsy and there is difficulty in the performance of fine tasks, picking up pins while sewing or threading a nut onto a bolt, for example. One patient noticed a sudden deterioration of his lifelong accuracy in casting with a fishing rod. Sometimes the weakness is in the legs, and the patient may trip over things easily because of a mild foot drop. Bulbar symptoms are said to be the initial complaint in up to one third of the patients,[4, 5] but only a few of the patients presenting in our clinic experienced bulbar symptoms initially although many said in retrospect that the bulbar symptoms were the first really troublesome complaints. Night cramps in the leg muscles are an early symptom. These pains, which are often in the calf or thigh muscles, may occur when the patient is resting in bed. There is a spasm and cramp of the muscles, often following a movement of the limb such as stretching.

Within weeks to months the disease spreads to involve almost all the muscles of the body. Distal involvement may be more severe than proximal, but this is not invariable. Fasciculations are often noticed early in the illness, may be prominent at night, and may even disturb the patient's sleep. Occasionally the patient will complain of sleep starts or myoclonic jerks when resting. Norris found that a relative absence of fasciculations is associated with slow progression of the illness.[6] Such is not always the case, and diffuse and abundant fasciculations have been associated with a relatively slow progression as with the severe disease.

The patient may complain of stiffness or of a "heavy," clumsy feeling in the legs, heralding the onset of upper motor neuron signs. Hyperreflexia can be so severe that ankle clonus is noted by the patient as, for example, when he presses his foot firmly on the brake pedal of a car.

Weakness of the bulbar musculature causes the patient to have difficulty with both speaking and swallowing. The speech is often difficult to evaluate and shares characteristics of both upper and lower motor neuron damage. Usually the upper motor neuron changes predominate, giving the speech a forced, monotonous quality. This abnormality progresses until in the terminal stages the patient may be completely mute or, at best, able to utter a strained, moaning sound. Difficulty in swallowing is also usually due to upper motor neuron damage. The patient has difficulty in initiating swallowing and will complain that solid foods lodge at the back of the throat. Saliva accumulates in the pharynx and causes choking spells. Some patients are bothered by a hyperactive cough reflex which causes the patient to cough when trying to talk or when stepping outside into cold air. Pseudobulbar affect may also be noticed in patients with the severe form of motor neuron disease associated with forced laughter or inappropriate crying. It should be borne in mind before the diagnosis of pseudobulbar affect is made that this disease is a devastating one and that frequently the patient has every reason to burst into tears.

The facial muscles are sometimes weak, but it is exceptional to find extraocular palsies or ptosis. Indeed, the occurrence of weakness in these muscles should give rise to some doubt about the diagnosis of motor neuron disease. Bladder and bowel problems are seldom noted. Urinary incontinence is rarely seen in patients with motor neuron disease and its basis is not clear.

With time, the patient becomes increasingly helpless. Confinement to a wheelchair often occurs within a matter of 12 to 18 months and finally the patient is bedridden, unable to move, talk, or swallow. Death occurs from respiratory failure, which may be ushered in by symptoms of anoxia such as nightmares and confusion. Survival from the onset of symptoms to death is just under three years in most cases.

The signs of damage to the lower motor neurons include wasting and weakness associated with fasciculations. Even when the patient's symptoms are localized to one area, the findings of fasciculations and weakness in more than one limb may indicate diffuse disease. Motor neuron disease is one of the rare situations in which wasted, weak muscles are associated with increased reflexes. Other upper motor neuron signs are surprisingly slight, and the plantar responses may be flexor even when the reflexes are abnormally brisk. The superficial abdominal reflexes are similarly preserved.

Examination of the bulbar muscles may reveal some facial weakness although, as was mentioned, the extraocular muscles are not involved. There may be atrophy of the tongue, which looks "scalloped," the indentations caused by the teeth becoming prominent along the edges. Fasciculations of the tongue may also be seen. They should be sought with the tongue resting quietly in the floor of the mouth, since the protruded tongue can be the site of quivering movements difficult to differentiate from fasciculations. Palatal weakness and poor movement of the posterior pharyngeal wall may also be noted. The upper motor neuron component of this weakness becomes obvious when the patient is asked to move his tongue rapidly from side to side; the movement is slow and stiff, and is often associated with a synkinetic movement of the lower jaw. Both neck extensors and flexors may be weak.

The diagnosis of motor neuron disease is made with some assurance if weakness, wasting, and fasciculations are found in three or more limbs, associated with hyperreflexia. If bulbar difficulties are also seen the diagnosis is even more likely. Sensory abnormalities are not a major part of the disease although careful quantitative sensory testing and pathological examination of the peripheral nerves shows abnormalities more frequently than was thought previously.[7]

Damage to other areas of the nervous system may be seen but should not be thought typical of the disease. Some patients have a clear cut dementia as part of the illness. Similarly, extrapyramidal tremor and rigidity have been noted on occasions. These patients differ from the form of motor neuron disease on Guam which is related to the Parkinsonism-dementia syndrome (see below). Perhaps sometimes the non-Guamanian ALS-Parkinsonism-dementia syndrome represents the chance association of two or three processes, particularly in the elderly patient with motor neuron disease. There seems to be no difference in the clinical course of this form of motor neuron disease from the classical variety.

The autonomic nervous system is spared; trophic changes in the limbs and pressure sores are not found. Sexual function is preserved.

Physicians in their hunt for eponymous fame have often collected patients with constellations of clinical findings, creating subclassifications within major disease groups. Motor neuron disease has not been exempt from this, and although such divisions are artificial they are hallowed by time and usage. When motor neuron disease involves the lower motor neurons of the spinal cord without upper motor neuron involvement, it is called progressive spinal muscular atrophy of Aran-Duchenne. Such patients have wasting and weakness of the arms, legs, and trunk with little hyperreflexia. Some patients with this form of the illness have a better prognosis than do patients with the other varieties. When the illness primarily causes difficulty with chewing and swallowing and other "bulbar" functions, it has been termed progressive bulbar palsy of Duchenne. The survival of these patients is expected to be shorter than the preceding group. The name amyotrophic lateral sclerosis was coined by Charcot in 1874. The term was used to denote the variety of illness which involved both upper and lower motor neurons supplying the trunk, extremities, and bulbar muscles. Because this is the most common and most diffuse form, the name is synonymous with motor neuron disease.

It was at one time thought that the differentiation into various syndromes had some prognostic significance. Such attempts at forecasting the outcome of the disease may equally well be based on common sense. Patients who have more severe disease are likely to die earlier than those with less severe disease, and those with involvement of the vital functions such as swallowing and breathing are inclined to have more trouble than those whose only difficulty is weakness of the arms and legs.

Laboratory Studies

Laboratory studies are helpful in the diagnosis of this illness and should be aimed at demonstrating denervation in widely separated areas of the musculature. Electromyography shows widespread fibrillations associated with giant polyphasic potentials and fasciculations. There may be slowing of motor nerve conduction velocities, although they are typically normal. The use of muscle biopsy in the evaluation of a patient with ALS is not governed by the usual criteria. Only the patients with early and predominantly lower motor neuron involvement give rise to much difficulty in diagnosis. The patient who presents with a weak hand or forearm may as easily have a local lesion of the brachial plexus as motor neuron disease. It is useful in such patients to biopsy the quadriceps muscle, even in the absence of clinical involvement. In motor neuron disease there is almost always pathological abnormality of all muscles whether or not clinical weakness is apparent. Evaluation of serum creatine phosphokinase (CPK) and other "muscle" enzymes is of less help in making the diagnosis, since in almost half of the patients with motor neuron disease the serum CPK may be increased to two and three times normal.[8, 9] Spinal fluid protein is usually normal but mild elevation, less than 100 mg per cent, may be seen.[10]

Although the typical picture of motor neuron disease is often easy to recognize, certain other illnesses may mimic some of the changes and should always be considered in the differential diagnosis. Thus, cervical spine disease with cord compression and root compression may give signs of widespread denervation in the arms together with upper motor neuron changes in the legs. In rare patients, widespread fasciculations are associated with cervical cord disease. A popular aphorism is that patients with motor neuron disease are not allowed to die before a myelogram is carried out. Although this may be an extreme statement, the possibility of a cervical lesion should always be considered. When myelography shows definite evidence of cervical spine disease, it is difficult to decide whether this alone is responsible for the symptoms or whether it is merely an incidental finding in a patient with real motor neuron disease. In my own experience I have erred on the side of enthusiasm and have recommended surgical exploration in such cases. Unhappily, my experience has not been reassuring. Some patients may improve temporarily after operation only later to resume their downhill course.

Heavy metal intoxication has been suggested as an occasional etiology for motor neuron disease.[11] Lead intoxication may present as a motor neuropathy in the absence of any sensory signs. The weakness is most marked in the wrist extensors. There may also be hyperreflexia and fasciculations. Usually there are other signs of systemic lead poisoning, but these may be subtle enough to be overlooked. Organic mercurial compounds were reported as a cause of motor neuron disease in a report of eleven patients poisoned by a fungicide used in wheat.[12] Although these patients had atrophy and fasciculations of the limbs there were sufficient differences to make the diagnosis of motor neuron disease doubtful. More recent and extensive case reports of organic mercurial poisoning have not described conditions which might be confused with motor neuron disease.[13] A retrospective study involving a small number of patients with ALS suggested that there was more often a history of exposure to mercury and lead than in normal people. It was also suggested that participation in athletics and the consumption of large amounts of milk distinguished patients with ALS from the others.[14]

The neuromuscular complications of hyperparathyroidism may sometimes include weakness, fatigability, and increased reflexes (see page 180). Hyperthyroidism may also be associated with muscle weakness and, in some cases, with either myokymia or fasciculations. Some authors have suggested that underlying malignancy might be a cause for motor neuron disease,[15] but recent experience has not confirmed this. There are patients with malignant tumors who do seem to have loss of anterior horn cells, but this does not present as the usual and classical motor neuron disease.

Etiology and Treatment

The etiology of the disease and its treatment will be considered together because various theories as to the cause have given rise to attempted therapy. It is easy to summarize the situation by saying that we know neither the cause of nor the cure for motor neuron disease. As is so often the case in such situations there have been many attempts at treatment, each of which has enjoyed popularity for a certain time. Defects of carbohydrate metabolism have been noted on several occasions. Abnormal glucose tolerance and tolbutamide tolerance and subnormal insulin secretion have also been found. Impairment of pancreatic exocrine function has been reported with decreased neutral fat uptake, mild steatorrhea, and an abnormal response to secretin stimulation.[16] These findings have been disputed by others[17, 18] and the possibility raised that some of these abnormalities may be due to decreased muscle mass and represent a secondary alteration in carbohydrate metabolism because of such profound wasting of muscle, one of the main tissues of the body. The hypothesis of pancreatic deficiency was the basis for the treatment of motor neuron disease with pancreatic extracts. Although certain patients seemed to derive some benefit from this, no consistent alteration of the illness has ever been demonstrated.[16, 19] Probably all physicians who treat motor neuron disease have seen the occasional patient whose illness seems to have been "arrested" by this or other medications, but the explanation is probably that we are treating one of the more benign forms. A hypothetical toxic cause has on occasion been suggested, particularly in Guamanian motor neuron disease.[4] Such a toxin, however, has never been identified. Wolfgram and Myers[20] found that the serum from patients with motor neuron disease was toxic and selectively killed the neurons grown in tissue culture from mouse anterior horn cells. They did not speculate on the nature of this toxic substance, and other workers could not confirm the findings.[21]

One of the early theories in motor neuron disease was that of a causative viral agent. The association between poliomyelitis and ALS was noted. Not only do the two diseases show a predilection for the anterior horn cell, but some patients who have had classical poliomyelitis may develop a chronically progressive form of motor neuron disease after a period of many years.[22, 23] The illness often begins in the limb affected by the poliomyelitis. There has never been any clear proof that a virus is involved in motor neuron disease. Virus like particles have been noted in the muscle of patients with ALS, but it is impossible to say whether they represented merely an incidental finding.[24] An increased incidence of HL-A3 antigen was found in patients with the severe form of ALS, perhaps indirectly pointing to an allergic or infectious cause.[25] Extracts of the central nervous system from patients with motor neuron disease were thought to produce a similar disease following intracerebral inoculation in monkeys, but attempts to reproduce this finding failed.[26, 27] The viral etiology of motor neuron disease remains unproven but not disproven. Therapeutic attempts with antiviral agents, however, have not awaited the proof of the theory. Thus, amantadine, idoxuridine, cytosine arabinoside, and isoprinosine have all been tried without success.[28-32] Guanidine, a drug which may be an antiviral agent but which also promotes the release of acetylcholine at the neuromuscular junction, has been employed. Initial encouraging results were not borne out on a long term controlled trial.[33]

Some patients with motor neuron disease demonstrate fatigability and respond to the use of anticholinesterases such as pyridostigmine. Edrophonium can be used as a diagnostic test to select those patients who might benefit from these drugs. Other drugs which have been used without benefit include levodopa,[34] vitamins E and B_{12}, and Elavil. Phthalazinol has also been used, but further studies are necessary before it can be properly evaluated.

It is apparent that the treatment of motor neuron disease is aimed at making the patient more comfortable. In addition to the need for supportive devices such as walkers, raised toilet seats, wheelchairs, and braces, the patient with motor neuron disease has at some stage three other problems. The first is difficulty with saliva pooling in the posterior pharynx. This produces choking spells and can be extremely disturbing. A portable suction device, properly used can make an enormous difference to the patient's comfort. The second problem occurs at a stage when it is difficult to swallow solid foods. Many times patients struggle on, trying to swallow solids, not realizing that homogenized foods can be swallowed relatively easily. The use of a blender should be urged at the appropriate time. Sometimes the question arises as to whether a gastrostomy should be performed in order to circumvent the dysphagia. There is certainly much to be said for this procedure in patients whose mealtimes are spent in paroxysms of choking. From a practical point of view, we have found that the patient for whom a gastrostomy is being considered should be admitted to the hospital for a few days to evaluate the caloric intake with a properly balanced diet which is pureed or homogenized. In such a situation, we have never had to perform a gastrostomy. During the hospitalization, the patient has always learned to take the semi liquid diet without too much problem. In one or two patients we have used feeding via nasogastric tube for brief periods of time. Recently cricopharyngeal myotomy has been used in selected cases when dysfunction of this muscle can be demonstrated.[35, 36] This simple procedure is far more acceptable to the patient than the unpleasantness of gastrostomy.

The last problem concerns sleep. Patients with motor neuron disease have their sleep disturbed by two symptoms, one of which occurs early and the other late. Night cramps are very troublesome and, although there is no real cure for them, they may be relieved by the use of quinine, Valium, or occasionally calcium gluconate. Late in the disease, when the respiratory involvement produces mild anoxia, sleep is disturbed by frequent arousals and nightmares. Portable oxygen by the bedside can make the difference between a terrifying and restless night and a sound night's sleep. In the classical form of motor neuron disease, death is inevitable and heroic efforts to keep the patient alive at all costs are a disservice. It is equally obvious that the patient and his relatives should be consulted in any decision with regard to management.

Slow Motor Neuron Disease

The existence of a form of motor neuron disease which is only slowly progressive has been known for some time. It has not been emphasized in the major texts because it was felt that only a small minority of the patients were thus affected. It now seems that slow motor neuron disease may be more common than was previously thought. Obviously, physicians who see a large number of patients with motor neuron disease will see a disproportionate number with the benign form; the mere fact of their survival ensures a steadily increasing population of such patients in the muscle clinic. This is in contrast to patients with the rapidly progressive illness, who die in a short time and, therefore, disappear from the clinic population. Nevertheless, it seems that about twenty per cent of patients with motor neuron disease will conform to the "benign" variety with survival in excess of five years. There is no basic difference between the slow form and the more classical variety of motor neuron disease except that bulbar symptoms and upper motor signs are often absent in the early phase of the illness. Wasting, weakness, and fasciculations of the limbs are found, often in a patchy distribution and frequently more distal than proximal. Some signs of denervation may be noted in the tongue. It is only to be expected that those patients with the mildest form of the disease should have the longest survival. Whether slow motor neuron disease is a different illness characterized by absence of bulbar findings or whether the absence of bulbar paralysis permits the patient with motor neuron disease to survive longer is thus an unanswerable question. Slow motor neuron disease may be differentiated from the Kugelberg-Welander form of juvenile spinal muscular atrophy by the characteristic proximal distribution of the latter disease.

Focal Motor Neuron Disease

An interesting but only tentatively identified form of motor neuron disease is one in which only one area of the body is attacked. The disease begins insidiously with wasting and fasciculations involving one group of muscles. The shoulder girdle is particularly susceptible, and I have also seen the small muscles of one hand and forearm and the thigh muscles involved. Typically, the disease is progressive for several months and may result in quite severe localized disability. The process then stops and the patient is left with a fixed deficit, from which he does not recover. We have seen some patients with atrophy of one shoulder girdle who have had an identical episode some years later involving the other shoulder girdle. Yet others with apparent focal motor neuron disease develop the slowly progressive variety after an interval of some years. No autopsy studies have been performed and, therefore, the diagnosis is still not proven pathologically. However, the muscle biopsy findings and EMG studies are characteristic of those seen in amyotrophic lateral sclerosis.

When there is such localized involvement, it is extremely important to rule out other possible diagnoses such as root compression, spinal cord tumors, or various forms of mononeuritis, diabetic and otherwise. Such lesions of the nerves or spinal cord are usually revealed by the presence of sensory abnormalities, although these may be slight. One patient, in whom the diagnosis of focal motor neuron disease was thought likely, developed some numbness of the lateral aspect of the shoulder six years after first noticing weakness of the shoulder. A benign tumor involving the C-5 root was found at exploratory surgery. When the shoulder girdle is involved, the possibility of brachial neuritis or neuralgic amyotrophy should be considered. This may be differentiated from focal motor neuron disease by the antecedent history of pain and by the tendency for recovery to occur following the episode of weakness. In summary, if focal motor neuron disease is to be considered as a diagnosis, great care should be taken to exclude other causes of focal atrophy. The final proof of its existence will depend upon autopsy studies.

OTHER MOTOR NEURON DISEASES

Since we neither know the cause of motor neuron disease nor have an absolute marker (such as a missing enzyme) with which to characterize the illness, it is difficult to decide whether the following diseases are merely variants of the classical form or whether they exist as clinical or pathological entities in their own right. At any rate, there are sometimes distinguishing characteristics which warrant inclusion in a separate category. Some of the syndromes occur recurrently in the literature and may have assumed an independent existence for that reason alone.

Guamanian Motor Neuron Disease[1, 4, 37]

Motor neuron disease occurs among the Chamorro population on the island of Guam. The incidence of the disease is about thirty times higher than in the rest of the world, and it is the cause of death in almost ten per cent of the adult population. There is some evidence that the incidence may now be declining. Another major illness in the same population is the Parkinsonism-dementia complex. These two syndromes may be related, although the nature of their association is not clear. Guamanian patients who present with motor neuron disease rarely develop the Parkinsonism-dementia complex, although patients with the latter illness may develop motor neuron disease terminally. The degree of involvement of the lower motor neurons in the Parkinsonism-dementia syndrome is rather mild, and it has been suggested that this is merely the type of muscular atrophy associated with a very ill patient. Thus, clinically, there seems to be no good correlation between Guamanian motor neuron disease and the Parkinsonism-dementia complex other than their occurrence in the same population as two major causes of death. Pathologically, however, both illnesses show similar changes, changes which are different from those seen in classical motor neuron disease.[38] Alzheimer's neurofibrillary degeneration has been described in various locations in the nervous system including the cerebral cortex, Ammon's horn, various basal ganglia, and some cranial nuclei of the brain stem. Granulovacuolar bodies were noted particularly in the pyramidal cells of Ammon's horn. Crystalloid inclusion bodies were also described. Guamanian ALS demonstrates a familial incidence of the disease in fifty-seven per cent of the patients. Interestingly, analysis of this does not reveal any particular form of inheritance and it is possible that the familial incidence represents an abnormal genetic stratum on which motor neuron disease develops from other causes, or possibly even an environmental cause for the illness.

Kii Peninsula Motor Neuron Disease[39–41]

Other geographical foci of motor neuron disease have been described. The most notable is that occurring on the Kii Peninsula in Japan. Alzheimer's neurofibrillary degeneration was found in these patients in a similar fashion to the Guamanian patients. The course of the disease and the clinical picture do not differ from the common classical variety.

Ryukyuan Muscular Atrophy

In a fascinating report, Kondo et al. outlined the historical, clinical, and pathological features of a neuromuscular disease with a high incidence in the Ryukyu Islands south of Japan.[42] The disease clinically resembled juvenile spinal muscular atrophy with a slowly progressive, predominantly proximal weakness in which the legs were more involved than the arms. Some patients had fasciculations. Kyphoscoliosis and pes cavus were features of the disease. Although the results were not clear cut, the authors felt that EMG and biopsy studies showed more evidence of neurogenic changes than of myopathic changes. The inheritance was through a recessive gene, attributed to a co-ancestor from northern Okinawa living in the 14th century.

Progressive Juvenile Bulbar Palsy (Fazio-Londe Disease)

This very rare disorder may be a variant of juvenile motor neuron disease. The disease is not present at birth which helps to differentiate it from other causes of facial diplegias such as myotonic dystrophy, infantile facioscapulo-humeral dystrophy, and Moebius syndrome. A progressive weakness of the facial, ocular, and bulbar muscles occurs in the first decade. As the disease progresses, there is atrophy and weakness of the trunk and limb muscles; the prognosis is similar to that in the more common motor neuron diseases, with death occurring in months to years. Post mortem examination shows loss of motor nuclei throughout the brain stem and also loss of anterior horn cells in the spinal cord.[43, 44] I have seen only one case of this illness. The pathological findings on muscle biopsy from a clinically unaffected limb were those of denervation.

Scapuloperoneal and Facioscapulohumeral Syndromes

There are several entities which by implication are thought to represent anterior horn cell disease, but the literature seems to be in some disarray. Part of the problem reflects the changes which have occurred in the last decade in the criteria by which denervation or myopathic abnormalities are ascertained. Some years ago, the classification of muscle biopsies into the two categories of "neurogenic" and "myopathic" seemed to be clear cut. Electro-myography showed an equally clear cut difference between the two groups. Recently this classical interpretation has been revised and the distinction blurred. Basophilia and phagocytosis may be seen in denervating diseases. Grouped fiber atrophy may, in fact, not be due to denervation but may reflect fiber type-specific atrophy. Fibrillation potentials may be seen in the dystro-phies and short, polyphasic potentials in neuropathies. About the only ac-ceptable evidence that an illness is of the anterior horn cell is the autopsy demonstration of selective damage to these neurons. Such reports are con-spicuously lacking from much of the literature.

A syndrome in which weakness of the anterior tibial and peroneal muscles is associated with weakness of the muscles around the shoulders has been termed the scapuloperoneal syndrome. This is a rather common combination in the muscle clinic, and about half of the patients seem to have an illness which is related to facioscapulohumeral dystrophy by its genetic, electromy-ographic, chemical, and pathological characteristics. The other patients may have any one of a number of illnesses ranging from central core disease to nemaline myopathy. Many reports suggest the existence of a form of the illness caused by anterior horn cell disease. Close analysis of these reports reveals some discrepancies between the findings and the conclusions. In one family with a dominant inheritance, only two out of twelve members had definite shoulder weakness, and both EMG and muscle biopsy studies showed "myopathic" changes in some instances and "neuropathic" in others. A single autopsy report showed changes only in the cranial nerve nuclei.[45] In another case, the published photograph of the muscle biopsy does not show convincing evidence of denervation, although the electromyogram revealed reduced motor unit activity with associated large potentials.[46] The child described by Emery et al.[47] developed severe and generalized weakness after the initial symptoms of peroneal weakness, and the disease resembled a progressive motor neuron disease. This paper was criticized by Meadows and Marsden,[48] who felt that the patient might have had Charcot-Marie-Tooth disease and cited one of their own patients with a similar clinical picture who later developed progressive slowing of the nerve conduction velocities. Feigenbaum and Munsat have pointed out in their paper on the subject the difficulties involved in determining the underlying pathology.[49]

Motor neuron disease has also been implicated as a cause of a facioscapulohumeral syndrome clinically identical to the more familiar dystrophic form.[50] Again, the evidence for this is disputable. The neuropathic etiology was based on the presence of small angulated fibers. Such fibers, however, have never been shown to be pathognomonic of denervation alone, and, in our experience, have been part of the picture of otherwise classical facioscapulohumeral dystrophy. The patient's EMG did not show any evidence of denervation. Although the girl's mother (who did not undergo a muscle biopsy) had an EMG which revealed fibrillations, this was only in the small hand muscles and not around the shoulders. I do not wish to imply that there are no scapuloperoneal syndromes caused by denervation. There may be such. It might be prudent, though, to await better definition of these cases before predicting their genetics and prognosis.

"Incidental" Motor Neuron Disease

Degeneration of motor neurons undoubtedly occurs as part of several other diseases. In such illnesses the brunt of the pathology is borne by other areas of the nervous system and the presenting symptoms reflect this. The motor neuron disease is only an incidental finding, although it is no less real.

In Jakob-Creutzfeldt disease there is widespread neuronal degeneration. It is of particular interest because transmission of the disease to the chimpanzee has been accomplished, indicating that the disorder is due to a transmissible agent.[27] The disease begins with an increasing dementia, sometimes heralded by depression and behavioral disturbances. Early on, the patient may become fidgety and jumpy, later developing frank myoclonic movements and abnormal startle responses. As the disease progresses, difficulty with the bulbar musculature affects swallowing and talking. The rapidly progressive dementia may be associated with either spasticity or rigidity; other cases have been described with cerebellar ataxia. The wasting of the muscles, which is particularly seen around the shoulders, occurs late in the disease, but gives the typical appearance of motor neuron disease with fasciculations, wasting, and weakness. The disease runs a rapid course, and usually death occurs in less than a year. The terminal patient is often obtunded, blind, and mute, with a decorticate posture. If brain biopsy is performed in an attempt to confirm the diagnosis, care should be taken in the handling of the specimen, since this is a transmissible disease.

BIBLIOGRAPHY

1. Kurland, L. T., Choi, N. W., and Sayre, G. P. Implications of incidence and geographic patterns on the classification of amyotrophic lateral sclerosis. In: *Motor Neuron Diseases*, edited by F. H. Norris and L. T. Kurland. Grune and Stratton, New York, 1969, pp. 28–48.
2. Bobowick, A. R., and Brody, J. A. Epidemiology of motor neuron diseases. New Engl. J. Med. *288:* 1047–1055, 1973.
3. Horton, W. A., Eldridge, R., and Brody, J. A. Familial motor neuron disease. Neurology *26:* 460–465, 1976.
4. Mulder, D. W., and Espinosa, R. E. Amyotrophic lateral sclerosis: Comparison of the clinical syndrome in Guam and the United States. In: *Motor Neuron Diseases*, edited by F. H. Norris and L. T. Kurland. Grune and Stratton, New York, 1969, pp. 12–19.
5. Brain, W. R., Croft, P., and Wilkinson, M. The course and outcome of motor neuron disease. In: *Motor Neuron Diseases*, edited by F. H. Norris and L. T. Kurland. Grune and Stratton, New York, 1969, pp. 20–27.
6. Norris, F. H. Adult spinal motor neuron disease. In: *Handbook of Clinical Neurology*, edited by P. J. Vinken and G. W. Bruyn. 1975, vol. 22, North Holland, Amsterdam, pp. 1–56.
7. Dyck, P. J., Stevens, J. C., Mulder, D. W., and Espinosa, R. E. Frequency of nerve fiber degeneration of peripheral motor and sensory neurons in amyotrophic lateral sclerosis. Neurology *25:* 781–785, 1975.
8. Welch, K. M. A., and Goldberg, D. M. Serum creatine phosphokinase in motor neuron disease. Neurology *22:* 697–702, 1972.
9. Williams, E. R., and Bruford, A. Creatine phosphokinase in motor neuron disease. Clin. Chim. Acta *27:* 53, 1970.
10. Kjellin, K. G., and Stibler, H. Isoelectric focusing and electrophoresis of cerebrospinal fluid protein in muscular dystrophies and spinal muscular atrophies. J. Neurol. Sci. *27:* 45–57, 1976.
11. Boothby, J. A., deJesus, P. V., and Rowland, L. P. Reversible forms of motor neuron disease: Lead "neuritis." Arch. Neurol. *31:* 18–23, 1974.
12. Kantarjian, A. D. A syndrome clinically resembling amyotrophic lateral sclerosis following chronic mercurialism. Neurology *11:* 639–642, 1961.
13. Rustam, H., and Hamdi, T. Methyl mercury poisoning in Iraq. Brain *97:* 499–510, 1974.
14. Felmus, M. T., Patten, B. M., and Swanke, L. Antecedent events in amyotrophic lateral sclerosis. Neurology *26:* 167–172, 1976.
15. Norris, F. H., and Engel, W. K. Carcinomatous amyotrophic lateral sclerosis. In: *The Remote Effects of Cancer on the Nervous System*, edited by W. R. Brain and F. H. Norris. Grune and Stratton, New York, 1965.
16. Quick, D. T. Pancreatic dysfunction in amyotrophic lateral sclerosis. In: *Motor Neuron Diseases*, edited by F. H. Norris and L. T. Kurland. Grune and Stratton, New York, 1969, pp. 189–198.
17. Engel, W. K., Hogenhuis, L. A. H., Collis, W. J., Schalch, D. S., Barlow, M. H., Gold, G. N., and Dorman, J. Metabolic studies and therapeutic trials in amyotrophic lateral sclerosis. In: *Motor Neuron Diseases*, edited by F. H. Norris and L. T. Kurland. Grune and Stratton, New York, 1969, pp. 199–208.
18. Charcaflie, R. J., Fernandez, L. B., Perec, C. J., Gonzalez, E., and Marzi, A. Functional studies of the parotid and pancreas glands in amyotrophic lateral sclerosis. J. Neurol. Neurosurg. Psychiatry *37:* 863–867, 1974.
19. Dorman, J. D., Engel, W. K., and Fried, D. M. Therapeutic trial in amyotrophic lateral sclerosis. JAMA *209:* 257–260, 1969.
20. Wolfgram, F., and Myers, L. Amyotrophic lateral sclerosis: Effect of serum on anterior horn cells in tissue culture. Science *179:* 579–580, 1973.
21. Horwich, M. S., Engel, W. K., and Chauvin, P. B. Amyotrophic lateral sclerosis sera applied to cultured motor neurons. Arch. Neurol. *30:* 332–333, 1974.
22. Kayser Gatchalian, L. Late muscular atrophy after poliomyelitis. Eur. Neurol. *10:* 371–380,

1973.

23. Mulder, D. W., Rosenbaum, R. A., and Layton, D. D. Late progression of poliomyelitis or forme fruste amyotrophic lateral sclerosis. Mayo Clin. Proc. *27:* 756–761, 1972.

24. Oshiro, L. S., Cremer, N. E., Norris, F. H., and Lennette, E. H. Viruslike particles in muscle from a patient with amyotrophic lateral sclerosis. Neurology *26:* 57–60, 1976.

25. Antel, J. P., Arnason, B. G. W., Fuller, T. C., and Lehrich, J. R. Histocompatibility typing in amyotrophic lateral sclerosis. Arch. Neurol. *33:* 423–425, 1976.

26. Zil'ber, L. A., Bajdakova, Z. L., Gardasjan, A. N., Konovalov, N. V., Burina, T. L., and Barabadze, E. M. Study of the etiology of amyotrophic lateral sclerosis. Bull. WHO *29:* 449, 1963.

27. Gibbs, C. J., and Gajdusek, D. C. Kuru – A prototype subacute infectious disease of the nervous system as a model for the study of amyotrophic lateral sclerosis. In: *Motor Neuron Diseases,* edited by F. H. Norris and L. T. Kurland. Grune and Stratton, New York, 1969, pp. 269–279.

28. Norris, F. H. Amantadine in Jakob-Creutzfeldt disease. Brit. Med. J. *2:* 349, 1972.

29. Liversedge, L. A., and Campbell, M. J. Motor neurone diseases. In: *Disorders of Voluntary Muscle,* edited by J. N. Walton. Churchill Livingston, London, 1974, p. 790.

30. Liversedge, L. A., Swinburn, W. R., and Yuile, G. M. Idoxuridine and motor neuron disease. Brit. Med. J. *1:* 755, 1970.

31. Brody, J. A., Chen, K. M., Yase, Y., Holden, E. M., and Morris, C. E. Inosiplex and amyotrophic lateral sclerosis: Therapeutic trial in patients on Guam. Arch. Neurol. *30:* 322–323, 1974.

32. Percy, A. K., Davis, L. E., Johnston, D. M., and Drachman, D. B. Failure of isoprinosine in amyotrophic lateral sclerosis. New Engl. J. Med. *285:* 689, 1971.

33. Norris, F. H., Calanchini, P. R., Fallat, R. J., Panchari, S., and Jewett, B. The administration of guanidine in ALS. Neurology *24:* 721–728, 1974.

34. Mendell, J. R., Chase, T. N., and Engel, W. K. Amyotrophic lateral sclerosis: A study of central monoamine metabolism and a therapeutic trial of levo dopa. Arch. Neurol. *25:* 320, 1971.

35. Calcaterra, T. C., Kadell, B. M., and Ward, P. H. Dysphagia secondary to cricopharyngeal muscle dysfunction. Arch. Orolaryngol. *101:* 726–729, 1975.

36. Smith, R. A., and Norris, F. H., Symptomatic care of patients with amyotrophic lateral sclerosis. JAMA *234:* 715–717, 1975.

37. Brody, J. A., and Chen, K. M. Changing epidemiological patterns of amyotrophic lateral sclerosis and parkinsonism-dementia on Guam. In: *Motor Neuron Diseases*, edited by F. H. Norris and L. T. Kurland. Grune and Stratton, New York, 1969.

38. Hirano, A., Malamud, N., Kurland, L. T., and Zimmerman, H. M. A review of the pathologic findings in amyotrophic lateral sclerosis. In: *Motor Neuron Diseases,* edited by F. H. Norris and L. T. Kurland. Grune and Stratton, New York, 1969, pp. 51–60.

39. Kurtzke, J. F. Comments on the epidemiology of amyotrophic lateral sclerosis. In: *Motor Neuron Diseases,* edited by F. H. Norris and L. T. Kurland. Grune and Stratton, New York, 1969, pp. 85–89.

40. Shiraki, H. The neuropathology of amyotrophic lateral sclerosis (ALS) in the Kii peninsula and other areas of Japan. In: *Motor Neuron Diseases,* edited by F. H. Norris and L. T. Kurland. Grune and Stratton, New York, 1969, pp. 80–84.

41. Kimura, K., et al. Epidemiological and geomedical studies on amyotrophic lateral sclerosis. Dis. Nerv. Syst. *24:* 155–159, 1963.

42. Kondo, K., Tsubaki, T., and Sakamoto, F. The Ryukyuan muscular atrophy: An obscure heritable neuromuscular disease found in the islands of southern Japan. J. Neurol. Sci. *11:* 359–382, 1970.

43. Gomez, M. R., Clermont, V., and Bernstein, J. Progressive bulbar paralysis in childhood. Arch. Neurol. *6:* 317–323, 1962.

44. Alexander, M. P., Emery, E. S., and Koerner, F. C. Progressive bulbar paresis in childhood. Arch. Neurol. *33:* 66–68, 1976.

45. Kaeser, H. E. Scapuloperoneal muscular atrophy. Brain *88:* 407–418, 1965.

46. Furukawa, T., Tsukagoshi, H., Sugita, H., and Toyokura, Y. Neurogenic muscular atrophy simulating facioscapulohumeral muscular dystrophy. J. Neurol Sci. *9:* 389–397, 1969.

47. Emery, E. S., Fenichel, G. M., and Eng, G. A spinal muscular atrophy with scapulopero-

neal distribution. Arch. Neurol. *18:* 129–133, 1968.

48. Meadows, J. C., and Marsden, C. D. Scapuloperoneal amyotrophy. Arch. Neurol. *20:* 9–12, 1969.

49. Feigenbaum, J., and Munsat, T. L. A neuromuscular syndrome of scapuloperoneal distribution. Bull. Los Angeles Neurol. Soc. *35:* 47–57, 1970.

50. Fenichel, G. M., Emery, E. S., and Hunt, P. Neurogenic atrophy simulating facioscapulohumeral dystrophy. Arch. Neurol. *17:* 257–260, 1967.

3

peripheral neuropathies

Diseases of the peripheral nerves are so numerous and their causes so diverse that their study involves many different disciplines. The cursory attention which is given to them in this chapter is no indication of their importance. Excellent reviews are available elsewhere for those who need a fuller explanation of the subject.[1-3]

The peripheral nerves running between the central axis of the nervous system and the muscles and sensory organs contain some of the most remarkable cells in the body. Axons up to 1 meter in length may depend for their integrity on a cell body only 50 micra in diameter. The metabolic problems that this presents have been solved by a complicated system of axonal transport. Concepts with regard to the functions of peripheral nerves are slowly changing and neurons are no longer considered passive conductors of electrical impulses. It is now apparent that they convey not only electrical impulses, but also nutrient and other trophic substances. They play a complex role in the maintenance of muscle tissue: not only do muscle fibers atrophy if their nerve supply is removed, but the type of muscle fiber, its biochemical and physiological properties, are partly determined by the activity of the nerve by which it is innervated. It is possible that trophic substances pass from the nerve across the neuromuscular junction to the muscle, although conclusive proof of this is lacking.

Peripheral nerves consist of both myelinated and unmyelinated fibers of various sizes. The Schwann cells are responsible for the formation of the myelin, which is arrayed in concentric layers around the axon. Each Schwann cell is associated with a short segment of myelin, and is separated by a node of Ranvier from its neighbor. The thickness of the myelin and the length of the segments vary proportionately with the size of the axon. The myelin acts as an insulating substance and allows rapid conduction of the electrical impulse down the nerve. This is made possible by the fact that the impulse "jumps" from node to node, the so-called "saltatory" type of nerve conduction. The largest myelinated fibers are the most rapidly conducting fibers, whereas small, unmyelinated fibers conduct relatively slowly. The nerves serving various functions may also be roughly grouped in sizes, although such grouping is not without exceptions. Among the largest myelinated fibers are those conducting impulses to the muscle and those transmitting the proprioceptive impulses of joint and position sense and touch pressure sensation back to the spinal cord. On the other hand, the small, unmyelinated fibers include autonomic fibers and some of the fibers conducting pain and temperature sensation.

SIGNS AND SYMPTOMS

The symptoms of peripheral nerve disease are weakness, due to damage of the motor nerves, and sensory alteration, due to damage of the afferent nerves. The sensory change may be either a loss of sensation or an abnormal sensation. In some forms of neuropathy the motor symptoms predominate, while in others sensory complaints are more noticeable. Most often it is the longest nerve fibers which are preferentially involved. Because of this, weakness and numbness of the hands and feet may be the presenting complaint. The various symptoms of weakness are not peculiar to peripheral neuropathy but depend on the distribution of the muscles involved in the weakness. Patients may have difficulty turning door handles or opening car doors. Undoing screw capped jars or manipulating small objects, such as coins or pins, may be a problem. Weakness of the feet may cause stumbling and tripping as the toes catch on the curb. The ankle may be sprained on frequent occasions, and walking over rough ground may be impossible because the ankle turns over. Impairment of sensation in the hands and feet is usually described as a sense of numbness, although the word "weakness" may be used for this feeling. Frequently, when the patient with sensory abnormality is questioned about the numbness, he will run his thumb lightly over the tips of his fingers while answering as though testing for himself the presence or absence of the symptom. The skin may feel as if a membrane overlies it. In severe sensory loss in the feet the patient may complain of a sensation of walking on sponge. The name "glove and stocking" hypesthesia has been given to the sensory loss seen in peripheral neuropathies, partly because the distribution of the numbness conforms to this area, but perhaps partly because the patient feels as if perpetually clad in gloves and stockings.

The symptoms are not limited to loss of sensory ability; there also occur abnormal sensations, dysesthesiae. When severe, there may be a constant burning pain in the hands and feet. At other times such pain is experienced only in response to a stimulus. This results in the paradoxical situation wherein a patient's ability to perceive touch or pin prick is impaired but, when the strength of the stimulus is increased until it is finally detected, the sensation is accompanied by an unpleasant burning quality and the patient feels it more than would a normal person. A moment's reflection on a common phenomenon may explain this. Stubbing one's toe hard against an object results in an immediate, sharp pain which is succeeded a fraction of a second later by the suffusion of an intensely unpleasant glow of pain. This second pain is due to conduction along the small unmyelinated fibers and may be preserved in patients with peripheral neuropathy. Thus, when pin prick is tested, they sense not the initial sensitive fast pain sensation, but only the second uncomfortable feeling. A common sensory complaint which is difficult to explain is the occurrence of paresthesiae. This varies from the feeling of "pins and needles" to such peculiar sensations as water running over the fingers or insects crawling across the limbs. Sometimes this tingling is spontaneous; at other times it is produced in response to rubbing or percussing the skin. The origin of these sensations is not clear.

Examination of the patient with a peripheral neuropathy reveals motor weakness which is predominantly distal and which is accompanied by sensory abnormalities. The detection of these sensory abnormalities may be quite difficult at times, and tests with greater and lesser degrees of sophistication have been designed. Touch sensation can be tested by stroking the skin lightly and inquiring whether the feeling is normal. In patients who are reliable this method, though simple, can be quite accurate. A more quantitative evaluation of touch can be gained by using Frey hairs. Other methods have been devised for the quantitative evaluation of touch-pressure and thermal sensation.[4, 5] In testing joint position sense, the normal subject should be able to perceive the smallest movement of the finger joints that can be made by the examiner, since in this way the examiner's proprioceptive mechanisms are being used to rate those of the subject. In testing position sense in the toes, larger movements of the joints must be made. The examination of vibration sense requires the use of a tuning fork at 128 Hz.

A rough evaluation of the conduction velocity of a nerve can be made clinically. The examiner holds a pin between the thumb and forefinger with the point slightly concealed. The dorsum of the patient's foot or hand is then tapped repetitively several times a second, using the pad of the index finger. At some moment the point of the pin is substituted for the finger but the rhythm is not changed. If the patient has been instructed to tell the examiner at the exact moment when he feels the pin prick, he will normally do this within a fraction of a second of the changeover. Patients with peripheral neuropathy, however, may show as much as a second's delay. A control test must always be done using the proximal part of the limb or the shoulder area for the same test. Unless there is a more rapid response with a proximal stimulus, the test is invalidated.

Since sensory testing involves the patient's cooperation, it is sometimes difficult to determine the validity of a sensory loss in a patient who has a vested interest in persuading the physician that it is real. There are, however, many ways that this can be done. The most banal is to ask the patient to close his eyes, touch the skin repetitively, instructing the patient to say "yes" when he feels a stimulus and "no" when he does not. Given the level of sophistication in this day and age, it is unlikely that patients will fall for that particular ruse. A variation on the theme can be played, however, using a pin. The patient is asked whether the pin feels sharp or dull, and the pin is then pressed only very lightly on the skin. Patients will almost uniformly say that the pin feels dull. Some minutes later the test is repeated after distracting the patient's attention with other matters. This time, although the stimulus is identical, the instruction is given to the patient to tell the examiner whether the touch is perceived. If the patient now denies feeling the light touch at all, this is a discrepancy not to be explained on anatomical grounds. Patients who have hysterical position sense loss may sometimes be baffled by the following maneuver. The patient is asked to lie down and then the examiner holds the patient's foot in the air with the knee slightly flexed. The patient is instructed to close his eyes and point at the big toe. Patients who feel that they should have position sense loss do not point at the toe but point off to one side. The examiner then moves the toe so that it is in line with the pointing finger, which upsets the patient who promptly moves the finger. Obviously, the ability of the patient to know where his toe is in space can be demonstrated by having him point away from the toe just as well as it can by having him point at the toe. Hysterical abnormalities of vibration sense are best detected by demonstrating differences on two sides of a bony structure such as the forehead or the sternum. Since the vibration is transmitted through the bone, this is, obviously, not a real defect. Two point discrimination can also be used to detect sensory loss which is not real. The two point threshold is determined on one occasion and then several minutes later is re-evaluated. Marked differences over the same site are unlikely to be due to organic disease.

Palpation and percussion of the peripheral nerves is an important part of the examination. Palpation of nerves should be carried out in normal patients as well as those suspected of having a neuropathy. Only after repeated examination of the normal does it become possible to decide when a nerve is truly hypertrophic. Percussion of the nerves at various points such as the carpal tunnel, the ulnar groove, and the lateral head of the fibula is also useful. Tinel's sign is the production of a tingling sensation in the sensory distribution of the nerve being percussed. Although originally used to follow the progress of a regenerating nerve (percussion over the newly regenerating region produces the tingling), it may be useful in some cases in demonstrating early degeneration of peripheral nerves.

CLASSIFICATION

Many systems of classification have been devised for peripheral neuropathies in the past, and perhaps new and more suitable ones will be devised in the future. For those who wish only a brief acquaintance with these diseases, it may be convenient to consider the parts of the peripheral nerve which can be affected. A disease can affect the axon, the Schwann cell and myelin sheath, the spaces between the nerve fibers (as for example, when the deposition of foreign material compresses the nerve fibers in amyloidosis), or the blood supply of the nerve. Unfortunately, in most neuropathies the damage is not limited to one of these areas but occurs secondarily throughout the nerve. It is then quite difficult to decide where the earliest change began or whether simultaneous damage to different structures has occurred. This reduces any system of classification based on the anatomical changes, at best, to an approximation.

Neuropathies following Trauma

Following a local crush injury a process known as Wallerian degeneration takes place. The axons distal to the injury degenerate. The surrounding myelin breaks into large ellipsoids and then finally into small fragments and droplets. Macrophages move in to remove the debris. In cases where the nerve crush is incomplete, axon sprouts grow back down the original pathways and are remyelinated by the Schwann cells which survive the general degenerative process. If the injury is a local crush injury without transection of the nerve, regeneration is usually complete. However, if there has been severe damage to the nerve or if transection of the nerve has resulted in a loss of apposition of the two cut ends, regeneration is much less complete and may not take place at all. Frank lacerations of the nerves will seldom be seen in a muscle clinic for obvious reasons, but sometimes patients with less overt damage are seen. Repeated trauma to the ulnar nerve in the ulnar groove may present with sensory and motor difficulties in the hand. The appropriate history may not be obtained unless the patient is questioned closely. One patient arriving in the muscle clinic with an ulnar palsy denied any history of trauma. While discussing his day to day activities, he mentioned that he was a truck driver and that, while driving, he had found the most comfortable position to be one with his elbow resting on the partly raised window on the side of his cab. He even commented that there seemed to be a little groove in the elbow into which the edge of the window fit. Other peripheral nerves are also susceptible to such damage. The median nerve may be compressed in the carpal tunnel in a variety of illnesses. The radial nerve may be compressed by the back of a kitchen chair on a Saturday night or the tops of crutches. The lateral popliteal nerve where it winds around the fibula may suffer from insults as various as ill fitting plaster casts or the sacks tied tightly around the legs of hop-pickers to protect them against thorns and brambles.

Neuropathies with Prominent "Axonal" Changes

Some peripheral neuropathies are primarily the result of axonal degeneration. Often a "dying back" phenomenon is noted, in which there is a progressive destruction of the axon beginning in its most peripheral portions. Usually, but not always, the longest neurons in the body are involved first. The cause of the phenomenon is not fully known. It seems reasonable to suspect some abnormality of the nutritional system in the neuron. The distal ends of the axon are maintained by a cell body and nucleus far removed and, in any abnormality affecting the "transport" systems of the axon, the terminal parts of the axon might be expected to suffer first. Many of the neuropathies produced by toxic substances are associated with this type of change. Man has produced an almost infinite variety of chemicals with which to poison himself. They range from industrial solvents to insecticides, from medicines to such well known compounds as triorthocresyl phosphate,[6, 7] acrylamide,[8] vincristine,[9] and thalidomide.[10] For a more complete list of these, other references should be consulted.[1–3]

Acute intermittent porphyria is associated with a peripheral neuropathy in which changes in the terminal portions of the axons are pronounced.[11] There may be associated changes in myelin but these are probably secondary. The patient suffers from an acute, often relapsing, neuropathy associated with a history of recurrent abdominal pain and not infrequently of psychotic episodes. These attacks may be precipitated by the use of drugs such as barbiturates or sulfonamides. The neuropathy of porphyria may affect proximal muscle groups, but patients with a typical peripheral distribution of weakness are also seen. The disease is predominantly a motor neuropathy and, although sensory complaints are seen, they are not as pronounced as those of weakness.

Thiamine deficiency also produces a distal sensorimotor neuropathy. The pathology probably affects both the myelin sheath and the axon, but experimental evidence suggests that the axonal damage is more pronounced than the destruction of myelin. Other vitamin deficiences such as those of B_6 (pyridoxine) and B_{12} are associated with peripheral neuropathy. Isoniazid also causes a neuropathy by interfering with the metabolism of pyridoxine.

The peripheral neuropathy associated with alcoholism is well known. The malnutrition so common in alcoholism plays an essential part in the development of the neuropathy, although whether it alone gives rise to the disease or whether there is some toxic effect of alcohol is uncertain. The symptoms of alcoholic peripheral neuropathy, like those of the neuropathy of diabetes, include painful burning sensations in the extremities. The hands and feet may be so sensitive that even the touch of bed clothes or the approach of the neurologist in quest of the Babinski response may cause the patient to wince.

Giant axonal neuropathy is an unusual form of axonal degeneration in which an apparent peripheral neuropathy commences in childhood and is progressive.[12, 13] The motor findings are more severe than the sensory abnormalities. Ballooning of the axons occurs, owing to the accumulation of neurofilamentous material. The hair of such patients is described as pale reddish and tightly curled, although no morphologic abnormality of the hair shaft has yet been noted. This distinguishes the disease from kinky hair disease, together with the sparse hair which is characteristic of the latter. Biochemical abnormalities were seen with a decrease in the number of disulfide groups and an increase in sulfhydryl groups in the hair. A similar axonal degeneration with the accumulation of neurofilamentous material has been reported in a patient with neuropathy secondary to "glue-sniffing," the glue containing *n*-hexane.[14]

Infantile neuroaxonal dystrophy is a progressive and fatal disease with severe involvement of the central nervous system as well as the peripheral nerves.[15–17] This clinical distinction is reinforced pathologically by the different ultrastructural characteristics of the axonal swellings which, in this disease, contain tubular material and glycoprotein.

Fabry's disease is a rare, inherited sphingolipidosis due to a deficiency of ceramide trihexosidase. Abnormal glycolipid, mostly ceramide trihexose, accumulates in different tissues. The illness occurs in males far more often than in females. Characteristic lesions of the skin of the lower trunk and thighs, consisting of small, telangiectatic papules, give rise to the alternate name for the illness, angiokeratoma corporis diffusa. Abnormalities of the blood vessels may be associated with renal, cerebral, and myocardial disease. Corneal opacities are noted, and dilated, tortuous blood vessels are seen in the retina and conjunctiva. A prominent part of the illness is the occurrence of severe lancinating or burning pain of an intermittent nature involving the hands and feet. Pathological studies have shown the primary change to be axonal affecting the small myelinated and unmyelinated fibers. Abnormal lipid deposition is seen in the dorsal ganglia cell bodies of the spinal roots.[18]

Tangier disease is yet another rarity. It is associated with low levels of high density lipoprotein and low levels of plasma cholesterol. Cholesteryl esters are deposited in many tissues, including the tonsils, which are enlarged and bright orange, the skin, and the rectal mucosa. Half the patients suffer from a peripheral neuropathy of varying severity, often demonstrating a propensity for loss of pain and temperature sensation before other modalities. Nerve biopsies show a loss of both myelinated and unmyelinated fibers.[19] Some of the damage may be mechanical, caused by the accumulation of cholesterol in the peripheral nerves.

A peripheral neuropathy is frequently part of the syndrome in Bassen Kornzweig's disease associated with a-beta-lipoproteinemia.

Neuropathies with Prominent Changes in the Schwann Cells or Myelin

Distinct from the illnesses in which the axon bears the brunt of the pathology are those in which segmental demyelination is found. This occurs when myelin is lost from the segment between two nodes of Ranvier, the territory of the Schwann cell. Whether myelin is lost from neighboring segments depends on whether there has been damage to neighboring Schwann cells. The difference is clearer in theory than in practice, but it does have several implications. In cases in which damage to the Schwann cell and myelin occurs, since myelinated fibers are preferentially involved, signs of motor disturbance and position and vibration sense loss might be expected. With loss of small unmyelinated axons, preferential loss of pain and temperature sensation might be anticipated. Unfortunately, this is not always accurate; a more reliable correlation is found in abnormalities of nerve conduction velocities. When loss of the myelin sheath occurs, it does so segmentally. The myelin associated with one Schwann cell between two nodes of Ranvier is lost, while neighboring segments may be quite intact. This results in a slowing of conduction of the nervous impulse, but does not obliterate such conduction. Each peripheral neuron may have many hundreds of nodes distributed along its length. If the involvement of the Schwann cells is random, then one would expect all the myelinated nerves to suffer at one or more points along their length. This will result in a slowing of conduction in all nerves. Electromyographic studies in which conduction velocity is estimated will demonstrate this slowing. In axonal damage, on the other hand, the axon is much more likely to stop conducting the impulse at all rather than to slow it down. Furthermore, if the axonal disease is random, some axons will be totally nonconductive and others will be spared, and those that are spared will conduct the impulse normally. Since the conduction velocity is measured from the fastest conducting fibers, marked slowing is not seen, although the amplitude of the evoked potential may be much less than normal.

Another aspect of the difference between axonal degeneration and segmental demyelination is the speed with which recovery takes place after nerve damage. If the axon is damaged, even when the factor causing the damage is removed, it takes a considerable time for the axon to grow back down to its termination. In segmental demyelination, on the other hand, recovery is much more rapid. Thus, when the noxious influence causing the segmental demyelination is removed, myelin is fairly swiftly laid down by the surviving Schwann cells. An experimental model which is often used to produce this change in animals is diphtheria. The organism produces a neurotoxin which becomes fixed to the nerves and which, after two to six weeks, may produce a severe neuropathy. Diphtheria may also cause a local paralysis of the palatal muscles without such delay. The illness is seldom seen these days because of the wide use of immunization and the sensitivity of the organism to antibiotics. Lead poisoning, another cause of segmental demyelination, may produce a peripheral neuropathy which is predominantly motor with a predilection for the extensor muscles of the forearm. These symptoms are usually, but not always, associated with abdominal cramps and central nervous system complications of lead intoxication. The diagnosis depends upon the demonstration of abnormal lead levels and may be suspected in the presence of basophilic stippling of the erythrocytes. Occasionally the so-called "lead line," a blue discoloration, may be seen close to the border of the gums.

That a neuropathy is associated with diabetes is well known, although the pathological changes which cause the symptoms are less well defined. There is evidence for the occurrence of both segmental demyelination and axonal changes in patients with diabetic peripheral neuropathy. A few authors have suggested that the proliferation of the endothelium in peripheral blood vessels together with abnormalities in the capillaries cause an ischemic change in the nerve. Clinically, the patient suffers from increasing distal sensory loss, usually experiencing painful and burning sensations. The numbness and tingling begin in the fingers and toes and gradually spread upwards. There are alterations in pain sensation and in autonomic function which may be associated with perforating ulcers of the feet and other trophic changes in the extremities. Distal neuropathy is only one of the neurological complications of diabetes. Episodes in which the function of a major proximal nerve trunk is impaired are not uncommon. These may occur quite suddenly, are often heralded by pain, and are probably due to ischemia. The brachial plexus is involved as is the femoral nerve. The latter provides such a distinct clinical picture that it was thought to be a separate complication of diabetes and was named diabetic amyotrophy. This usually occurs in an elderly male whose diabetes is out of control. The onset of the illness is heralded by pain, and there ensues an asymmetric proximal wasting of the anterior muscles of the thigh. The sensory involvement in this and other proximal lesions of the nerve trunk may be quite minor. In many patients the weakness associated with these proximal syndromes improves as the diabetes is brought under control. In this regard it is unlike the peripheral neuropathy, which often persists in spite of adequate treatment of the diabetes. Other ischemic complications of diabetes involve peripheral nerves. Sequential involvement of major peripheral nerves (mononeuritis multiplex) or of the oculomotor nerves is not uncommon.

In acute idiopathic polyneuropathy and polyradiculopathy, usually known as the Guillain-Barré syndrome, the most severe change is in the proximal part of the nerve roots rather than in the peripheral nerve. A brisk inflammatory response is followed by segmental demyelination which also affects peripheral nerves.[20] The disease often begins about one to three weeks after a preceding upper respiratory infection or other "viral" illness. The initial symptom is almost always a numb or tingling sensation in the arms and legs. In spite of the symptoms there are rarely any sensory findings. Shortly after this a progressive weakness of the muscles of the limbs develops which may rapidly spread to involve truncal muscles. The facial nerves may also be involved, and varieties of the disease affecting other cranial nerves have been described. The weakness may become worse for about two to three weeks and then levels off. If the patient survives the period of greatest weakness, in which respiratory paralysis may occur, recovery ensues. The recovery may be incomplete in some cases. The most helpful laboratory investigation is examination of the cerebrospinal fluid which, at some stage in the disease, demonstrates albuminocytologic dissociation, an elevated protein with normal cell counts. In those patients in whom such elevation of protein is not found the excuse is often used that the lumbar puncture is performed too soon, before the protein becomes abnormal, or too late, after it has again fallen to normal. The similarity between this illness and experimental allergic neuronitis, a disease of animals produced by the injection of peripheral nerve extract and Freund's adjuvant, has suggested an autoimmune etiology. This seems likely, although the response to steroids is equivocal.

There are other diseases of myelin besides those of segmental demyelination. In sulfatide lipidosis (metachromatic leukodystrophy) the peripheral nerves are involved, both clinically and as demonstrated by electromyography, in addition to the more severe abnormalities in the central nervous system. The disease is due to a deficiency of aryl sulfatase a. This results in an abnormal breakdown of myelin owing to the fact that cerebroside sulfate cannot be degraded, and the accumulation of this lipid in the nervous tissue gives rise to the metachromatic staining properties. The diagnosis may be made by estimation of the enzyme itself, by the demonstration of metachromatic degeneration of myelin, or by the presence of metachromatic granules in the urine. Clinically, it is one of the causes of severe neurologic deficit (spasticity, ataxia, dementia) associated with a peripheral neuropathy. In the infantile variety the emphasis is on the progression of these neurologic deficits. In the adult, intellectual deterioration and psychiatric disorders may predominate.

Other Neuropathies

Nerves may be damaged by the infiltration of foreign substances into the nerve trunk, as is seen in amyloidosis. Some forms of amyloidosis are secondary to other general medical diseases. A form of primary amyloidosis occurs as an autosomal dominant. It is prevalent in northern Portugal, afflicts young adults, and is progressive, with survival for about ten years. The peripheral neuropathy is predominantly sensory. This correlates with the fact that the smallest fibers are lost first. There is also loss of autonomic function; the systemic signs of this include gastrointestinal problems, impotence, postural hypotension, anisocoria, and cardiac abnormalities. Amyloid deposits occur in the kidneys, and renal function becomes progressively impaired.

In another form the disease is much milder, occurs later in life, and is only slowly progressive. It is also inherited as an autosomal dominant and often begins in the hands as a carpal tunnel syndrome because of infiltration of the flexor retinaculum with amyloid material. Later the symmetrical polyneuropathy develops. Renal involvement and autonomic abnormalities may occur late in the disease, and some families have vitreous opacities. Other varieties of amyloidosis have also been described. (For review see Reference 21.)

Inflammatory diseases of the nerve are rarely seen except in tropical countries, although leprosy is still a very common cause of neuropathy worldwide. There are two forms. In the lepromatous type of disease, a characteristic skin lesion with hypertrophy and disfiguration is common. A peripheral sensory neuropathy occurs, and the peripheral nerves are heavily infested by the bacteria. The loss of pain sensation is severe and, because of the loss of this protective mechanism, trauma and infection of various parts of the body lead to severe disfiguration with loss of fingers, penetrating ulcers, and disorganized joints. The tuberculoid form of leprosy is associated with patches of depigmented and atrophic skin. There is some thickening of the nerves, and the picture is very often that of a mononeuritis rather than a diffuse peripheral neuropathy. The bacilli are not commonly found in the nerve. Intermediate forms between the two clinical extremes are seen.

Peripheral nerves may be damaged by ischemia, and neuropathies, particularly mononeuritis multiplex, are associated with the many "collagen vascular" diseases, probably because of the occlusion of small vessels. Malignant disease is also associated with a neuropathy—carcinomatous neuropathy—which is difficult to characterize. Often the sensory changes have a fleeting, evanescent character that can be very puzzling.

Chronic Familial Peripheral Neuropathies (Hereditary Motor and Sensory Neuropathies[1])

There is a group of patients with peripheral neuropathies which is seen with great frequency in the muscle clinic. This is not because the disease is more common than the other varieties but perhaps because superficially it resembles muscular dystrophy. Such patients experience a slow progression of weakness with but minor sensory abnormalities. There is often a family history of the illness. The most common example is the variety of peripheral neuropathy described by Charcot and Marie and by Tooth. Although long regarded as a single disease, the existence of at least two separate entities now seems likely.[22, 23] In both there is a distal weakness of the legs with a predilection for involvement of the muscles innervated by the peroneal nerves, particularly the evertors of the foot (Figures 3.1 to 3.4).

In one form the nerves are hypertrophic and, although the disease is usually an autosomal dominant with fairly marked penetrance, it may also occur sporadically.[23] As in so many diseases which are slowly progressive, it is difficult to ascertain the time of onset. Generally, within the first twenty years, some deformity of the feet is noted. The foot is often high arched with the toes flexed at the interphalangeal joints. The metatarsophalangeal joint is dorsiflexed, which causes the toe to be drawn back towards the dorsum of the foot. Initially the foot is quite flexible, and upward pressure with one finger over the ball of the foot may cause the deformity to disappear. The ball of the foot is made especially prominent by the structural change and may become painful owing to the pounding it receives as the patient walks. Early on in the illness the walk is noted to be clumsy, with frequent tripping and a marked tendency to sprain the ankles. Walking over rough surfaces, such as a plowed field, gives particular trouble. The weakness spreads, and involvement of the plantar flexors and then of the more proximal muscles in the legs is not uncommon. Patients who have weakness of both extensors and plantar flexors of the foot have great difficulty standing still because of loss of stability of the ankle joint. It is in such patients that a triple arthrodesis of the ankle can be of great help. Patients seldom complain of dysesthesiae. The painful sensations and the "pins and needles" feelings which are so common in some of the other peripheral neuropathies are absent from Charcot-Marie-Tooth disease. As the weakness progresses in the legs, the hands also become involved and difficulty with the manipulation of small objects is noted. At a later stage, the disability is severe enough to cause a marked slap-footed gait.

Examination of the patient in the early stages may show no more than the pes cavus. A little later, wasting and weakness of the peroneal musculature are noted. Careful inspection almost always reveals atrophy of the extensor digitorum brevis on the dorsum of the foot, even in the early stages of the disease. This is useful in differentiating Charcot-Marie-Tooth disease from some of the "non-neurogenic" causes of anterior tibial weakness in which this same muscle may be hypertrophied. In the moderately advanced stage of the disease, severe distal atrophy is noted in both hands and feet, producing a tapered appearance to the limb. Dyck and Lambert point out that the

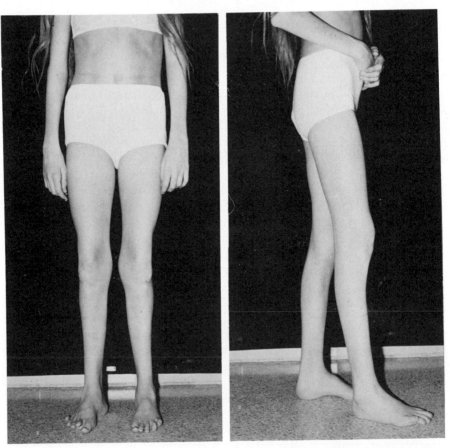

Figures 3.1 and 3.2. Hereditary motor neuropathy (Charcot-Marie-Tooth). Distal wasting of the leg muscles. In the anterior view, wasting of the lower part of the quadriceps muscle is seen. The lateral bulge of this muscle is much higher up the thigh than normal.

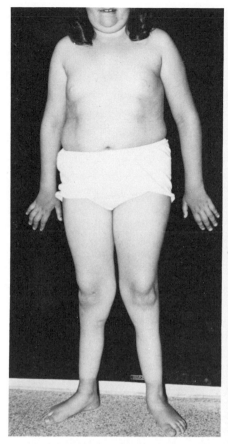 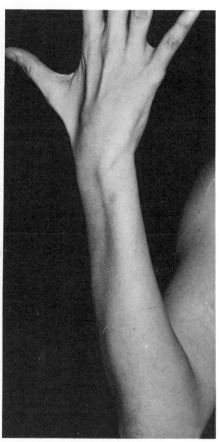

Figure 3.3 (*left*). Hereditary motor neuropathy (Charcot-Marie-Tooth). Distal wasting of the muscles of the leg is associated with a knock kneed appearance. The feet are flat rather than high arched.

Figure 3.4 (*right*). Wasting of the hand and the distal part of the forearm in a patient with hereditary motor neuropathy. There is hollowing of the interosseous spaces and between the radius and ulna.

classical stork leg configuration, with an almost total loss of muscle bulk below the knee, is not seen in this type of Charcot-Marie-Tooth disease. Loss of the deep tendon reflexes occurs, beginning at the ankle jerks, then involving the quadriceps, and later the deep tendon reflexes of the arms. Sensory examination shows diminution of all sensory modalities, but particularly of vibration, joint position, and light touch. Again, the sensory changes are relatively slight compared to the motor abnormalities. The nerves are palpably abnormal (hypertrophic) in about one quarter of the cases.

Electromyography and nerve biopsy are the most useful studies for the diagnosis of this illness. Conduction velocities are approximately one half the normal value, and the distal latency may be increased to three times normal. Even early in the disease, before clinical troubles become marked, there is reduction in the conduction velocity and in some relatives of patients with the dominant form of Charcot-Marie-Tooth disease there may be reduction in the conduction velocity with only mild abnormality in the clinical picture. Muscle biopsy in patients with Charcot-Marie-Tooth disease shows abnormalities which, in our experience, are uniformly present even in a muscle that is quite strong. We often biopsy the biceps muscle and find the changes of type grouping and other mild changes of denervation and reinnervation. A sural nerve biopsy, however, is more useful in the evaluation of this illness. There is an increase in the fascicular cross-sectional area with some reduction in the number of nerves. The largest myelinated nerves are smaller than normal. Evidence of repetitive demyelination and remyelination is seen in the formation of "onion bulb" structures. Similar evidence for segmental demyelination is found in teased nerve preparations where the usually regular internodal length can become quite variable. Sometimes the entity is associated with a static tremor of the hands, and the eponym Roussy-Levy has been given to this. Some feel that these two diseases are the same and any distinction based on the presence or absence of tremor is artificial.

The second form of Charcot-Marie-Tooth disease has been termed the "neuronal" variety.[23] It is also inherited with an autosomal dominant pattern and differs from the hypertrophic type of Charcot-Marie-Tooth disease in that the pathology involves not segmental demyelination but neuronal changes. Thus, the conduction velocities are only slightly reduced and the nerve fibers do not show evidence of the segmental demyelination or hypertrophic changes seen in the first variety. Clinically, the disease begins later. The first symptoms are often noticed in early adult life or even in middle age. The distal weakness of the legs is more severe and the characteristic stork leg is more frequently seen in this variety. Weakness of the plantar flexors of the feet is more marked in this illness than in the previous variety. The hands, conversely, are less affected and the sensory changes are even less pronounced. Otherwise, the disease behaves similarly and the progression of the weakness can be observed over many years. Interestingly, most patients are able to function in their daily activities in spite of the most severe atrophy of muscles. It is startling to watch the patient with Charcot-Marie-Tooth disease walk when almost no muscles are visible below the knee, whereas a patient with motor neuron disease and the same degree of wasting would be totally disabled.

A third type of Charcot-Marie-Tooth disease, possibly a variant of the "neuronal" type, has been suggested as a form of spinal muscular atrophy. This diagnosis is based on the absence of any sensory findings in a patient who seems to have Charcot-Marie-Tooth disease. Hypertrophic nerves are not present. This variety may be related to the disease described under slow motor neuron disease or focal motor neuron disease in the previous chapter.

One of the most severe peripheral neuropathies is that originally described by Déjèrine and Sottas. This disease is a sensorimotor neuropathy which is present at or shortly after birth. The onset of walking is almost always delayed, and the patients are usually confined to a wheelchair by the time they reach adult life. Some may have truncal ataxia and choreic movements of the outstretched hands. Most often, however, these are the "piano playing" movements of severe position sense loss seen when the patient tries to discover exactly where his fingers are in space by moving them from time to time. All of the patients with Déjèrine-Sottas disease have markedly slow conduction velocities, indeed, among the slowest ever encountered. The disease is inherited as an autosomal recessive; the diagnosis can be made by nerve biopsy. In addition to the onion bulb formations, there is frequent segmental demyelination. The disease may differ from Charcot-Marie-Tooth in that the myelin surrounding the nerve is often thinned. It used to be thought that the presence of onion bulb formations was rather specific for this type of neuropathy. They are seen, however, in all conditions in which segmental demyelination and remyelination are continuing processes.

Another familial form of peripheral neuropathy is Refsum disease. In this condition, which is inherited as an autosomal recessive disease, there is an accumulation of phytanic acid in the body. The clinical picture is of a peripheral neuropathy associated with cerebellar abnormalities (ataxia, nystagmus), retinal degeneration with night blindness, nerve deafness, ichthyosis, and cardiac abnormalities. Treatment of this illness has been attempted by dietary reduction of the amount of phytol, from which phytanic acid is derived. Although this results in considerable improvement, the disease is by no means cured.

The chronic familial neuropathies seem to be one end of a spectrum, the other pole of which is occupied by the familial spinocerebellar degenerations. It is not uncommon to find clinical signs of peripheral nerve disease in patients with Friedreich's ataxia, and electrical evidence of damaged peripheral nerves is the rule. One also sees mixed pictures in which the predominant abnormality is a peripheral neuropathy but in which fragments of the spinocerebellar disorders are expressed. This has led to a confusing array of clinical pictures in which it seems that no two families have exactly the same disease. A noteworthy attempt to reduce this chaos is a classification proposed by Dyck. In summary, within the category of hereditary motor and sensory neuropathies, he proposed seven types. Type I is equivalent to the dominantly inherited hypertrophic form of Charcot-Marie-Tooth disease, and Type II to the neuronal variety. Type III is the hypertrophic neuropathy of infancy (Déjèrine-Sottas disease) and Type IV is Refsum disease. Type V is an illness in which the major problem is a spastic paraplegia often inherited as an autosomal dominant. In these patients the peripheral neuropathy may be found only on electromyographic or pathological studies or it may be overt. Type VI is proposed for the association of optic atrophy and peroneal muscular atrophy, and Type VII indicates patients with retinitis pigmentosa.[1]

Neuralgic Amyotrophy (Brachial Neuralgia)

Neuralgic amyotrophy is characterized by the onset of shoulder weakness following an attack of acute pain in the shoulder. Most cases are sporadic; these often follow an episode of trauma or infection, or they may be preceded by a vaccination. The disease may also begin during the acute stage of serum sickness. In the sporadic variety men are more frequently affected than women by a ratio of 2.4 to 1. The disease may occur at any age, but the majority occur between the third and seventh decades.[24]

The illness is ushered in by a sudden and acute pain in the shoulder. The pain is intense and is described as stabbing, aching, or throbbing. It may be sharply localized to the shoulder or it may be more diffuse with radiation to the neck or down the arm. On occasion it is difficult for the patient to state exactly where the pain is. As the pain subsides the muscles of the shoulder girdle lose their strength. In most patients, this occurs within two weeks of the onset of the pain. The muscles supplied by the upper trunks of the brachial plexus are often preferentially involved. The deltoid, serratus anterior, supra- and infraspinatus, and trapezius are especially susceptible. Occasionally, a specific peripheral nerve such as the radial or the long thoracic will be involved. Paralysis of the diaphragm due to phrenic nerve involvement has also been seen. More unusually the muscles supplied by the lower part of the brachial plexus become weak. Recovery is the rule but may be delayed up to two or more years from the onset of the pain. In one series 80% recovered fully and only 2 of 84 patients had noted no improvement since the onset of their weakness.[24] In addition to the motor findings, two-thirds of the patients have sensory abnormalities. It is not uncommon to find a patch of hypesthesia over the lateral aspect of the deltoid or over the radial side of the forearm. The disease is usually unilateral, but up to a third of the patients may have bilateral symptoms. It is important to exclude local pathology with nerve compression as a possible reason for shoulder atrophy.

Laboratory studies show definite evidence of denervation, although the site of the pathology is not clearly delineated. Nerve conduction studies may show decreased conduction velocity in the affected nerves. Corticosteroids have been used in the treatment of this illness, but do not seem to have any noticeable effect.

In addition to the sporadic cases, neuralgic amyotrophy may occur on a familial basis and is often recurrent. Bradley et al.[25] suggested that the familial variety be divided into those with recurrent attacks restricted to the brachial plexus, those who had recurrent attacks with additional lesions outside the brachial plexus, some of whom had associated hypotelorism, and those with familial pressure sensitive neuropathy without any predominance for the brachial plexus.

The illness seems to occur as an autosomal dominant. It is seen in a younger age group, and the disease has no preference for either sex. Pregnancy is particularly associated with exacerbations. The sensory changes are more commonly seen over the radial aspect of the forearm; evidence for involvement of other nerves includes dysphonia and Horner's syndrome.[26] Pathological examination of the sural nerve in two cases showed a reduction in the number of myelinated fibers and focal thickening of the myelin sheaths. In recurrent acute neuropathy without a family history, no such changes were noted but there was evidence of old segmental demyelinization with variation of the internodal length.

BIBLIOGRAPHY

1. Dyck, P. J., Thomas, P. K., and Lambert, E. H. *Peripheral Neuropathy*. Saunders, Philadelphia, 1975.
2. Bradley, W. G. *Disorders of Peripheral Nerves*. Churchill-Livingstone, Oxford, 1975.
3. Goldstein, N. P., and Dyck, P. J. Diseases of peripheral nerves. In: *Clinical Neurology*, edited by A. B. Baker and L. H. Baker. Harper & Row, New York, 1973.
4. Dyck, P. J., Schultz, P. W., and O'Brien, P. C. Quantitation of touch-pressure sensation. Arch. Neurol. *26:* 465–473, 1972.

5. Dyck, P. J., Curtis, D. J., Bushek, W., and Offord, K. Description of "Minnesota thermal disks" and normal values of cutaneous thermal discrimination in man. Neurology *24:* 325–330, 1974.

6. Cavanagh, J. B. The toxic effects of triorthocresyl phosphate on the nervous system. J. Neurol. Neurosurg. Psychiatry *17:* 163–172, 1954.

7. Vasilescu, C. Motor nerve conduction velocity and electromyogram in triorthocresyl-phosphate poisoning. Rev. Roum. Neurol. *9:* 345–350, 1972.

8. Morgan-Hughes, J. A., Sinclair, S., and Durston, J. H. J. The pattern of peripheral nerve regeneration induced by crush in rats with acrylamide neuropathy. Brain *97:* 235–250, 1974.

9. Casey, E. B., Jellife, A. M., Le Quesne, P. M., and Millett, Y. L. Vincristine neuropathy: Clinical and electrophysiological observations. Brain *96:* 69–86, 1973.

10. Fullerton, P. M., and O'Sullivan, D. J. Thalidomide neuropathy: A clinical, electrophysiological, and histological follow-up study. J. Neurol. Neurosurg. Psychiatry *31:* 543–551, 1968.

11. Ridley, A. The neuropathy of acute intermittent porphyria. Quart. J. Med. *38:* 307–333, 1969.

12. Asbury, A. K., Gale, M. K., Cox, S. C., Baringer, J. R., and Berg, B. O. Giant axonal neuropathy—A unique case with segmental neurofilamentous masses. Acta Neuropathol. *20:* 237–247, 1972.

13. Carpenter, S., Karpati, G., Andermann, F., and Gold, R. Giant axonal neuropathy. Arch. Neurol. *31:* 312–316, 1974.

14. Korobkin, R., Asbury, A. K., Sumner, A. J., and Nielsen, S. L. Glue sniffing neuropathy. Arch. Neurol. *32:* 158–162, 1975.

15. Martin, J. J., and Martin, L. Infantile neuroaxonal dystrophy. Europ. Neurol. *8:* 239–250, 1972.

16. Berard-Badier, M., Gambarelli, D., Pinsard, N., Hassoun, J., and Toga, M. Infantile neuroaxonal dystrophy or Seitelberger's disease. Acta Neuropathol. (Suppl.) *5:* 30–39, 1971.

17. Liu, H. M., Larson, M., and Mizuno, Y. An analysis of the ultrastructural findings in infantile neuroaxonal dystrophy (Seitelberger's disease). Acta Neuropathol. *27:* 201–213, 1974.

18. Kahn, P. Anderson-Fabry disease: A histopathological study of three cases with observations on the mechanism of production of pain. J. Neurol. Neurosurg. Psychiatry *36:* 1053–1062, 1973.

19. Kocen, R. S., King, R. H. M., Thomas, P. K., and Haas, L. F. Nerve biopsy findings in two cases of Tangier disease. Acta Neurol. Pathol. *26:* 317, 1973.

20. Asbury, A. K., Arnason, B. G., and Adams, R. D. The inflammatory lesion in idiopathic polyneuritis. Medicine *48:* 173–215, 1969.

21. Cohen, A. S., and Benson, M. D. Amyloid neuropathy. In: *Peripheral Neuropathy,* edited by P. J. Dyck, P. K. Thomas, and E. H. Lambert. Saunders, Philadelphia, 1975, pp. 1067–1091.

22. Dyck, P. J., and Lambert, E. H. Lower motor and primary sensory neuron diseases with peroneal muscular atrophy. I. Neurologic, genetic and electrophysiologic findings in hereditary polyneuropathies. Arch. Neurol. *18:* 603–618, 1968.

23. Dyck, P. J., and Lambert, E. H. Lower motor and primary sensory neuron diseases with peroneal muscular atrophy. II. Neurologic, genetic and electrophysiologic findings in various neuronal degenerations. Arch. Neurol. *18:* 619–625, 1968.

24. Tsairis, P., Dyck, P. J., and Mulder, D. W. Natural history of brachial plexus neuropathy. Arch. Neurol. *27:* 109–117, 1972.

25. Bradley, W. G., Madrid, R., Thrush, D. C., and Campbell, M. J. Recurrent brachial plexus neuropathy. Brain *98:* 381–398, 1975.

26. Geiger, L. R., Mancall, E. L., Penn, A. S., and Tucker, S. H. Familial neuralgic amyotrophy. Brain *97:* 87–102, 1974.

4 diseases of the neuromuscular junction

MYASTHENIA GRAVIS

In 1672 Thomas Willis, writing upon palsies, made the following comments:

> There is another kind of this disease depending on the scarcity and fewness of the Spirits, in which the motion fails wholly in no Part or Member, yet it is performed weakly only, or depravedly by any; — those who be in trouble with a scarcity of Spirits, will force them as much as they may to local Motions, are able at first rising in the Morning to walk, move their Arms this way and that, or to lift up a weight with strength; but before Noon, the stores of the Spirits which influenc'd the Muscles being almost spent, they are scarce able to move Hand or Foot.
>
> I have now a prudent and honest Woman in cure, who for many years has been obnoxious to this kind of bastard Palsey not only in the Limbs, but likewise in her Tongue; this person for some time speaks freely and readily enough, but after long, hasty, or laborious speaking, presently she becomes mute as a fish and cannot bring forth a word, nay, and does not recover the use of her Voice till after an hour or two.[1]

In the intervening three centuries our knowledge of the disease has increased considerably, although our descriptive eloquence seldom matches that of Willis. The illness that he chronicled is likely to have been that which we now know as myasthenia gravis. It is a reflection upon the puzzling nature of the disease that not only has it baffled physicians throughout the course of history but even today presents many diagnostic problems.

Clinical Aspects

The characteristic signs and symptoms of myasthenia are consequent upon the abnormal susceptibility of the patient's muscles to fatigue. Fatigability is a normal phenomenon, as may be witnessed by anyone who has tried to carry a 100 pound suitcase for more than a few blocks. The hand grip cannot be sustained as the muscles of the forearm become exhausted. The degree of fatigue varies enormously from individual to individual. The trained athlete is capable of sustained exertion far beyond the reach of the rest of us. Patients with myasthenia gravis, however, may find the effort of holding up their eyelids to be overwhelming. In the ranges between these two extremes lie the hysterics whose asthenia overwhelms them when the pressures of their lives become too great and the myasthenic whose disease is slight enough that his symptoms are present only under situations of exertion. It is small wonder that the one is frequently confused with the other and that the myasthenic can spend many months or years being labelled an hysteric whereas the hysteric may equally unfairly enjoy the mistaken diagnosis of myasthenia gravis. In spite of those in whom the diagnosis is difficult, there are certain characteristics of the disease and of the laboratory abnormalities associated with it that may reliably lead to the diagnosis.

The illness is seen more frequently in women than in men, by a ratio of about 3:2. It usually occurs in sporadic fashion with an incidence of approximately 1 in 20,000.[2] About 5 per cent of the cases have a family history, although there is no clear cut pattern of inheritance. The onset may be at any time, but there are two ages of peak incidence: for women the third decade and in males the fifth and sixth decades. The onset is sometimes difficult to date, and I have seen patients with an apparently recent history of myasthenia who insist that their strength after treatment with thymectomy and steroids is better than at any time in their lives; they may have had sub-clinical myasthenia for many years. This is particularly true of the younger myasthenic.

Generally, the symptoms begin in one of three groups of muscles: those of the eyes, of the bulbar musculature, or of the limbs and trunk. In about half of the patients the eyes are initially involved, in a third the disease presents with difficulty in speaking, swallowing, or chewing, and in about one fifth of the patients the predominant early symptoms are of generalized weakness of the limbs.[3]

When ptosis is an early sign, it may be quite variable. It is frequently very asymmetric and on occasions is unilateral. Like the other symptoms of myasthenia gravis, it may be worse towards the end of the day and improve after a night's rest. Another curious feature of the myasthenic ptosis is that it can alternate from one side to the other on successive examinations. It may also be exacerbated by a sudden exposure to bright light. The other muscles of the eyes, with the exception of the pupillary muscles, are frequently involved. The abnormalities may be so slight as to produce only a blurring of vision, or they may be severe enough that bizarre and dramatic paralyses are seen. It is usually easy to differentiate the myasthenic extraocular palsies from those due to peripheral nerve lesions because the pattern of weakness does not conform to any anatomical distribution of peripheral nerves.

The bulbar muscles also suffer from the effects of myasthenia. The facial muscles are often weak, and a peculiar difficulty with the muscles of the lower part of the face converts the normally pleasant smile into an unsightly snarl. This may be so embarrassing that the patient will hide his mouth behind his hand while laughing. Weakness of the palate and tongue can render speech unintelligible. The patient's enunciation may be distinct as he begins to talk, but after some time the voice becomes hollow, echoing, and totally without consonants. Difficulty with swallowing and choking spells are noted, but a more frequent problem is found in chewing food. When chewing meat, particularly if it is tough, the patient may have to support the chin with the hand in order to complete the task. Weakness of the muscles of the neck is not at all uncommon and is generally of the neck extensors so that the head tends to flop uncontrollably forward. This leads to the characteristic posture adopted by such patients who support the head with the hand tucked under the chin.

The symptoms of the disease when it involves the limbs and the trunk differ only by the nature of the fatigability from symptoms seen in other diseases in which weakness occurs. The weakness may be exacerbated by heat, and many patients complain that taking a hot shower or bath is a debilitating experience. The respiratory muscles are often involved, particularly when the illness is advanced, and respiratory distress is a very real problem for the myasthenic. Sensory symptoms are unusual although aching of the muscles can occur, bearing some relationship to the introspection which is natural to such patients.

Frequently the myasthenic tends to be demanding and rather querulous, particularly when the disease has been long-standing. It should be remembered, however, that the terrors of this disease are appreciated only by those who have suffered from it. The patient with myasthenia awakes to an uncertain day, not knowing whether some mild increase in weakness may not be the harbinger of a devastating crisis. It is not surprising in such situations that patients may lose their equanimity.

The clinical course of myasthenia is often a relapsing, remitting one. Overall, about a third of the patients eventually improve and half of these will have no signs of the disease nor will they be taking any medications. The other two thirds will be either unchanged or worse. In general, as in all other neuromuscular diseases, the worse the patient's weakness, the worse the prognosis. The potentially fatal complication in myasthenia gravis is respiratory failure.

One subcategory of myasthenia deserves special mention. Ocular myasthenia, in which the eye muscles alone are affected, is a relatively benign disease. Only a minority of the patients (11%) progress to develop weakness of other muscles.[3] If a patient with ocular myasthenia remains stable for two years after the onset of the disease, it is almost certain that he will have no further progression.[4] At the opposite end of the scale, other patients with generalized myasthenia experience such a rapid progression that they decline from perfectly normal health to severe weakness with respiratory insufficiency in a matter of weeks.

Fluctuations in the severity of the disease occur unpredictably, but certain situations are so consistently associated with worsening of myasthenia that it is wise to consider their possibility in any patient who presents with an exacerbation. Perhaps the commonest cause of an apparent worsening of myasthenia gravis is due not to the disease but to the medication used in its treatment. Those who feel that their strength is not as it should be often take increasing doses of anticholinesterase medications. An overdose of these may itself induce weakness which the patient interprets as further indication of the need for more medicine. A vicious cycle is then established in which the patient takes increasing amounts of the drug, eventually provoking a cholinergic crisis. Other causes that precipitate a worsening of myasthenia are infections, either viral or bacterial, and either hypo- or hyperthyroidism. Pregnancy is commonly associated with changes in myasthenia gravis. These may be in the direction of either improvement or deterioration. There is no constant relationship but, in general, the disease tends to exacerbate more frequently in the first trimester and may improve in the last two trimesters. Occasionally there is a post-partum myasthenic crisis. Emotional disturbances of all kinds make the patients feel weaker. It is not uncommon to find myasthenics whose immediate reaction to such stress is to take increasing amounts of medication to the point of overdosage. Electrolyte imbalance, particularly hypokalemia or hypocalcemia, may markedly worsen myasthenic symptoms.

Myasthenia may occur in childhood, when it presents with the same signs and symptoms as in the adult. An unusual form of myasthenia is seen in approximately 15 per cent of babies born to mothers with myasthenia gravis. This neonatal myasthenia is present at birth but lasts no more than twelve weeks. For this reason, the diagnosis and treatment of the illness are extremely important. The baby usually presents as a hypotonic child with difficulty breathing. The baby may have considerable difficulty sucking, and his chin may have to be supported while nursing in the same way as the adult myasthenic has to support his own chin while chewing. The disease may be due to the influence of maternal antibodies and disappears when the infant's own immune system supervenes. Passive transfer of a factor which blocks neuromuscular transmission has been accomplished from myasthenic patients to the mouse.[5] The neonatal myasthenia may be a natural equivalent to this experiment.

The diagnosis of myasthenia gravis may be suspected from the clinical examination by the demonstration of pathological fatigability. A fatigable ptosis is demonstrated by asking the patient to sustain upward gaze. The eyelids begin a slow drift downwards with the passage of time. This test is often used in conjunction with an edrophonium (tensilon) test by timing the point at which the lids cross the border of the pupil. Fatigability of the limbs can be demonstrated by having the patient sit with outstretched arms or by having him grasp a dynamometer repetitively and measuring his grip strength.

A phenomenon sometimes known as the Walker phenomenon has been described in patients with myasthenia. When a cuff is inflated around the upper arm and the arm exercised ischemically, the muscles fatigue. This fatigability is limited to the arm. When the cuff is released, a subsequent dramatic deterioration in the myasthenic signs in the rest of the body has been reported.[6] Thus a patient may develop a marked ptosis following such arm exercise. This does not seem to be a constant finding, and many physicians have never seen it. Recent studies have suggested that the worsening may be due to production of lactate and the subsequent reduction of available calcium.[7]

If pathological fatigue is demonstrated, the effect of edrophonium should be investigated. This anticholinesterase drug when injected intravenously acts within 30 seconds to 1 minute. Its effect is over within 5 to 10 minutes. After establishing the level of fatigue in the untreated patient, a test injection of 1 mg. of edrophonium is given intravenously. If there is no untoward effect from this test injection, up to 10 mg. may be given, although a clear cut result is usually seen with 6 mg. if any effect is to be found. Obviously, in children the dose should be appropriately smaller. The patient's fatigability is then tested again to determine any change. It is particularly important to quantitate such testing since relying on the patient's, or even the examiner's, impression can be misleading. A control injection of normal saline is useful on occasions, although once the patient has experienced the effect of edrophonium and its side effects, he is in doubt as to which is the active drug and which is the control. If there is no response to edrophonium it is important to evaluate the effect of prostigmin, since some patients, especially those with ocular myasthenia, may not improve with edrophonium.

Patients with myasthenia may have marked atrophy of muscles, but this is unusual and is seen only in those whose myasthenia is long-standing.

Laboratory Studies

Because of the coincidence of myasthenia gravis and thymomas, a chest x-ray and, preferably, tomograms are an important part of the evaluation. Approximately 10 per cent of myasthenic patients have a thymoma, and the prognosis in these patients is significantly worse than in those without tumor.

Electrical testing is most useful in the diagnosis of myasthenia gravis and is designed to demonstrate the defect in neuromuscular conduction. When surface recording electrodes are placed over a muscle belly, the electrical potential which is evoked following stimulation of the motor nerve gives some measure of the number of muscle fibers which are being activated. If there is a progressive failure in neuromuscular transmission, the amplitude of the evoked potential will become progressively smaller. In normal subjects, repetitive stimulation at frequencies below 10 cycles per second produces little change in the amplitude of the evoked potential (less than 10 per cent). In myasthenia gravis there is a decrement of more than 10 per cent in the amplitude of evoked potentials at such frequencies. This reduction in potential reaches its maximum on the fourth evoked potential, and further decrement is not seen after the sixth evoked potential.[8] Indeed, with sustained repetitive stimulation there may be some increase in the amplitude, or fluctuations may occur which are difficult to interpret. This abnormality may be seen in only one of several muscles. The proximal muscles are more likely to be affected than the distal ones. This presents a practical problem, since the proximal muscles are not as easy to stimulate. However, with some practice, stimulation over the brachial plexus at Erb's point can be used to produce evoked potentials in the deltoid muscles. Although intracellular recordings have given much information as to the nature of myasthenia gravis, the standard needle EMG is really of little help in the diagnosis of this disease.

With the recent development of single fiber electromyography, a phenomenon known as "jitter" has been analyzed.[9] Muscle fibers innervated by the terminal branches of the same motor unit will be depolarized more or less synchronously. It is the investigation of this "more or less" aspect which has given rise to the concept of jitter. Because of slight differences in the lengths of the terminal nerve branches and because of some differences in conduction properties, the individual muscle fibers of a motor unit are not actually depolarized simultaneously. If one takes the action potential from a single muscle fiber as a reference potential, a similar potential from a muscle fiber in the same motor unit will occur a fraction of a second after the first. In normal muscle, this second motor unit potential will always occur when the first is seen. The time interval between the two motor unit potentials can be ascertained and is relatively constant. However, there is a certain variability in this time interval, and this is known as jitter. In patients with myasthenia gravis not only is the jitter increased, but there may be occasions on which the second motor unit may disappear entirely, probably because of a failure of neuromuscular transmission.[10]

The curare provocative test may be of great help in making the diagnosis of myasthenia gravis, particularly with its recent modification, the regional curare test.[11, 12] Patients are particularly susceptible to the paralyzing action of curare, and the test is not without hazard. It should never be done unless intubation and respiratory support can be carried out immediately should it become necessary. Thus, the test is usually performed with an anesthesiologist in attendance. Electromyography should be carried out concurrently and the evoked potential from a suitable muscle obtained. The stimulating and recording electrodes should be adjusted until a consistent potential is produced and its amplitude measured. In addition, various tests of the patient's strength can be carried out. Although many anesthesiologists feel that there is no "normal" curarizing dose, approximately 0.15 mg. of curare per kilogram of body weight will paralyze most patients. The normal curarizing dose for the patient is calculated, and one-fifth of this is diluted in 10 ml.; 1 ml. of this is given intravenously, and the patient's strength and the evoked potential are studied after one minute. After two minutes a second injection of 2 ml. is given and the test is repeated. Similarly, 3 ml. are injected after a further two minutes, and finally 4 ml. The test is discontinued at any stage if the patient's strength deteriorates or the evoked potential starts to fall.

Because of the hazards of a severe paralysis associated with standard curare test, a modification termed the regional curare test has been designed.[11, 12]

In this test 0.125 mg. of curare is diluted in 20 ml. of saline. A cuff is placed around the upper part of the forearm and inflated above systolic pressure, the arm being held vertically in such a way as to promote venous drainage. The curare is then injected intravenously at the wrist, and this injection is followed by 5 ml. of saline. The total time of the injection is 1 minute; the cuff is deflated after a further $4^1/_2$ minutes. The repetitive evoked potentials are then recorded from the abductor pollicis brevis at 5, 15, and 20 minutes after the injection. Normally there is little or no diminution of the evoked potentials compared to those obtained before the injection. In patients with myasthenia there is considerable reduction in the amplitude of the evoked potential (usually more than 20 per cent), and this reduction persists longer than in the normal subject. The amount of curare reaching the rest of the circulation will not be sufficient to cause a generalized paralysis.

In the past the decamethonium test has been recommended as useful for the diagnosis of myasthenia gravis. Patients with myasthenia seem to be resistant to the effects of this drug. However, a recent article which commented on the necessity of general anesthesia during this test did little to reassure physicians about its utility.[13]

Routine muscle biopsy has been of less use in the diagnosis of myasthenia gravis, unless the morphology of the end plates is investigated by electron microscopy or intravital staining with methylene blue. The routine muscle pathology usually shows signs of Type 2 fiber atrophy, which is sometimes focal, or of mild denervation. Lymphorrhages were originally thought to be commonly associated with myasthenia gravis, but in our experience they have been quite rare and are seen in no more than 10 per cent of the patients.

Pathology and Etiology

The abnormality which causes the symptoms in myasthenia gravis lies at the neuromuscular junction, but the fundamental process that causes such change is less clear. In order to provide a background against which the abnormalities of myasthenia gravis may be understood, it is necessary to review the normal neuromuscular junction. Where the motor nerves contact the muscle, they lose their myelin and the terminal expansions of the axons come into direct contact with the muscle. At an ultrastructural level, many small vesicles are found in the terminal expansions. These vesicles contain acetylcholine, and it is their discharge through the presynaptic membrane that releases the small quanta of acetylcholine. The gap between the nerve terminal and the underlying end plate region is known as the primary synaptic cleft. Acetylcholine must travel across this gap to reach the receptor sites in the postjunctional part of the apparatus. Postjunctionally, the membrane is dimpled and folded producing secondary synaptic clefts. In addition to the acetylcholine receptor sites, the end plate zone is also the location of acetylcholinesterase. When an electrical impulse travels down the motor nerve, the terminal expansions are depolarized, causing a massive release of acetylcholine from the presynaptic vesicles. This transmitter substance travels across to the postsynaptic receptors and causes a depolarization at the end plate region, which results in a propagated electrical potential and eventual contraction of the muscle fiber. The acetylcholine is broken down by the acetylcholinesterase and the depolarization reversed. Even during the resting state there is a continuous discharge of the presynaptic vesicles, although not in sufficient quantities to cause a propagated depolarization of the entire muscle fiber. They can, however, be recorded by intracellular electrodes as miniature end plate potentials (MEPPS).

Normal neuromuscular function depends upon many things. For example, it is necessary that acetylcholine be synthesized and stored. Certain substances such as calcium are implicated in the release of acetylcholine. Cyclic AMP facilitates neuromuscular transmission, and stimulators of adenyl cyclase such as noradrenaline and ephedrine (which increase the cellular level of cyclic AMP by increasing its formation) may facilitate neuromuscular transmission.[14] Cyclic AMP may be linked with calcium in its action in neuromuscular transmission since the compound is important in the mobilization of calcium in living cells.[15]

Abnormalities of the motor end plates were noted by Coers and Woolf in their study of motor point biopsies from patients with myasthenia gravis.[16] Both the end plates and the subneural apparatus were found to be elongated. Engel and Santa, in a careful study of the ultrastructure of the end plate region, found that the nerve terminals were rather small, that the primary cleft between the nerve and the subneural apparatus was widened, and, most strikingly, that the secondary synaptic clefts were shallow and sparse.[17] They showed that the area which was reactive for acetylcholinesterase was reduced in size, with multiple small reactive areas appearing along an extended length of the fiber. There was no abnormality in the number or size of synaptic vesicles. This last finding is important because other studies had shown a decrease in the amplitude of the miniature end plate potentials and the suggestion had been made that the packets of acetylcholine released from the synaptic vesicles were abnormally small.[18]

In any patient taking medication, the possibility exists that this may produce some of the changes seen in the muscle. Engel, Lambert, and Santa studied the effect of long term anticholinesterase therapy in rats to see whether the end plates of these animals were subject to changes similar to those of human myasthenics.[19] Changes were, indeed, noted, but were limited to the soleus and the diaphragmatic muscles. The postsynaptic pinocytotic vesicles became quite abundant and the primary synaptic cleft became wider. The Schwann cell processes proliferated terminally, partially covering up the presynaptic membrane. The same type of changes were thus produced as seen in myasthenia gravis but with important differences. In myasthenia gravis all muscle fiber types are involved. Additionally the nerve terminal area in myasthenia gravis is reduced as well as the postjunctional part of the end plate. However, the experiment did suggest that prolonged administration of anticholinesterase may have an adverse effect on the neuromuscular junction. Others have commented on a similar adverse effect with both physiological and anatomical changes.[20]

It is likely that the abnormality of neuromuscular transmission is secondary to some other cause. The search for this has been a fascinating study over the years. The possible relationship of myasthenia gravis to "autoimmune" diseases was pointed out by Simpson.[21] Although rheumatoid arthritis is the commonest of these and occurs in 3 per cent of patients, many others including systemic lupus erythematosus, Sjögren's syndrome, and pernicious anemia have been described. A fifth of myasthenics have a positive test for anti nuclear antibodies and in the presence of one other autoimmune disease, this antibody is found in all patients.[22] Strauss and others showed that in almost one half of the patients with myasthenia gravis there was a circulating antibody (a 7S gamma globulin) which bound to the A bands of skeletal muscle.[23] It is difficult to understand why this should be significant, since the pathology of myasthenia gravis lies not in the A bands but in the neuromuscular junction. Careful attempts to demonstrate binding of this antibody to the neuromuscular junction were unsuccessful.[24] This same antibody, however, showed reactivity to cells in the thymus, and this may be a more important finding. In patients with thymomas the majority (12 of 13 patients in one series)[25] demonstrate such antibodies whereas in the general population of myasthenics it is seen in only a quarter to a half of the patients.

It has been claimed that the sera of myasthenic patients contain an immunoglobulin that reacts with the nuclei of neurones, particularly with Purkinje cells in the cerebellum.[26] An attempt to reproduce these findings was not successful, however.[27]

The whole concept of the role of immunity in myasthenia gravis widened following the purification of the nicotinic acetylcholine receptor protein from the electric eel, a technical tour de force in itself. When the receptor protein was injected into rabbits in conjunction with Freund's adjuvant, the animals became sensitized. A second injection of receptor protein, after 15 days, caused the majority of the animals to develop severe weakness, very similar to that of myasthenia gravis, which was responsive to anticholinesterase medications.[28] An antibody to the receptor protein was demonstrated in the serum of these animals. Experimental myasthenia gravis has now been produced in monkeys[29] and in rats and guinea pigs.[30]

Two separate studies have shown that about 80% of patients with myasthenia also possess antibodies against the acetyl choline receptor protein.[31, 32]

Alpha bungarotoxin is a component of snake venom with a specific affinity for the acetylcholine receptor site. Myasthenic endplates demonstrate reduced binding of this substance,[33] indicating that the amount of receptor protein on the postjunctional surface is reduced. A serum globulin present in myasthenic patients inhibits the binding of alpha bungarotoxin to the endplate receptor site,[34, 35] suggesting that there is a circulating compound which might inhibit the normal functioning of the postsynaptic part of the neuromuscular junction. This same immunoglobulin may be involved in the passive "transfer" of myasthenia from man to mouse which has been accomplished by injecting the animal with an ammonium sulfate-precipitated immunoglobulin fraction.[36]

Although there remains little doubt that a circulating immunoglobulin is a significant part of the illness, there is strong evidence for altered cellular immunity in the disease. In about 70% of patients thymic hyperplasia is present.[37] Normally there is a progressive involution of this organ following the first decade. In patients with myasthenia, hyperplastic changes of the lymphoid tissue are often associated with the presence of germinal centers. It has been suggested that the germinal centers themselves represent areas of active proliferation of forbidden clones of immunocompetent cells.[38] In 10 per cent of patients, thymomas are found.[37]

Using stimulation with phytohemagglutinin, Armstrong et al. showed that in the majority of patients with myasthenia gravis there was a population of thymic lymphocytes that was cytotoxic to cultured muscle.[39] Using phytohemagglutinin and pokeweed, Abdou et al. showed a greater stimulation of thymocytes from myasthenic patients, both with and without thymomas.[40] In mixed cultures of peripheral leukocytes and thymocytes, the same authors showed a stimulation of the peripheral blood lymphocytes by autologous thymocytes. They also found an increased number of B cells, which are responsible for humoral immunity, and that these B cells carried Igm. A tentative suggestion was made that the increased number of B cells and the new antigenic determinants on their surface might represent persistent stimulation by a virus.[41]

The stimulation of lymphocytes by exposure to purified acetylcholine receptor protein has been reported.[42, 43] These studies indicated an abnormally high degree of stimulation in patients with myasthenia, and also suggested that prednisone was effective in reducing this.[44] In experimental myasthenia of guinea pigs the disease was passively transferred to other animals by injection of washed lymph node cells.[45]

The "transplantation" antigens, the HL-A antigens from lymphocytes, are abnormal in patients with myasthenia. HL-A 8, which occurs in 18 per cent of a control population, is found in 38 per cent of myasthenics.[25, 46] It is often associated with HL-A1, the latter probably being a secondary change.[47] The presence of HL-A 8 seems to be more characteristic of women under the age of 35 who suffer from the disease, 60 to 80 per cent of whom have HL-A 8 antigen.[48–50] HL-A 8 and 1 are associated with an increased rejection of transplants in other studies.

Whatever the exact nature of the pathological process, it is likely that an altered immune state lies at its heart. Humoral immunity certainly seems to be indicated in the reduction of available receptor sites characteristic of the disease, but the complex interactions between B and T— cells make it difficult to isolate one system or the other as a primary culprit.

Treatment

Anticholinesterase Medications. The early observations that myasthenia gravis resembled curare poisoning led Walker to try the use of anticholinesterase medications. The two most common ones are neostigmine bromide (Prostigmin) and pyridostigmine (Mestinon). Pyridostigmine is probably the choice of most physicians and patients because it has less of the cholinergic side effects and a slightly longer action. It is more likely to give patients relief from bedtime until morning than is neostigmine. The drug begins to act within half an hour of oral administration, and the length of its action is between four and six hours. It is commonly administered at four to six hour intervals. There is really no "correct" dose. Enough of the drug is given to counteract the effects of myasthenia as nearly as possible. In some patients this may be as little as $1/2$ tablet (30 mg.) every six hours. Others take 20, 30, or more pills per day. Mestinon is also available in a slow release form (Timespan). This contains 180 mg. of the medication and is well tolerated by some patients. Many, however, find the effect of this preparation to be somewhat unpredictable.

Another anticholinesterase drug which is less frequently used is ambenomium (Mytelase). This drug is said to be more effective in peripheral weakness. It should be started in low doses (5 mg.), and it may have to be discontinued because of the development of headaches. If a patient is being given ambenomium, he should be cautioned against the use of phospholine iodide, a long term esterase inhibitor which is used in glaucoma and which markedly potentiates the effect of ambenomium.[2] Other useful preparations are liquid preparations of pyridostigmine, which are easily administered by nasogastric tube in patients who cannot swallow, and parenteral preparations of neostigmine. The following are roughly equivalent doses: 15 mg. neostigmine, 60 mg. pyridostigmine, and 25 mg. ambenomium by mouth, and 1 mg. neostigmine by intramuscular injection. The patient who is being given anticholinesterase medication should be warned about the cholinergic side effects and the possibility of overdosage. It should be stressed that weakness is one of the chief side effects. It is often impossible to distinguish the weakness due to myasthenia from that due to overmedication. Although the latter is frequently associated with abdominal cramping pains and diarrhea as well as with wide spread fasciculations, the absence of these side effects does not necessarily mean that the patient is having an exacerbation of myasthenia.

Anticholinesterase medications may not be an unmixed blessing, since there is evidence that they may cause structural abnormalities at the neuromuscular junction. With the increasing use of thymectomy and of corticosteroid medications, it is possible that the use of anticholinesterase medication in the future will become much less popular.

Adjuvant medications which are used from time to time are all agents which directly or indirectly affect neuromuscular transmission. Ephedrine is commonly used in doses of 25 mg. thrice daily. Aldactone, spironolactone, guanidine, and the veratrum derivates germine mono and diacetate[51] have all been used in the treatment of myasthenia gravis, although the results have been equivocal.

Corticosteroids. The use of corticosteroids and ACTH in myasthenia gravis is receiving theoretical support from recent work on the etiology of the disease. ACTH was formerly recommended in short intensive courses which were sometimes repeated at intervals.[52] The usual course consisted of daily injections of 100 units of ACTH for 10 days. Frequently an initial worsening of the disease was seen, followed by a gradual recovery which was usually not sustained. Early reports on the use of oral corticosteroids emphasized the worsening of the disease which may occur with such medication. With recent years, however, the emphasis has changed. Although it is well recognized that the use of prednisone or similar steroids may cause an initial increase of the weakness, this is often outweighed by the dramatic improvement which is seen with the long term use of suppressive doses of these medications. The use of prednisone 100 mg. on alternate days given in a single morning dose has been recommended. This was combined with the administration of a low-sodium, high-protein diet with appropriate antacid medications together with the daily administration of 20 to 30 meq. of potassium as replacement therapy.[53] Engel and others reported that of nineteen patients with severe myasthenia gravis who were treated in this fashion, seven had total remissions and only three, all young women, had no response.[37] The side effects were said to be minimal. In our experience, the commonest side effect has been the development of cataracts after a year or so.

The patients should be admitted to the hospital for the administration of steroids. Skin tests and chest x-ray should be obtained to rule out the possibility of tuberculous infection, and respiratory function should be evaluated. If the patient is taking anticholinesterase therapy, the dose of medication should be halved or, if possible, discontinued. Close watch is kept on the respiratory function and assisted respiration is started if the patient appears to be deteriorating in the early stages of steroid therapy. The most usual time for exacerbations to occur has been during the first three weeks. Engel and co-workers believe that part of this exacerbation may be due to increased sensitivity of the patient to his anticholinesterase medication. Others have implicated an enhancement of lymphocyte reactivity.

Perhaps because we have been treating patients in the early stages of myasthenia, we have not had to assist respirations during the initial period of treatment and have noticed very little worsening. We usually monitor the vital capacity every four hours and have not had to institute any other measures. Attempts should be made to discontinue the anticholinesterase medication as soon as this is feasible. Very frequently the patient notices a difference in muscle strength between the day off prednisone and the day on prednisone. The patient is usually weaker on the "off" day but occasionally may be stronger. This difference usually disappears after three to four weeks on prednisone; if it persists beyond the fourth week of treatment, it may be helpful to add a small amount of prednisone on the "off" day. In patients with severe myasthenia, in whom the potential dangers of the phase of worsening may be life threatening, Seybould and Drachman have recommended slowly increasing the dose of prednisone from 25 mg. every other day to 100 mg. by 12.5 mg. steps at each third dose.[54]

Suppressive doses of steroids should be continued for two years or more; otherwise, relapses are common. Withdrawal of the medication should be very gradual.

Thymectomy. Removal of the thymus gland has been used as a form of therapy for myasthenia gravis since the changes of hyperplasia and thymoma were noted in the thymus. Recent series attest to the benefit obtained from such a procedure.[55-58] Both patients with and without thymoma are helped, although the presence of a tumor is associated with a worse prognosis. At least three quarters of the patients improve after thymectomy, and in a third of the patients the improvement continues all the way to total remission of the disease. One unusual aspect of the improvement after thymectomy is that it may continue up to 7 to 10 years. Perhaps this prolonged recovery time is due to the survival of abnormal lymphocytes in the circulation. Some have suggested that the presence of germinal centers in the thymus may be associated with slower improvement,[55] although others have found this not to be true.[59] Younger patients seem to do better than older ones, and females are more likely to be helped than males. One series indicates that the less severe the myasthenia the better the prognosis.[57] The operative mortality is less than 1 per cent. The use of irradiation in addition to surgical removal of the thymus has also been suggested,[60] but is not widely practiced.

Combined Therapy. There is some discussion over the selection of patients for thymectomy, as there is for those to be treated with steroids. Traditionally, one does not use either of these two forms of treatment until the patient has moderately severe difficulty from the myasthenia gravis. There lies in this, however, more than a grain of illogic. In thymectomy and steroid treatment we have two forms of therapy which are ultimately of benefit but which may initially make the patient worse. Instead of using these early in the disease, when the patient's general condition enables him better to withstand the threat of major surgery and the side effects of a potentially dangerous medication, we have waited until the patient is already severely debilitated and frequently in respiratory crisis. It is not surprising that the complications involved in such treatment have been pronounced. It seems much more logical to use both thymectomy and steroids early in the disease. If myasthenia gravis or treatment with anticholinesterase drugs produces permanent changes in the muscle, it would be unwise to allow the disease to continue if its eradication is a practical possibility. The question whether the treatment with thymectomy and steroids does, in fact, eradicate the disease during its early stages is not yet answered. In our clinic we have used the combined approach of thymectomy and steroids as soon as the diagnosis of myasthenia is made, unless the myasthenia is limited totally to the eyes. After a complete evaluation of the patient's disease, thymectomy is performed. The anticholinesterase medications are reduced or discontinued before surgery. As soon as is practical after the surgery (usually on the fourth or fifth day) the patient is started on high dose, alternate day prednisone therapy, and this is continued for approximately 6 months to a year.

Patients who were placed on steroids without thymectomy often had a relapse of their illness if steroids were withdrawn within the year. The worsening usually occurred 6 to 12 weeks after cessation of the medication. Our patients who have had a thymectomy can be withdrawn from steroids at an earlier date without such relapse and, therefore, the side effects of steroids are reduced. In comparison to the large series of patients reported elsewhere, our own experience is so small as to be anecdotal, but the therapy seems particularly effective in the young myasthenic with a short history of the illness. Out of eleven such patients, all except one are in remission and the remaining patient is only mildly handicapped. The longest period during which we have followed such patients is only six years.

Management of Crisis. Patients with myasthenia gravis not infrequently arrive in the emergency room with an acute exacerbation of weakness. It is often difficult to know whether they are in myasthenic crisis or cholinergic crisis. The edrophonium test has been recommended as a means of distinguishing between the two. The advantage of edrophonium is that if the patient is, in fact, in cholinergic crisis, its action is short-lived and any worsening of the patient's condition is rapidly reversed. If there is a clear cut improvement with edrophonium, the patient's medication can be adjusted accordingly and sometimes the patient will be well enough to return home. This, however, is the exception and on many occasions it is difficult to know whether there has been any improvement with edrophonium; if improvement is noted, this may be slight. In such a situation, it may be worth considering discontinuing all medication. The only way of dying from myasthenia gravis itself is from respiratory failure, and assisted respirations are a routine procedure in the intensive care unit. The patient should be admitted to such a unit and intubation or tracheostomy carried out if necessary. All medications are withdrawn and a suction machine provided to remove the saliva that pools in the nasopharynx. The patient is maintained in this fashion for between four to ten days and then anticholinesterase medications are reinstated in small doses. Very often, there is a dramatic increase in the sensitivity of the patient to cholinergic medications after this "drying out" period, and management may once again be instituted on an out-patient basis.

Usually the patient undergoes cycles of these crises so that he seems to need more and more anticholinesterase medicines to control his disease and eventually he will once again be resistant to the effects of the medicine.

Obviously, any patient who is seen in myasthenic crisis may be suffering from some other condition (such as intercurrent infection) which may be exacerbating the condition as discussed earlier.

Drugs To Be Used with Caution. Certain drugs have an adverse effect on neuromuscular transmission and should be used only with caution or not at all in patients with myasthenia. These include quinine, quinidine, and procainamide,[61] propranolol and other β-adrenergic blockers,[62] antibiotics such as neomycin and streptomycin, and diphenylhydantoin.

BIBLIOGRAPHY

1. Guthrie, L. B. Myasthenia gravis in the 17th century. Lancet *1:* 330, 1903.
2. Osserman, K. E., and Genkins, G. Studies in myasthenia gravis: A review of a 20 year experience in over 1,200 patients. Mt. Sinai J. Med. N.Y. *38:* 497–537, 1971.
3. Perlo, V. P., Poskanzer, D. C., Schwab, R. S., Viets, H. R., Osserman, K. E., and Genkins, G. Myasthenia gravis: Evaluation of treatment in 1,355 patients. Neurology *16:* 431–439, 1966.
4. Osserman, K. E. *Myasthenia Gravis.* Grune and Stratton, New York, 1958.
5. Toyka, K. V., Drachman, D. B., Pestronk, A., and Kao, I. Myasthenia gravis: Passive transfer from man to mouse. Science *190:* 397–399, 1975.
6. Walker, M. B. Myasthenia gravis: Case in which fatigue of forearm muscles could induce paralysis of extraocular muscle. Proc. Roy. Soc. Med. *31:* 722, 1938.
7. Patten, B. M., Oliver, K. L., and Engel, W. K. Effect of lactate infusions on patients with myasthenia gravis. Neurology *24:* 986–990, 1974.
8. Ozdemir, C., and Young, R. R. Electrical testing in myasthenia gravis. Ann. N.Y. Acad. Sci. *183:* 287–302, 1971.
9. Ekstedt, J., Nilsson, G., and Stahlberg, E. Calculation of the electromyographic jitter. J. Neurol. Neurosurg. Psychiatry *37:* 526–539, 1974.
10. Stahlberg, E., Ekstedt, J., and Broman, A. Neuromuscular transmission in myasthenia gravis studied with single fiber electromyography. J. Neurol. Neurosurg. Psychiatry *37:* 540–547, 1974.
11. Brown, J. C., Charlton, J. E., and White D. J. K. A regional technique for the study of sensitivity to curare in human muscle. J. Neurol. Neurosurg. Psychiatry *38:* 18–26, 1975.
12. Brown, J. C., and Charlton, J. E. A study of sensitivity to curare in myasthenia disorders using a regional technique. J. Neurol. Neurosurg. Psychiatry *38:* 27–33, 1975.
13. Meadows, J. C., Ross-Russel, R. W., and Wise, R. P. A re-evaluation of the decamethonium test for myasthenia gravis. Acta Neurol. Scand. *50:* 248–256, 1974.
14. Hokkanen, E., Vapaatalo, H., and Anttila, P. On the possible role of cyclic AMP in the neuromuscular transmission and in the treatment of myasthenia gravis. Acta Neurol. Scand. (Suppl.) *51:* 375, 1972.
15. Takamori, M., Ishii, N., and Mori, M. The role of cyclic 3'5'-adenosine monophosphate in neuromuscular disease. Arch. Neurol. *29:* 240–242, 1973.
16. Coers, C., and Woolf, A. L. *The innervation of Muscle.* Blackwell, Oxford, 1959.
17. Engel, A. G., and Santa, T. Histometric analysis of the ultrastructure of the neuromuscular junction in myasthenia gravis and in the myasthenic syndrome. Ann. N.Y. Acad. Sci. *183:* 46–63, 1971.
18. Elmqvist, D., Hoffmann, W. W., Kugelberg, J., and Quastel, D. M. J. An electrophysiological investigation of neuromuscular transmission in myasthenia gravis. J. Physiol. *174:* 417–434, 1964.
19. Engel, A. G., Lambert, E. H., and Santa, T. Study of long term anticholinesterase therapy: Effects on neuromuscular transmission and motor end plate fine structure. Neurology *23:* 1273–1281, 1973.
20. Ward, M. D., Forbes, M. S., and Johns, T. R. Neostigmine methylsulfate: Does it have a chronic effect as well as a transient one? Arch. Neurol. *32:* 808–814, 1975.
21. Simpson, J. A. Myasthenia gravis and myasthenic syndromes. In: *Disorders of Voluntary Muscle*, 3rd edition, edited by J. N. Walton. 1974, pp. 653–692.
22. Rule, A. H., and Kornfeld, P. Studies in myasthenia gravis: Biological aspects. Mt. Sinai J. Med. N.Y. *38:* 538–572, 1971.
23. Strauss, A. J. L., Siegal, B. C., Hsu, K. C., Burkholder, P. M., Nastuk, W. L., and Osserman, K. E. Immunofluorescence demonstration of a muscle binding, complement

fixing, serum globulin fraction in myasthenia gravis. Proc. Soc. Exp. Biol. *105:* 184, 1960.

24. McFarlin, D. E., Engel, W. K., and Strauss, A. J. L. Does myasthenic serum bind to the neuromuscular junction? Ann. N.Y. Acad. Sci. *135:* 656–663, 1971.

25. Feltkamp, T. E. W., Van den BergLoonen, P. M., Nijenhuis, L. E., Engelfriet, C. P., VanRossum, A. L., Vanloghem, J. J., and Oosterhuis, H. J. G. H. Myasthenia gravis autoantibodies and HL-A antigens. Brit. Med. J. *1:* 131–133, 1974.

26. Martin, L., Herr, J. C., Wannamaker, W., and Kornguth, S. Demonstration of specific antineuronal nuclear antibodies in sera of patients with myasthenia gravis: Indirect and direct immunofluorescence. Neurology *24:* 680–683, 1974.

27. Whitaker, J. N., and Engel, W. K. A search for antibodies to neuronal nuclei in the serum of patients with myasthenia gravis. Neurology *24:* 61–63, 1974.

28. Patrick, J., and Lindstrom, J. Autoimmune response to acetylcholine receptor. Science *180:* 871–872, 1973.

29. Tarrab-Hazdai, R., Aharonov, A., Silman, I., Fuchs, S., and Abramsky, O. Experimental autoimmune myasthenia induced in monkeys by purified acetylcholine receptor. Nature *256:* 128–130, 1975.

30. Lennon, V. A., Lindstrom, J. M., and Seybold, M. E. Experimental autoimmune myasthenia: A model of myasthenia gravis in rats and guinea pigs. J. Exp. Med. *141:* 1365–1375, 1975.

31. Aharonov, A., Abramsky, O., Tarrab-Hazdai, R., and Fuchs, S. Humoral antibodies to acetylcholine receptor in patients with myasthenia gravis. Lancet *2:* 340–342, 1975.

32. Appel, S. H., Almon, R. R., and Levy, N. Acetylcholine receptor antibodies in myasthenia gravis. New Engl. J. Med. *293:* 760–761, 1975.

33. Fambrough, B. M., Drachman, D. B., and Satyamurti, S. Neuromuscular junction in myasthenia gravis: Decreased acetylcholine receptors. Science *182:* 293–295, 1973.

34. Almon, R. R., Andrew, C. G., and Appel, S. H. Serum globulin in myasthenia gravis: Inhibition of alphabungarotoxin binding to acetylcholine receptors. Science *186:* 55–57, 1974.

35. Bender, A. N., Ringel, S. P., Engel, W. K., Daniels, M. P., and Vogel, Z. Myasthenia gravis: A serum factor blocking acetylcholine receptors of the human neuromuscular junction. Lancet *1:* 607–608, 1975.

36. Toyka, K. V., Drachman, D. P., Pestronk, A., and Kao, I. Myasthenic gravis: Passive transfer from man to mouse. Science *190:* 397–399, 1975.

37. Engel, W. K., Festoff, B. W., Patten, B. M., Swerdlow, M. L., Newball, H. H., and Thompson, M. D. Myasthenia gravis. Ann. Intern. Med. *81:* 225–246, 1974.

38. Papatestas, A. E., Osserman, K. E., and Kark, A. E. The effects of thymectomy on the prognosis in myasthenia gravis. Mt. Sinai J. Med. N.Y. *38:* 586–593, 1971.

39. Armstrong, R. M., Nowak, R. M., and Falk, R. E. Thymic lymphocyte function in myasthenia gravis. Neurology *23:* 1078–1083, 1973.

40. Abdou, N. I., Lisak, R. P., Zweiman, B., Abrahamsohn, I., and Penn, A. S. The thymus in myasthenia gravis: Evidence for altered cell population. New Engl. J. Med. *291:* 1271–1275, 1974.

41. Editorial. New Engl. J. Med. *291:* 1304, 1971.

42. Abramsky, O., Aharonov, A., and Webb, C. Cellular immune response to acetylcholine receptor rich fraction in patients with myasthenia gravis. Clin. Exp. Immunol. *19:* 11–16, 1975.

43. Richman, D. P., Patrick, J., and Arnason, B. G. W. Cellular immunity in myasthenia gravis. New Engl. J. Med. *294:* 694–698, 1976.

44. Abramsky, O., Aharonov, A., Teitelbaum, D., and Fuchs, S. Myasthenia gravis and acetylcholine receptor. Arch. Neurol. *32:* 684–687, 1975.

45. Tarrab-Hazdai, R., Aharanov, A., Abramsky, O., Yaar, I., and Fuchs, S. Passive transfer of experimental autoimmune myasthenia by lymph node cells in inbred guinea pigs. J. Exp. Med. *142:* 785–789, 1975.

46. Fritze, D., Herrmann, C., Naeim, F., Smith, G. S., and Walford, R. L. HL-A antigens in myasthenia gravis. Lancet *1:* 240–242, 1974.

47. Pirskanen, R. Genetic associations between myasthenia gravis and the HLA system. J. Neurol. Neurosurg. Psychiatry *39:* 23–33, 1976.

48. Möller, E., Hammarstrom, L., Smith, E., and Matell, G. HL-A8 and LD-8a in patients with

myasthenia gravis. Tissue Antigens 7: 39–44, 1976.
49. Hammarström, L., Smith, E., Möller, E., Franksson, C., Mattell, G., and Von Reis, G. Myasthenia gravis: Studies on HL-A antigens and lymphocyte subpopulations in patients with myasthenia gravis. Clin. Exp. Immunol. *21:* 202–215, 1975.
50. Kaakinen, A., Pirskanen, R., and Tiilikainen, A. LD Antigens associated with HL-A8 and myasthenia gravis. Tissue Antigens *6:* 175–182, 1975.
51. Flacke, W. E., Blum, R. P., Scott, W. R., Foldes, F. F., and Osserman, K. E. Germine monodiacetate in myasthenia gravis. Ann. N.Y. Acad. Sci. *183:* 316–333, 1971.
52. Liversedge, L. A., Yuill, G. M., Wilkinson, I. M. S., and Hughes, J. A. Benefit from adrenalcorticotrophin in myasthenia gravis. J. Neurol. Neurosurg. Psychiatry *37:* 412–415, 1974.
53. Warmolts, J. R., and Engel, W. K. Myasthenia gravis: Benefit from alternate day prednisone. New Engl. J. Med. *286:* 17–20, 1972.
54. Seybould, M. E., and Drachman, D. B. Gradually increasing doses of prednisone in myasthenia gravis. New Engl. J. Med. *290:* 81–84, 1974.
55. Perlow, V. P., Arnason, B., Poskanzer, D., Castleman, B., Schwab, R. S., Osserman, K. E., Papatestas, A., Alpert, A. L., and Kark, A. The role of thymectomy in the treatment of myasthenia gravis. Ann. N.Y. Acad. Sci. *183:* 308–315, 1971.
56. Cohn, H. E., Solit, R. W., Schatz, N. J., and Schlezinger, N. Surgical treatment of myasthenia gravis. J. Thorac. Cardiovasc. Surg. *68:* 876–885, 1974.
57. Mulder, D. G., Herrmann, C., and Buckberg, G. D. Effect of thymectomy in patients with myasthenia gravis: A 16 year experience. Am. J. Surg. *128:* 202–206, 1974.
58. Genkins, G., Papatestas, A. E., Horowitz, S. H., and Kornfeld, P. Studies in myasthenia gravis: Early thymectomy. Am. J. Med. *58:* 517–524, 1975.
59. Sambrook, M. A., Reid, H., Mohr, P. D., and Boddie, H. G. Myasthenia gravis: Clinical and histological features in relation to thymectomy. J. Neurol. Neurosurg. Psychiatry *39:* 38–43, 1976.
60. Schultz, M. D., and Schwab, R. S. Results of thymic (mediastinal) irradiation in patients with myasthenia gravis. Ann. N.Y. Acad. Sci. *183:* 303, 1971.
61. Kornfeld, P., Horowitz, S. H., Genkins, G., and Papatestas, A. E. Myasthenia gravis unmasked by antiarrhythmic agents. Mt. Sinai J. Med. *43:* 10–14, 1976.
62. Herishann, Y., and Rosenberg, P. β Blockers and myasthenia gravis. Ann. Intern. Med. *83:* 834–835, 1975.

MYASTHENIC SYNDROME (EATON-LAMBERT SYNDROME)

The defect of neuromuscular transmission seen in the myasthenic syndrome is quite different from that of myasthenia gravis.[1-5] The symptoms of the illness are equally distinct and perhaps the name "myasthenic" syndrome implies more common ground between this disease and myasthenia gravis than actually exists. The disease occurs more frequently in men than women by a factor of 5 and is usually found over the age of 40. The association of the myasthenic syndrome with small cell carcinoma of the bronchus is well recognized; over half of the patients have such neoplasms. Up to 70 per cent of the patients have a malignancy of one kind or another, and only 30 per cent when followed over a long period of time remain free of cancer. It is remarkable that the symptoms of the myasthenic syndrome may occur many months before the malignancy becomes apparent. The initial symptom is usually a feeling of weakness and tiredness around the hip which gives the patient predictable difficulty in arising from a chair or climbing stairs. Mild and non-specific aching of the back and thighs may be found at this stage. The weakness differs from that of myasthenia gravis in being worst soon after arising in the morning, having a tendency to improve as the day goes on. Exercise may help rather than hinder the patient's strength for a brief time, although fatigue again supervenes after prolonged effort. The weakness may spread to involve muscles of the legs, shoulders, and arms, but rarely does it involve the muscles of the head and neck. While some mild difficulty with swallowing is noted in about a third of the patients, and a few have noticed transient blurring of vision or ptosis, the severe involvement of extraocular and bulbar muscles which is so characteristic of myasthenia gravis is lacking in the myasthenic syndrome.

Another unusual symptom is that of a peculiar taste or dryness of the mouth. Perhaps the fact that the majority of patients have small cell carcinoma of the bronchus and that this is associated with cigarette smoking may partly explain this symptom.

The clinical examination may show mild weakness or no weakness at all. Sometimes the increase in strength following exercise is noted on examination. Thus, when the patient attempts to raise the legs straight off the examining couch he may intially be unable to withstand any resistance to the movement on the part of the examiner. After a few attempts, however, the strength gradually returns to the legs and may be almost normal. This increasing strength may impart to the examiner a sensation similar to drawing up water from a well with a hand pump; with each movement the resistance needed to overcome the patient's strength increases. Prolonged sustained activity of the muscles, however, causes the weakness to appear again. The deep tendon reflexes are usually depressed, particularly at the knees. Since the illness is one of the remote effects of cancer, and since the various syndromes associated with cancer seldom occur in isolation, the myasthenic syndrome may co-exist with symptoms of cerebellar ataxia, or the fleeting, changing paresthesiae and hypesthesiae of carcinomatous neuromyopathy.

The only laboratory examination which is useful in the diagnosis of the myasthenic syndrome is the EMG, in particular the response of evoked potentials to repetitive stimulation. The amplitude of the initial evoked response is very small when a single stimulus is given. With repetitive stimulation at rates of 3 cycles per second or less there is a further decrease in the amplitude of the evoked potential. However, with repetitive stimulation of from 10 to 50 cycles per second, facilitation of the response occurs and the amplitude may increase to 20 times the resting amplitude. Repetitive stimulation at 40 cycles per second causes the amplitude of the evoked potential to become normal in a few seconds. Within 2 seconds after a 10 second period of maximum voluntary contraction, the evoked potential is also markedly increased, up to 12 times the resting level. This increase decays over the next 20 to 30 seconds and within 2 to 4 minutes after the contraction the evoked potential is less than the resting value. Single fiber electromyography demonstrates a block in neuromuscular transmission that worsens following rest.[6]

Intracellular recordings[3, 7] show that, although the frequency and size of the miniature end plate potentials recorded in the muscle are normal, the end plate potential produced by an evoked response is less than it should be. This may be due to a decrease in the number of packets of acetylcholine being released from the nerve terminal following the arrival of the nerve impulse. The abnormality in neuromuscular transmission in the myasthenic syndrome is similar in this regard to that produced by magnesium ions, botulinum toxin, and neomycin. Since the release of acetylcholine is calcium dependent, the possibility that some unknown substance is interfering with the utilization of calcium has been entertained. Takamori et al. have suggested that the defective calcium dependent acetylcholine release in the Eaton-Lambert syndrome can be partially corrected by calcium, epinephrine, aminophylline, or caffeine.[8]

The muscle biopsy in myasthenic syndrome shows rather nonspecific findings with histochemical or light microscopic techniques. Some Type 2 fiber atrophy is seen and an occasional inflammatory response. With electron microscopic examination of the neuromuscular junction, Engel and Santa have shown overdevelopment of the postsynaptic region; this is in contrast to the changes seen in myasthenia gravis.[9]

Treatment of the illness begins with a search for malignancy. When one is found, the myasthenic syndrome sometimes improves after treatment of the underlying cancer. Since the myasthenic syndrome may precede the appearance of the tumor, the search for malignancy should be repeated every three to six months. The fatigue of the myasthenic syndrome is usually only poorly responsive to therapy with the cholinesterase inhibitors. Guanidine, on the other hand, may be very effective. Daily doses of from 20 to 30 mg. per kilogram of body weight are employed. Usually a third of this dose is administered every eight hours. It is wise to start the drug out in small doses and gradually to increase them. Possible side effects include nausea, vomiting, some dizziness, and tingling of the fingers. Liver and blood toxicity may also be noted.

BIBLIOGRAPHY

1. Eaton, L. M., and Lambert, E. H. Electromyography and electric stimulation of nerves in diseases of motor units: Observations on myasthenic syndrome associated with malignant tumors. JAMA *163:* 1117–1124, 1957.
2. Elmqvist, D., and Lambert, E. H. Detailed analysis of neuromuscular transmission in a patient with the myasthenic syndrome sometimes associated with bronchogenic carcinoma. Mayo Clin. Proc. *43:* 689–713, 1968.
3. Lambert, E. H., and Rooke, E. D. Myasthenic state and lung cancer. In: *The Remote Effects of Cancer on the Nervous System,* edited by W. Brain and F. H. Norris. Grune & Stratton, New York, 1965.
4. Herrmann, C. Myasthenia gravis and the myasthenic syndrome. Calif. Med. *113:* 27–36, 1970.
5. Lambert, E. H. Defects of neuromuscular transmission in syndromes other than myasthenia gravis. Ann. N. Y. Acad. Sci. *135:* 367–384, 1966.
6. Schwartz, M. S., and Stalberg, E. Myasthenic syndrome studied with single fiber electromyography. Arch. Neurol. *32:* 815–817, 1975.
7. Lambert, E. H., and Elmqvist, D. Quantal components of end plate potentials in myasthenic syndrome. Ann. N. Y. Acad. Sci. *183:* 183–199, 1971.
8. Takamori, M., Ishii, N., and Mori, M. The role of cyclic 3′,5′-adenosine monophosphate in neuromuscular disease. Arch. Neurol. *29:* 420–424, 1973.
9. Engel, A. G., and Santa, T. Histometric analysis of the ultrastructure of the neuromuscular junction in myasthenia gravis and in the myasthenic syndrome. Ann. N. Y. Acad. Sci. *183:* 46–63, 1971.

BOTULISM

It is a testimony to the potency of the botulinum toxin that its fame is celebrated in the lay literature as much as in medical texts. Botulism is caused by the exotoxin of *Clostridium botulinum,* an anaerobic organism which may contaminate improperly canned food. Home canned vegetables have been the most common culprits; of these, peppers seem particularly noteworthy.

Recent outbreaks have been caused by commercially canned foods, and fish products have also been been known to harbor toxin. Since the bacillus and the exotoxin it produces are destroyed by heat, proper boiling of food before canning and during the preparation of the food for the table should eliminate attacks. At high altitudes water boils at a lower temperature, and this may account for a greater frequency of botulism.[1, 2] The use of a pressure cooker at such altitudes may solve the problem. Contaminated food may be suspected if the can is buckled or "blown," or if home prepared food has a strong and unpleasant smell. A second source of the botulinum toxin is the infection of a wound by the organism. Most cases of wound botulism occur between spring and fall and are generally subsequent to wounds sustained in open fields or on farms.

There are several distinct types of *C botulinum,* but the three major ones associated with botulism are A, B, and E. Types A and B are more frequently found in cases from the Eastern United States and are more often the causal agent in botulism due to canned vegetables, whereas outbreaks due to Type E have been due to contaminated fish products. The mortality following Type B botulism may be less than in Types A or E.[3] The majority of cases of wound botulism have been due to Type A.

The exact mode of action of the toxin is not known, but the site of its action lies at the neuromuscular junction. A recent study indicates that the toxin interferes with the release of acetylcholine[4] by blocking exocytosis. Clinically the symptoms begin within 2 hours to 7 days of ingestion of contaminated food. With wound botulism the incubation time is somewhat longer, up to 14 days.[5] This is probably due to the time lag necessary for the development of the bacillus in the wound.

The symptoms usually begin in the bulbar muscles. Blurring of vision, diplopia, and difficulty with chewing and swallowing are noted. When the disease is due to ingested toxin, nausea, gastric discomfort, or vomiting may occur. The weakness becomes rather rapidly widespread, and paralysis of the arms, legs, and the respiratory muscles ensues. Death occurs from respiratory failure, and the mortality rate is as high as 25 per cent. If the patient does not die, full recovery may be expected although this may take many months. Examination reveals a flaccid and areflexic patient; the extraocular muscles are involved, and there may be paralysis of the pupil. Such pupillary paralysis was long considered to be the hallmark of the disease, but a recent series of studies suggested it is by no means as common as was previously thought.[2] Sensory abnormalities are not seen. The normal spinal fluid protein serves to differentiate botulism from the Guillain-Barré syndrome, which it may closely resemble. Mild cases of botulism have additional interesting features. Although fatigability of the type seen in myasthenia gravis is not usually part of the clinical picture, it sometimes exists and may even respond to anticholinesterase drugs. Electrophysiologically, the defect in botulism approximates that of the Eaton-Lambert syndrome. There is initially a low amplitude evoked response which is potentiated by repetitive stimulation at frequencies of 50 Hz. That type A botulinum toxin does not cross the placental barrier may be deduced from the case of an unaffected child delivered by a mother who suffered from botulism at the time.

The diagnosis may be established by using the mouse toxin neutralization test. The type of botulinum toxin is established by its lethal effect on mice and by neutralization of the toxin with the specific antitoxin. From 10 to 20 ml of the patient's serum should be sent to the nearest competent laboratory. Further information can be obtained from the Center for Disease Control in Atlanta, Georgia. Samples of the gastric content should also be examined for the toxin, and 50 grams of feces should also be collected and similarly analyzed.

The main principles of treatment are the same as for any patient with a severe respiratory paralysis. Proper care and respiratory support, including tracheostomy, will give the patient the best chance of recovery. After the collection of specimens, botulinum antitoxin may be administered to the patient. However, its efficacy has not really been proven and the incidence of side effects associated with the administration of a foreign protein are frequent enough to cause some hesitation in its use. It has also been suggested that gastric lavage and the administration of enemas will help eliminate the bacillus and the toxin from the GI tract. The use of guanidine and germine has been suggested and may have been of benefit in some patients, but their usefulness requires confirmation.

BIBLIOGRAPHY

1. Cherington, M. Botulism: Clinical and therapeutic observations. Rocky Mt. Med. J. *69:* 55–58, 1972.
2. Cherington, M. Botulism: Ten year experience. Arch. Neurol. *30:* 432–437, 1974.
3. Merson, M. H., Hughes, J. M., Dowell, V. R., Taylor, A., Barker, W. H., and Gangarosa, E. J. Current trends in botulism in the United States. JAMA *229:* 1305–1308, 1974.
4. Kao, I., Drachman, D. B., Price, D. L., Botulinum toxin: Mechanism of presynaptic blockade. Science *193:* 1256–1258, 1976.
5. de Jesus, P. V., Slater, R., Spitz, L. K., and Penn, A. S. Neuromuscular physiology of wound botulism. Arch. Neurol. *29:* 425–431, 1973.

TICK PARALYSIS

The association of a progressive symmetrical paralysis with a tick bite is a rare occurrence, but if the possibility is not considered the patient's life may be unnecessarily placed in hazard. The paralysis is probably due to a neurotoxin which the tick injects while embedded in the skin. The mode of action is not precisely known but seems to be at the myoneural junction.[1, 2] Ticks in the higher elevations and in dry parts of the country thrive in the spring and early summer when they may occasionally be ubiquitous. As the summer's heat advances and the vegetation dries, the creatures disappear until the next year. In more humid areas they persist throughout the summer. It is probably not illuminating to say that ticks may be recognized by the fact that they look like ticks, but verbal descriptions are not very helpful. They have eight legs, as opposed to flies, beetles, and other insects, and a flattened hard abdomen almost impossible to crush in the non-engorged state. Most cases of tick paralysis are in children and the majority of these are girls. It is necessary for the tick to be embedded for 5 to 6 days before the paralysis begins. Although social habits are continually changing, many young girls have long hair and the tick, which is usually embedded near the hairline, is unnoticed. When the paralysis begins it rapidly becomes generalized. Bulbar symptoms include difficulty with speech and swallowing, weakness of the face, and, occasionally blurring of vision. The paralysis of arms and legs is associated with areflexia and occasionally sensory symptoms are noted, with numbness and tingling of the extremities and of the face. When an engorging tick is found in such a situation it should be removed. The emergency room physician who finds himself faced with an embedded tick and is new to the situation should resist the temptation to grasp the abdomen of the insect and yank it out. This will probably leave the head firmly embedded in the patient, and the danger of secondary infections is apparent. There are many ways of removing ticks but the initial step is to cause the tick to withdraw from the skin. This may be done by applying a lighted match or cigarette to the tick. I disapprove of this method since it seems a little incendiary and the risk to the patient's hair is a real one. Another favorite method is to cover the creature with vaseline; presumably the anoxia produced by this causes the tick to withdraw. The abdomen may then be grasped with forceps and the tick may be withdrawn by turning it gently. A hot debate rages in Colorado as to whether the tick should be turned clockwise or anticlockwise to permit the easiest withdrawal. As far as I know, no controlled study has been done.

BIBLIOGRAPHY

1. Editorial: Tick paralysis. Brit. Med. J. *3:* 314–315, 1969.
2. Cherington, M., and Snyder, R. D. Tick paralysis: Neurophysiologic studies. New Engl. J. Med. *278:* 95–97, 1968.

5

muscular dystrophies

DUCHENNE'S MUSCULAR DYSTROPHY (PSEUDOHYPERTROPHIC MUSCULAR DYSTROPHY)

"I thought humanity to be inflicted with enough evils already. I do not congratulate you, sir, upon the new gift that you have made to it." In these words, one of Duchenne's acquaintants commented upon the description in 1868 of the "Pseudohypertrophic Muscular Paralysis."[1] In the intervening century his friend would have been dismayed by the number and variety of other neuromuscular ailments that have been uncovered. Yet Duchenne's dystrophy remains the best known of all of them to the extent that its name has become almost synonymous with muscular dystrophy.

Clinical Aspects

The disease is usually inherited as an x-linked recessive gene; the disease is passed to boys by their relatively unaffected mothers. Between 20 and 30 out of every 100,000 boys born will suffer from the disease and the prevalence rate in the total population is about 3 per 100,000.[2] Up to one third of the cases appear to be due to a spontaneous mutation either in the patient or his mother. Many of the mothers of isolated cases (i.e. boys with the illness, in whose family occur no other cases of muscular dystrophy) demonstrate abnormalities of membrane function similar to that of their affected sons.[3] This may indicate that the true incidence of spontaneous mutation is very much lower than was previously believed.

Although there is histological and laboratory evidence that the disease exists in children from birth, the clinical manifestations are usually seen in the second year of life. The child's early development and such milestones as his ability to raise his head and sit upright are normally attained. It is when he begins to stand and to walk that his difficulty becomes apparent. At first this is so slight that he is thought to be clumsy. His frequent falls, the slightly waddling walk, or the accentuation of the normal thud of the heel upon the ground are not considered abnormal in a child who has just recently started walking. There may be some early difficulty in arising from the floor, but the transient hand support upon his knee is shrugged off as an idiosyncrasy by parents and physician alike. The boy is often well muscled with the oddly compact and rubbery muscles characteristic of the illness. It is, therefore, hard to believe that any trouble with his strength could arise from abnormalities of the muscle. Shortly after the first difficulties are noted, the child begins to walk with heels slightly off the ground, often with the feet externally rotated and wide based (Figures 5.1–5.3). Sometimes an orthopedic problem is suspected and corrective shoes are provided. However, the inevitable discovery of the child's weakness comes by the time he is three to four years of age and is betrayed by his inability to keep up with his peers, by the difficulty he has climbing stairs (which are taken one at a time, usually with the same foot leading for each step) and by an increasing rolling movement to the hips while walking. Running is never well accomplished, and at best the patient achieves a clumsy lope. There are similar difficulties with jumping. Often in the early stage of the disease the patient will complain of leg pains. The history of these pains is seldom volunteered but can be elicited on questioning. They are usually in the calf muscles, come on fairly abruptly, and last for two to three days, after which time they gradually subside. They do not resemble the night cramps of patients with motor neuron disease, and their cause remains obscure. It is also during this stage of the illness, between three to seven years, when the boy may appear to improve. The inexorably progressive weakness produced by the disease is counterbalanced by the child's natural growth and development. He may, therefore, acquire motor skills at this time and false hopes may be raised that the diagnosis is in error or that he is responding to some particular form of medication. Such improve-

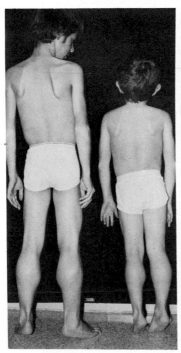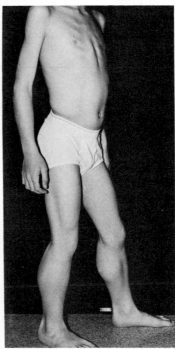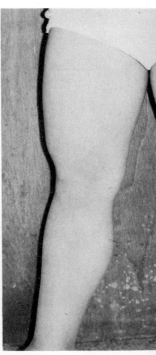

+ *Figures 5.1 (left)* and 5.2 *(center)*. Two brothers who had pseudohypertrophy of the calf muscles and stood and walked on their toes. The mother felt this was a "habit" since both boys could stand with their heels on the ground when so instructed, as in Figure 5.2.

Figure 5.3 *(right)*. Pseudohypertrophy is not limited to calf muscles. In this boy, the quadriceps were enlarged.

ment, however, is short lived and the disease resumes its downward march. Progressive difficulty occurs in arising from the floor, and the boy uses increasing amounts of hand support to push himself to an upright position. The accentuation of the lumbar lordosis associated with the forward thrust of the abdomen, the tendency to lock the knee backwards to prevent the collapse of that joint, and the shortening of the posterior muscles of the calf combine to give the child the appearance of being perched precariously on his toes, even during quiet standing (Figures 5.4 and 5.5). Frequent falls are no longer dismissed as the ordinary tumbles of a clumsy child and now become a serious problem. If the boy gets off balance the leg muscles lack the strength to make correcting movements and the knees collapse abruptly, pitching the patient on the ground. The boy ceases to be able to climb stairs, and six months to a year after this he is no longer able to walk independently and needs a wheelchair. Once in the wheelchair, contractures develop and joints may freeze in the position in which the boy sits. The hips, knees, and elbows are flexed. The feet turn downwards and inwards with a marked curve to the instep which prevents the child wearing normal shoes (Figure 5.6). A progressive kyphoscoliosis develops, further hampering an already weakened respiratory system. In the terminal stages, the boy sits in his wheelchair

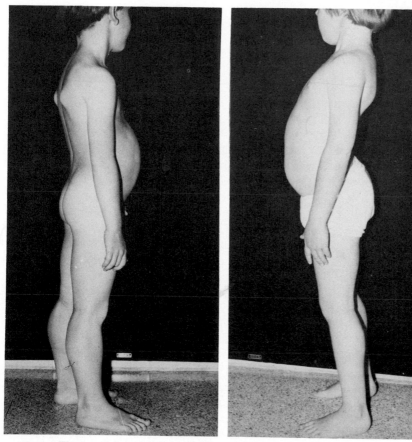

Figures 5.4 and 5.5. A lordosis is associated with the illness.

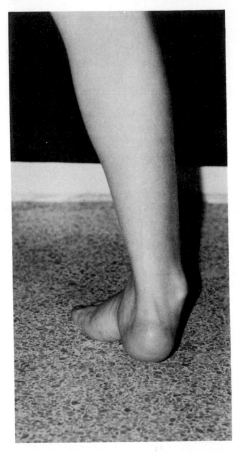

Figure 5.6. The foot assumes a position of inversion and plantar flexion. This is associated with tightening of the heel cords although it is not necessarily caused by that.

twisted like a pretzel, barely able to move any of his muscles. Even the face muscles are involved, and lack of neck support causes the head to loll against the back of the chair. The tongue is often enlarged and may protrude from a slack mouth. Because of poor pulmonary excursions, simple colds have a tendency to be complicated by secondary infection and pneumonia is the terminal event. Rarely, cardiac failure may be seen; when it does occur it may not respond to digitalization. The ankle edema seen in the late stage of Duchenne's dystrophy is probably due more to venous stasis in inactive legs than to congestive failure.

Mentally these children are often somewhat dull, although occasionally a child with Duchenne's dystrophy may be above average intelligence. There are particular problems in the perceptual area and in the development of visual concepts. In general the I.Q. is below the level of matched controls.[4] Perhaps some of the retardation could be due to physical handicap preventing the child from being in a proper learning situation, but children with spinal muscular atrophy who are equally handicapped do not suffer the same mental retardation and, if anything, seem unusually bright. The child with Duchenne's dystrophy often goes through two phases during which he may be anxious and depressed. Perhaps the surprising thing about the depression is not that it occurs but that it does not occur more often. Around the age of 5 the child realizes for the first time that there is something wrong with him, and he may become withdrawn and shy. This is not helped by the fact that his playmates at school often delight in pushing him over on the playground merely for the interest of seeing him get up again. The second phase during which children may become very depressed is shortly after they start using a wheelchair. To some extent this depends on the manner in which the wheelchair is offered to the boy. If the entire aim of treatment is presented to the child as keeping him out of the wheelchair, then the necessity for this device represents a failure. If, on the other hand, the wheelchair is approached simply as another form of treatment, the problems associated with it may be less. However, there is frequently some depression at this stage and many of the children respond with a period of bowel and bladder incontinence. This is only partially due to the fact that the help they need in going to the bathroom is sometimes unavailable. Usually parents can be reassured that this incontinence will disappear in a few months.

The findings on examination will vary, of course, depending on the stage of the disease. In younger boys mild proximal weakness, more of hips than of shoulders, is associated with rubbery, hard muscles and some contracture of the ankles. Deep tendon reflexes tend to disappear early. Later in the illness more florid changes are seen, and the weakness may involve all the muscles of the body except the extraocular muscles. Children in the advanced stages of Duchenne's dystrophy tend to be either very thin or very fat. The latter state is easy to understand in view of the muscular inactivity and the undiminished appetite, but the cause of loss of weight in Duchenne's dystrophy is less simple. It is not due to loss of muscle bulk alone, and the mechanical difficulties with swallowing are rarely severe enough to provide an adequate explanation. Other neurological abnormalities are rare in Duchenne's dystrophy. Although patients have been noted with extensor plantar responses, this finding should cast some doubt on the diagnosis.

Laboratory Studies

Laboratory tests which are of value in Duchenne's dystrophy include the serum creatine phosphokinase (CPK), the EKG, EMG, and muscle biopsy. Elevated levels of creatine phosphokinase are always seen in the early stages of the illness. When the patient is manifesting a slight waddle and is having mild difficulty in arising from the floor, one may expect to see CPK levels of several thousand. The serum CPK level may be even higher in the first year of life, when the disease is not yet clinically manifest. Indeed, the highest CPK levels we have ever seen have been in patients of two to three months of age who later went on to develop muscular dystrophy. In our experience, a child with a normal level of CPK during the first few months of life will not develop Duchenne's muscular dystrophy later, and a normal CPK level at this age is strong evidence against the possibility of the disease. As the disease progresses the serum CPK falls, although it never attains a normal value, remaining in the hundreds even in the patient who is severely handicapped and in a wheelchair.

Abnormalities in the EKG are common in Duchenne's muscular dystrophy, perhaps in the neighborhood of 70 per cent.[5, 6] There are tall, right precordial R waves and deep limb lead and precordial Q waves.[7] This results in an abnormally high value for the algebraic sum of the R and S waves (R-S) in V_1.[8] Arrhythmias and persistent tachycardias have been noted in patients with Duchenne's. Many different explanations have been postulated for these changes but none has been entirely satisfactory. The suggestions of right ventricular hypertrophy or abnormal right ventricular conduction are not confirmed by vectorcardiographic analyses.[9] Other explanations, such as the persistence of an infantile pattern of the vectorcardiogram or a genetically determined disorder in the electrical activity in part of the myocardium, remain as yet unconfirmed.

Electromyography shows the small polyphasic potentials and increased recruitment of the motor units with effort associated with myopathies, and advanced disease may show additional changes of fibrillations. The muscle biopsy is rather characteristic even early in the disease, with increased fibrosis, small groups of basophilic fibers, and a persistence of undifferentiated Type 2C muscle fibers.

Treatment

At the present time Duchenne's muscular dystrophy is an incurable disease. In spite of many therapeutic trials of substances as diverse as estrogens, steroids, and Vitamin E, no effective drug is available. Incurable and untreatable are not, however, synonymous and much can be done to make the life of a patient more comfortable. Sometimes the parents of dystrophic children faced with the problem of illness in their child manifest one of two reactions. They either try to ignore the child, or they build things for his aid so that he becomes encased in mechanical contraptions. Physicians on occasion have been known to have the same reactions, and the two extremes are equally to be avoided. It does not help the family to be told that there is nothing to be done and they should return home to await the inevitable end. On the other hand, bracing the child too early or recommending major reconstructive surgery inappropriately may salve the physician's hurt, but can do the patient a great deal of harm. The proper management of Duchenne's dystrophy depends on a team approach to management such as that outlined by Vignos et al.[10] The ideal situation is where the neurologist, the orthopedic surgeon, the physical and occupational therapists, and the social worker all take an active part in the clinic. In the early stages of the illness, passive stretching of the muscles is all that is required. Early attention should be given to two areas. The Achilles tendon should be stretched once, or preferably twice, daily in these patients. If practiced regularly, this can do much to impede the equinovarus deformity which otherwise develops. The application of light bivalve casts at night or of night splints may further retard the development of the foot deformity. The iliotibial band should also be stretched daily. Active exercises are usually unnecessary in children, since they run around to the best of their ability anyway. There is no solid evidence that exercise either injures the muscle in Duchenne's dystrophy or helps patients, but both of these points of view have their adherents. A sensible compromise is perhaps to tell parents that their children can take as much exercise as they wish, but should not exercise to the extent where muscle pains are noted. While the child is still walking, major surgery is probably inadvisable. There are only two exceptions to this. Sometimes the contractures of the posterior calf muscles are severe enough to make walking difficult. If it is felt that this is the only reason that walking is impeded (and this is an unusual circumstance), a release of the Achilles tendon or, perhaps better, a transplantation of the posterior tibial muscle may be helpful. Contractures of the iliotibial bands may also impair walking, and release of these on occasions may be necessary. It is vital that patients who undergo surgery be mobilized as soon as possible. All of us have had the disastrous experience of watching a patient, whose operation was supposed to help him walk, fail to recover his ability to do so following the prolonged bedrest associated with the surgery.

The phase during which surgery may be usefully recommended is at the point when the patient is about to cease walking. This implies a degree of prescience on the part of the physician, but there are some indications from the patient's history and examination. When the patient can no longer climb stairs or step up onto a small step, he is probably six months to a year away from using a wheelchair all the time. Another indication is when the patient can no longer straighten his knee out against gravity. At this stage, considera-tion should be given to a transposition of the posterior tibial muscle. The posterior tibial muscle is detached from its insertion and the tendon threaded between the tibia and fibula to be attached to the dorsum of the foot. This is associated with appropriate Achilles tendon lengthening and gives the patient a stable foot which is held at a right angle and which develops the equinovarus deformity less readily than following a simple Achilles tenotomy. This surgery usually necessitates the use of long leg braces thereafter. The long leg braces should be supplied with a pelvic band just under the ischial tuberosity and should be as light as possible. The knee joint should be provided with a spring loaded lock. The security of a knee lock is essential because should this brace give way disastrous injury may result. The best type of shoe to use with this brace is a high top boot with laces. Using this type of surgical approach, independent walking may be prolonged for two years or more.[11]

When the patient is confined to a wheelchair the tendency to develop contractures is accelerated and frequently a kyphoscoliosis starts to develop. It is difficult to prevent these deformities and equally difficult to decide how much energy to put into their correction. Contractures of the hips and knees may make life miserable for the patient, since he is unable to sleep in any position except on his side and cannot comfortably be supported in any position other than a sitting one. Stretching exercises which were previously designed to prevent Achilles shortening should now be expanded to prevent flexion contractures of the hip and knees. The development of a kyphosco-liosis may be impeded by the use of suitable back supports. Accessory pads on the back of the wheelchair may be of value; others prefer the use of light, plastic body jackets, or the full Milwaukee style brace. A word of caution is necessary with regard to bracing. The Milwaukee brace is very difficult for patients with muscle weakness to tolerate, and usually a body jacket is more successful. Some of the treatment failures from the use of braces stem from the fact that the brace spends more time in the closet than it does on the patient. Physicians, however, are the last ones to be told this. A child has to get used to a brace. The brace should be used initially for periods of half an hour or so, with the time gradually lengthened until the child is able to tolerate the brace all day. When the neck muscles become weak, the use of a head support can increase the boy's comfort. This can take the form of an extension to the back of a wheelchair, may be attached to the body jacket, or may simply be a plastic collar. The patient whose spine is hyperextended (with an increased lordosis) has less tendency to develop the lateral curvatures of those whose spines bow into an early kyphosis[12]. It is worthwhile when applying a body jacket to do so with the spine in extension. Additionally, a wheelchair back which is slightly reclined may be used further to promote the lordosis. Ensuring that the patient's pelvis is level may also help retard the spinal deformity and a firm board, suitably padded should be substituted for the slack seat upholstery of the average wheelchair.

When the curvature is becoming worse in spite of attempts at bracing, surgery should be considered. Surgery of the back has not been a popular method of treatment in the past because of the long hospital stay, the associated discomfort and the limited lifespan of the patient with Duchenne's dystrophy. If present trends continue though, it is likely to find increasing acceptance in the management of patients[13].

Ancillary devices are also helpful. When the child is having difficulty feeding himself because of weakness of the shoulders, a ball bearing forearm support, or ball bearing feeder, is helpful. The use of a gel cushion may prevent the development of pressure sores over the buttocks. When the child is no longer able to turn over in bed, the sleep of the entire family is disturbed since they have to get up and turn him every couple of hours. In this situation an alternating air mattress (alternating pressure pad) with a pump attached can give the family, as well as the patient, some much needed rest. When the child can no longer walk independently, pulmonary care becomes increasingly important[14] and daily postural drainage should be carried out by the family. Occasionally, the intranasal administration of oxygen at night can be helpful in giving the patient a comfortable night's rest.

Etiology

The interests of brevity and accuracy are both properly served by a simple statement that we do not know the etiology of Duchenne's muscular dystrophy. There has been so much discussion in the last few years challenging the traditional concept of muscular dystrophy as a primary illness of the muscle, that perhaps some elaboration is in order even if the search for the primary abnormality is returning to the muscle itself. An early suggestion that circulatory difficulties might be responsible for some of the findings in muscular dystrophy[15] was reinforced by the description of an experimental myopathy appearing in rabbit muscle subsequent to injection of the femoral arteries with small dextran particles. The findings in the rabbit muscle bore striking pathological similarities to the changes seen in Duchenne's dystrophy.[16] A combination of aortic ligation and the intraperitoneal injection of 5-hydroxytryptamine in rats produced a similar change.[17] Parker and Mendell[18] used 5-hydroxytryptamine in combination with imipramine, a compound capable of blocking the uptake of biogenic amines. They felt that the similarity between the experimental myopathy so produced and Duchenne's dystrophy was substantiated not only by the pathological changes in the muscle but also by the increase of CPK in the serum. The search for abnormalities in catecholamine metabolism was accelerated by the finding that there was a reduced initial rate of accumulation of serotonin in platelets from patients with Duchenne's muscular dystrophy.[19]

Those opposed to the vascular hypothesis of Duchenne's dystrophy have pointed out that morphological identity between Duchenne's dystrophy and the experimental myopathies does not necessarily prove an identical etiology. More recent studies of blood flow in muscles of patients with Duchenne's dystrophy have failed to demonstrate any abnormality.[20] Electron microscopic and morphometric studies of the capillaries in muscle from patients with the disease have been similarly unrevealing.[21]

The work of McComas and associates suggested that the muscle fibers in Duchenne's dystrophy were not being lost in a random fashion but were disappearing in groups associated with the loss of motor units. They proposed that Duchenne's dystrophy might have its origin in the malign influence of a sick motor neuron upon the muscle fibers.[22] Unfortunately, other laboratories have been unable to duplicate McComas' findings in Duchenne's dystrophy[23, 24] and, although the disease may be associated with an abnormal neural influence, this hypothesis is at the present time without much support.

Changes in the behavior of various cell membranes have been described in Duchenne's dystrophy. Thus, an abnormal surface deformation of erythrocytes was reported to have been produced by washing the red blood cells of patients with Duchenne's dystrophy in saline[25]. Attempts by others to reproduce this finding have been unsuccessful or have suggested that it may be a nonspecific result[26, 27]. The direct study of the properties of isolated membranes is difficult. Any attempt to isolate membranes results in a disturbance of the complex relationship between the membrane and the cell which it surrounds. It is thus not surprising that the evidence for altered membrane function remains at best circumstantial. The behavior of some of the enzymes which are associated with the sarcolemmal or erythrocyte membrane are anomalous. Thus, the activity of Na, K ATPase of erythrocyte membranes in patients with Duchenne's dystrophy is stimulated by ouabain, rather than being inhibited as in the normal situation[28]. A later study showed that a factor present in the patient's serum may contribute to this alteration[29]. The endogenous phosphorylation of a group of membrane proteins, so-called "protein kinase" activity, is also abnormally high in erythrocyte membranes[31]. Adenyl cyclase, an enzyme associated with sarcolemmal membranes, is also abnormal[32]. Ordinarily, the enzyme is stimulated by epinephrine and sodium fluoride but in patients with Duchenne dystrophy this stimulation is less than normal. Ultrastructural abnormalities of the membrane were found in a recent study by Engel and colleagues[30]. The earliest change detectable with the electron microscope is small, abnormal areas in the sarcolemmal membrane.

Carrier Detection

As in any x-linked recessive disease, genetic counseling depends upon the identification of potential carriers. The patient's mother, sisters and maternal aunts are most immediately at risk, but obviously all females on the maternal side of the family should be considered. Much work has been carried out on the identification of the carrier state but at the present time we are probably able to identify no more than 80 per cent of definite carriers. The identification of such carriers is based upon the fact that they manifest some parts of the disease which afflict the boys. This is perhaps due to inadequate suppression of the abnormal X chromosome, as suggested by Lyon's hypothesis. Occasionally there may be clinical evidence of the carrier state. In most reports this is found in less than 5 per cent of carriers and, when present, varies from gastrocnemius hypertrophy, which is often asymmetric, to the development of overt proximal weakness.[33] Occasionally all the carriers in a given family will demonstrate such weakness, giving rise to the suspicion that there may be some additional genetic factor which allows the disease to surface in the females.

Most of the efforts in carrier detection have been directed to the detection of subclinical abnormalities. Muscle biopsy has been suggested as one method. In carriers of Duchenne's one may see foci of necrotic fibers, moth eaten and whorled changes in the intermyofibrillar network pattern, and an abnormal number of internal nuclei.[34, 35] These changes may be noted in normal patients who are not carriers, particularly if the gastrocnemius muscle is biopsied, but their presence in patients who are at risk is strong presumptive evidence of the carrier state. The electrocardiogram may also be abnormal. The algebraic sum of the R and S waves in the V1 lead of the EKG has been found to be greater in carriers than in normal women.[36] Others have noted the same changes, but at least one study has failed to confirm the finding.[6] Thus at present the EKG has not proved a useful means of detecting carriers.

Abnormalities of the electromyogram in the carrier state have been described, with the focal appearance of short, low amplitude polyphasic potentials. The use of routine electromyography in this fashion, however, did not increase the possibility of carrier detection.[37, 38] A refinement of the technique with frequency analysis or computerized analysis of the potentials may sharpen the accuracy of this method,[39] but has not found wide acceptance. The search for biochemical abnormalities, not only in Duchenne's dystrophy but also in the carrier state, has ranged far and wide. Substances as esoteric as rubidium have been implicated, only to have later studies refute the finding[40]. An abnormality in ribosomal protein synthesis has been described in Duchenne's dystrophy[41]. Isolated ribosomes were found to synthesize increased amounts of collagen. A similar finding was noted in the carriers[42]. Ribosomes in the latter cases were found to synthesize abnormally high amounts of non-collagenous protein as well as collagen. The increased ability of the erythrocyte membrane to phosphorylate protein, which has been described as a feature of Duchenne's dystrophy, is also found in carriers of the illness[3]. The mean values for the groups of definite, probable and possible carriers were similar and different from the mean value for matched controls. This suggested that the spontaneous mutation rate must be very low, since if there were non-carrier mothers in the possible and probable groups, their normal values of protein kinase should have reduced the mean value of these two groups compared to the definite carriers. Unfortunately, in individual instances, the variability in the value makes the test unsuitable for use in carrier detection at present.

There is one basic problem in the detection of the carrier state that should always be borne in mind. There are three levels of certainty of the carrier state: definite, probable and possible. For a woman to be a definite carrier she must not only have an affected son but also one affected brother, maternal uncle or other male member of the maternal family. Probable carriers have two or more affected sons but there are no other affected members in the maternal family. Possible carriers are mothers of isolated cases or female relatives (e.g., sister) of affected males. The definite carriers, and to a lesser extent the probable carriers, are the group of women used to obtain data about the chemical abnormalities of the carrier state. It should be noted that an affected son is an essential part of the definition of definite and probable carriers. Many of these children are quite severely handicapped and require considerable physical exertion in their care. Morphologically this is expressed by an increase in the size of Type 2 fibers from biopsies of carriers[43] and perhaps it may also account for some of the differences between carriers and a population of mothers with normal children. However, not all of the abnormalities described in the literature are due to this.

The most reliable test at present is the CPK determination. Blood is drawn for evaluation on three or four separate occasions at least a week apart. If any one of these values is abnormally high the mother should be advised that she is most probably a carrier. If all values are normal there may still be a 10 to 20% possibility of the patient being a carrier. It is important to obtain blood samples from possible carriers before the age of 10 years whenever feasible because the levels of CPK are likely to be more abnormal in the first decade[44]. During pregnancy the CPK levels may also fall, limiting the usefulness of the test at this stage[45, 46]. The odds are somewhat modified by considering the rest of the family history, the number of female relatives who have had normal CPK values, the number of male relatives who were at risk and yet did not develop the disease, and the proximity of the known cases of muscular dystrophy to the girl whose carrier state is being evaluated. All of these are taken into account in genetic counseling and quite elaborate charts are drawn up to sharpen the accuracy of prediction. Changing the odds, however, from 15% to 5% really makes little difference to the possible carrier's decision about family planning. Those who have a close acquaintance with dystrophic children usually retain their reluctance to embark on a possible tragic pregnancy, whereas those whose acquaintance with muscular dystrophy is more remote, proceed undeterred.

Amniocentesis has been performed at 15 weeks of pregnancy and a determination of the sex of the fetus made. If the fetus is female, the child will not suffer the clinical symptoms of Duchenne's dystrophy. If the fetus is male, the mother may elect to have the pregnancy terminated. Analysis of amniotic fluid CPK has not proved useful in detecting whether a male fetus has the illness or not. With the technical feasibility of obtaining fetal blood at eighteen weeks during fetoscopy[47] prenatal diagnosis of the illness may be possible in the future.

BIBLIOGRAPHY

1. Duchenne de Boulogne. De la paralysie musculaire pseudohypertrophique ou paralysie myosclerosique. (Extrait des Archives generales de Médecine) Asselin, Paris, 1868.
2. Gardner-Medwin, D. Mutation rate in Duchenne type of muscular dystrophy. J. Med.

Genet. *7:* 334–337, 1970.

3. Roses, A. D., Roses, M. J., Miller, S. E., Hull, K. L., and Appel, S. H. Carrier detection in Duchenne muscular dystrophy. N. Engl. J. Med. *294:* 193–197, 1976.

4. Cohen, H. J., Molnar, G. E., and Taft, L. T. The genetic relationship of progressive muscular dystrophy (Duchenne type) and mental retardation. Dev. Med. Child Neurol. *10:* 754–765, 1968.

5. Fitch, C. W., and Ainger, L. E. The Frank vectorcardiogram and the electrocardiogram in Duchenne progressive muscular dystrophy. Circulation *35:* 1124–1140, 1967.

6. Jeliett, A. B., Kennedy, M. C., and Goldblatt, E. Duchenne pseudohypertrophic muscular dystrophy. A clinical and electrocardiographic study of patients and female carriers. Aust. N.Z. J. Med. *4:* 41–47, 1974.

7. Perloff, J. K., Roberts, W. C., de Leon, A. C., and O'Doherty, D. The distinctive electrocardiogram of Duchenne's progressive muscular dystrophy. Am. J. Med. *42:* 179–188, 1967.

8. Skyring, A., and McKusick, V. A. Clinical, genetic and electrocardiographic studies in childhood muscular dystrophy. Am. J. Med. Sci. *242:* 534–547, 1961.

9. Ronan, J. A., Jr., Perloff, J. K., Bowen, P. J., and Mann, O. The vectorcardiogram in Duchenne's progressive muscular dystrophy. Am. Heart J. *84:* 588–596, 1972.

10. Vignos, P. J., Spencer, G. E., and Archibald, K. C. Management of progressive muscular dystrophy in childhood. JAMA *184:* 89–96, 1963.

11. Spencer, G. E. Orthopaedic care of progressive muscular dystrophy. J. Bone Joint Surg. *49:* 1201–1204, 1971.

12. Wilkins, K. E., and Gibson, D. A. The patterns of spinal deformity in Duchenne muscular dystrophy. J. Bone Joint Surg. *58A:* 24–32, 1976.

13. Bonnett, C., Brown, J. C. Perry, J., Nickel, V., Walinski, T., et al. Evolution of treatment of paralytic scoliosis at Rancho Los Amigos Hospital. J. Bone Joint Surg. *57A:* 206–215, 1975.

14. Inkley, S. R., Oldenburg, F. C., and Vignos, P. J. Pulmonary function in Duchenne's muscular dystrophy related to stage of disease. Am. J. Med. *56:* 297–306, 1974.

15. Demos, J., and Ecoiffier, J. Troubles circulatoire au cours de la myopathie. Etude arteriographique. Rev. Franc. Etud. Clin. Biol. *2:* 489–494, 1957.

16. Hathaway, P. W., Engel, W. K., and Zellweger, H. Experimental myopathy after microarterial embolization. Arch. Neurol. *22:* 365–378, 1970.

17. Mendell, J. R., Engel, W. K., and Darrer, E. C. Duchenne muscular dystrophy: Functional ischemia reproduces its characteristic lesions. Science *172:* 1143–1145, 1971.

18. Parker, J. M., and Mendell, J. R. Proximal myopathy induced by 5-HT-imipramine simulates Duchenne dystrophy. Nature *247:* 103–104, 1974.

19. Murphy, D. L., Mendell, J. R., and Engel, W. K. Serotonin and platelet function in Duchenne's muscular dystrophy. Arch. Neurol. *28:* 239–242, 1973.

20. Paulson, O. F., Engel, A. G., and Gomez, M. R. Muscle blood flow in Duchenne type muscular dystrophy, limb-girdle dystrophy, polymyositis and in normal controls. J. Neurol. Neurosurg. Psychiatry *37:* 685–690, 1974.

21. Jerusalem, F., Engel, A. G., and Gomez, M. R. Duchenne dystrophy. I. Morphometric study of the muscle microvasculature. Brain *97:* 115–122, 1974.

22. McComas, A. J., Sica, R. E. P., and Currie, S. An electrophysiological study of Duchenne dystrophy. J. Neurol. Neurosurg. Psychiatry *34:* 461–468, 1971.

23. Panayiotopoulos, C. P., Scarpalezos, S., and Papapetropoulos, T. Electrophysiological estimation of motor units in Duchenne muscular dystrophy. J. Neurol. Sci. *23:* 89–98, 1974.

24. Ballantyne, J. P., and Hansen, S. New method for the estimation of the number of motor units in a muscle. 2. Duchenne, limb-girdle and facioscapulohumeral, and myotonic muscular dystrophies. J. Neurol. Neurosurg. Psychiatry *37:* 1195–1201, 1974.

25. Matheson, D. W., and Howland, J. L. Erythrocyte deformation in human muscular dystrophy. Science *184:* 165–166, 1974.

26. Miale, T. D., Frias, J. L., and Lawson, D. L. Erythrocytes in human muscular dystrophy. Science *187:* 453, 1975.

27. Miller, S. E., Roses, A. D., and Appel, S. H. Erythrocytes in human muscular dystrophy. Science *188:* 1131, 1975.

28. Brown, H. D., Chattpadhyag, S. K., and Patel, A. B. Erythrocyte abnormality in human

myopathy. Science *157:* 1577–1578, 1967.

29. Peter, J. B., Worsfold, M., and Pearson, C. M. Erythrocyte ghost adenosine triphosphatase (ATPase) in Duchenne dystrophy. J. Lab. Clin. Med. *74:* 103–108, 1969.

30. Mokri, B., and Engel, A. G. Duchenne dystrophy: electron microscopic findings pointing to a basic or early abnormality in the plasma membrane of the muscle fiber. Neurology *25:* 375, 1975.

31. Roses, A. D., Herbstreith, M. H., and Appel, S. H. Membrane protein kinase alteration in Duchenne muscular dystrophy. Nature *254:* 350–351, 1975.

32. Mawatari, S., Takagi, A., and Rowland, L. P. Adenyl cyclase in normal and pathologic human muscle. Arch. Neurol. *30:* 96–102, 1974.

33. Moser, H., and Emery, A. E. H. The manifesting carrier in Duchenne muscular dystrophy. Med. Genet. *5:* 271–284, 1974.

34. Pearce, G. W., Pearce, J. M. S., and Walton, J. N. The Duchenne type muscular dystrophy: Histopathological studies of the carrier state. Brain *89:* 109–120, 1966.

35. Roy, S., and Dubowitz, V. Carrier detection in Duchenne muscular dystrophy. J. Neurol. Sci. *11:* 65–79, 1970.

36. Emery, A. E. H. Abnormalities in the electrocardiogram in female carriers of Duchenne muscular dystrophy. Brit. Med. J. *2:* 418–420, 1969.

37. Gardner-Medwin, D. Studies of the carrier state in the Duchenne type of muscular dystrophy. 2. Quantitative electromyography as a method of carrier detection. J. Neurol. Neurosurg. Psychiatry *31:* 124–134, 1968.

38. Gardner-Medwin, D., Pennington, R. J., and Walton, J. N. The detection of carriers of X-linked muscular dystrophy genes. A review of some methods studied in Newcastle upon Tyne. J. Neurol. Sci. *13:* 459–474, 1971.

39. Moosa, A., Brown, B. H., and Dubowitz, V. Quantitative electromyography carrier detection in Duchenne type muscular dystrophy using a new automatic technique. J. Neurol. Neurosurg. Psychiatry *35:* 841–844, 1972.

40. Hilditch, T. E., Sweetin, J. C., and Thomson, W. H. S. Rubidium and detection of Duchenne carriers. Lancet *2:* 323, 1973.

41. Ionasescu, V., Zellweger, H., and Conway, T. W. Ribosomal protein synthesis in Duchenne muscular dystrophy. Arch. Biochem. Biophys. *144:* 51–58, 1971.

42. Ionasescu, V., Zellweger, H., Shirk, P., and Conway, T. W. Identification of carriers of Duchenne muscular dystrophy by muscle protein synthesis. Neurology *23:* 497–501, 1973.

43. Brooke, M. H., and Engel, W. K. The histographic analysis of human muscle biopsies with regard to fiber types. I. Adult male and female. Neurology *19:* 221–233, 1969.

44. Munsat, T. L., Baloh, R., Pearson, C. M., and Fowler, W. Serum enzyme alterations in neuromuscular disorders. JAMA *226:* 1536–1543, 1973.

45. Blyth, H., and Hughes, B. P. Pregnancy and serum CPK levels in potential carriers of severe X-linked muscular dystrophy. Lancet *1:* 855–856, 1971.

46. Emery, A. E. H., and King, B. Pregnancy and serum-creatine-kinase levels in potential carriers of Duchenne X-linked muscular dystrophy. Lancet *1:* 1013, 1971.

47. Hobbins, J. C., and Mahoney, M. J. In utero diagnosis of hemoglobinopathies. Technic for obtaining fetal blood. N. Engl. J. Med. *290:* 1065–1067, 1974.

SLOWLY PROGRESSIVE (BECKER'S) VARIETY OF X-LINKED MUSCULAR DYSTROPHY

A form of X-linked recessive dystrophy bearing a close resemblance to the Duchenne's variety was outlined by Becker.[1] The patient develops the same proximal weakness of the hips and shoulders, with a tendency to walk on the toes and with the characteristic hypertrophy (Figures 5.7 and 5.8). The onset of the disease is much delayed, and survival is prolonged until middle adult life. The existence of the Becker's variety of dystrophy as a separate entity is supported by genetic analysis.[2–4] Although the number of families reported in the literature is not large, Becker's variety and the Duchenne type of dystrophy are rarely found in the same pedigree, suggesting that they do not, in reality, represent the two extremes in the spectrum of progression of a single

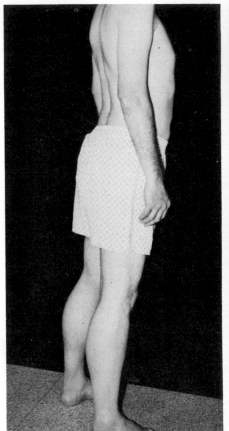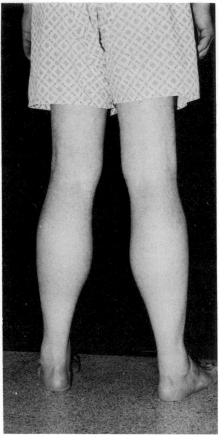

Figures 5.7 and 5.8. Beckers or mild variety of pseudohypertrophic dystrophy. This man was able to walk although he had some difficulty in standing from a low chair. The calf muscles were large and the heel cords tight.

disorder. Mental retardation is also less common in Becker's dystrophy than in Duchenne's. Except for the age of the patient and the degree of weakness, the physical examination in the two diseases is almost identical. There is perhaps less tendency for contractures to develop in Becker's dystrophy and the skeletal deformities are not as marked, but the gait, the manner of arising from the floor, and other aspects of the disease are similar. Laboratory studies show large increases in the levels of the serum CPK. The cardiogram may also show changes similar to those seen in Duchenne's dystrophy. As for carrier detection, the elevation of CPK is noted in only about 50% of the definite carriers of Becker's dystrophy and, when present, is not as pronounced as in carriers of Duchenne's disease.[5]

BIBLIOGRAPHY

1. Becker, P. E. Two new families of benign sex linked recessive muscular dystrophy. Rev. Can. Biol. *21:* 551–566, 1962.
2. Shaw, R. F., and Dreifuss, F. E. Mild and severe forms of X-linked muscular dystrophy. Arch. Neurol. *20:* 451–460, 1969.
3. Zellweger, H., and Hanson, J. W. Slowly progressive X-linked recessive muscular dystrophy

(Type IIIb). Arch. Intern. Med. *120:* 525–535, 1967.

4. Markand, O. N., North, R. R., D'Agostino, A. N., and Daly, D. D. Benign sex linked muscular dystrophy. Neurology *19:* 617–633, 1969.

5. Emery, A. E. H., Clark, E. R., Simon, S., and Tyalor, J. L. Detection of carriers of benign X-linked muscular dystrophy. Brit. Med. J. *4:* 522, 1967.

FACIOSCAPULOHUMERAL DYSTROPHY

The common concept of facioscapulohumeral dystrophy as a rather benign and slowly progressive weakness of muscles of the face, shoulder, and upper arm is only partially correct. There is marked variability in the severity of symptoms from patient to patient, as there is in the age of onset. What follows in the initial paragraphs relates to the classical concepts of facioscapulohumeral dystrophy and will be amplified later to cover the whole gamut of patients with this illness.

Clinical Aspects

The disease is inherited as an autosomal dominant. There is strong penetrance, and the incidence of the illness has been estimated at between 3 and 10 cases per million population.[1] As in so many muscle diseases, this incidence is probably erroneously low owing to the large number of undiagnosed cases. Typically, the disease is first noticed towards the end of the first decade or during the second. Facial weakness is present and an inability to whistle is often a symptom, although it may appear to the patient as no more than a mild quirk of nature. During sleep the eyes may remain slightly open and, because the extraocular muscles are unimpaired, a prominent Bell's phenomenon is seen displaying the sclera through partially opened lids. Drinking through a straw or blowing up balloons may be impossible but may again be dismissed by the patient as an idiosyncrasy rather than a true abnormality. The muscles of the upper arm and shoulders are usually involved simultaneously with the facial muscles, and this gives rise to predictable difficulty in handling heavy objects at a level above the shoulders. When the patient sits in a straight backed chair the protruding shoulder blades may catch on the back of the chair. The illness spreads slowly to other muscle groups, including those of the hips. Bilateral foot drop may be present. Occasionally this is one of the initial symptoms and it is then difficult to know whether to call the disorder facioscapulohumeral dystrophy or scapuloperoneal dystrophy. The overall progression takes place over many decades, interspersed with periods of relatively rapid deterioration.

Although the appearance of the patient with the fully developed illness is characteristic (Figures 5.9–5.14 and 5.17–5.20), the milder varieties may be overlooked. The patient's face is smooth and the forehead usually unlined. The mouth loses the normal contour and appears widened with a more horizontal appearance due to the loss of the normal upward curvature of the lower lip. When viewed from the side, the lips have a pouting appearance ("bouche de tapir"). On either side of the angles of the mouth, a dimple appears, often the only mark on the patient's face. The Mona Lisa illustrates a mild form of this dimpling but it may become pronounced. It also deepens when the patient smiles or attempts to bare the teeth. When the patient is asked to purse his lips, instead of forming the normal "moue," both upper

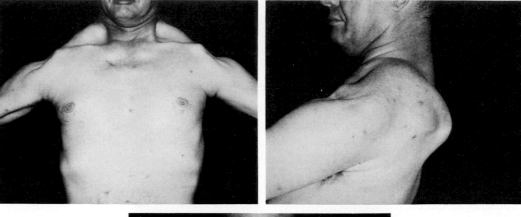

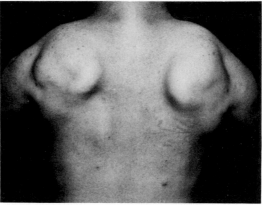

Figures 5.9–5.11. Facioscapulohumeral dystrophy. In this disease the shoulders have a characteristic appearance. When the arms are abducted, the trapezius mounds up and a "step" is formed at the point of the shoulder (Figure 5.9, *left*). The scapulae slide upwards and laterally and the inferomedial corner juts out posteriorly (Figures 5.10 (*right*) and 5.11 (*center below*).

and lower lips move horizontally in opposite directions. The blink is usually slowed and is frequently incomplete.

There is wasting of the neck muscles, and the medial ends of the clavicles jut forward, forming a distinct step at the base of the neck. Part of this prominence is due to a reorientation of the clavicles. Normally, these bones run slightly upwards and backwards from their medial ends. In facioscapulo-humeral dystrophy, there is a droop to the shoulders which causes the clavicles to run horizontally or to slope downwards. When the patient attempts to abduct the arms, the scapulae, having lost their fixation, ride upwards over the back and the upper borders may be seen rising up into the normal location of the trapezius muscle. Viewed from the side or the back, the scapulae are only loosely apposed to the thorax. The inferior medial angle is the most prominent and juts backwards on attempted movement. Although the term facioscapulohumeral dystrophy would imply that all the muscles of the shoulder and upper arm are atrophic, the deltoid is surprisingly well preserved in many cases. This may be overlooked, however, because poor

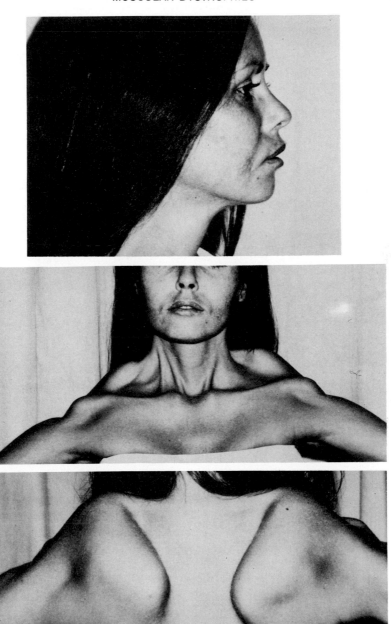

Figures 5.12–5.14. Facioscapulohumeral dystrophy. From the lateral view, the lips have a slight pout (Figure 5.12, *top*). When seen full face, there is a dimple lateral to the angles of the mouth. The identical appearance of this patients shoulders to those shown in Figure 5.9 should be noted. The posterior view shows the scapulae riding over the lateral part of the thorax (Figure 5.14, *bottom*).

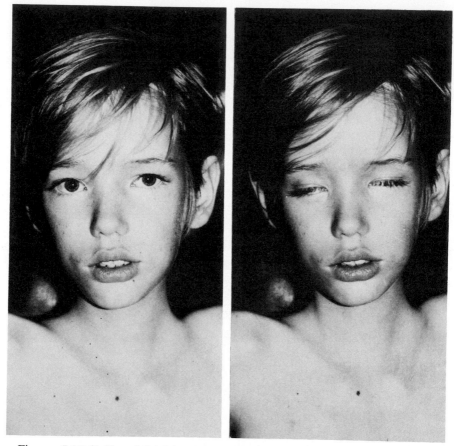

Figures 5.15 (*left*) and 5.16 (*right*). Infantile facioscapulohumeral dystrophy. This boy has had marked weakness of the face since birth. When he attempts to close his eyes tightly and to bare his teeth (Figure 5.16), the sclera are still showing and he could not move his mouth at all.

scapular fixation prevents the deltoid from exerting its maximal effect. Therefore, in testing the muscle it is well to have the patient lying down with the examiner's hand pressing the thorax backwards into the couch in order to prevent the scapula from moving. When the deltoid is examined in this fashion, it is often of normal strength or only slightly weak. Both the triceps and biceps are involved early and may waste rapidly. The slender stick-like upper arm is contrasted with the relative bulk of the forearm and a descriptive term for this type of abnormality is the "Popeye" arm. A remarkable discrepancy is seen in the strength of the forearm muscles. In severe cases, particularly the infantile or juvenile variety of facioscapulohumeral dystrophy, there is a marked weakness of the wrist extensors, producing a wrist drop. The wrist flexors, on the other hand, may maintain normal strength even when most of the other muscles of the body, including those of the hips and lower legs, are atrophic. The inability to extend the wrist results in another characteristic posture adopted by patients with this illness, the so-called "praying mantis" position. When asked to extend the arms, the patient holds the arms forward,

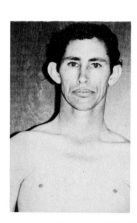 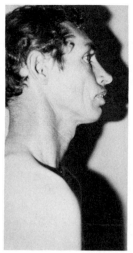 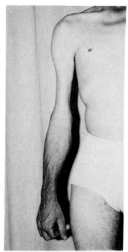 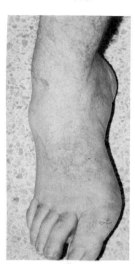

Figures 5.17–5.20. Facioscapulohumeral dystrophy. The facial weakness often gives the lips a flattened rectangular appearance when viewed full face (Figure 5.17, *left*). The lateral view, once again shows the pouting appearance of the mouth (Figure 5.18, *left center*). Preservation of the deltoid muscle with marked atrophy of the biceps and triceps is seen in Figure 5.19 (*right, center*). The muscles of the forearm are not atrophic and this is given rise to the appellation "Popeye" arm which is well illustrated in this patient. In spite of the fact that this man has a marked foot drop, the extensor digitorum brevis is hypertrophic as shown in this photograph where it appears as a mound on the lateral surface of the foot (Figure 5.10, *right*).

flexed at the elbows and wrists with the shoulder blades jutting backwards. The pattern of shoulder and arm weakness in facioscapulohumeral dystrophy is different from that of limb girdle dystrophy. The selective weakness of the biceps and the involvement of the deltoid in limb girdle dystrophy are helpful in making the differentiation.

Weakness of the hips may be found quite early in facioscapulohumeral dystrophy, although it may remain unnoticed by the patient until after he has noticed the weakness of the face and shoulders. There is often a compensatory lordosis, and this differs from other illnesses. Dorsal kyphosis is unusual, and associated scoliosis is also less common. The thoracic spine may remain as straight as a ramrod, but the lordosis which is seen in the lumbar region is much more marked than usual. In extreme cases, the sacrum forms a platform which runs almost horizontally, exaggerating the small of the back into a deep pit. The precarious gait of patients with this form of abnormality is remarkable. In the lower legs the same difference is seen between the plantar flexors and dorsiflexors of the ankle as is noted in the arms. The calf muscles are usually much stronger than the anterior tibial and peroneal group. The extensor digitorum brevis, on the other hand, is often hypertrophied and usually maintains its normal strength. Deep tendon reflexes are decreased early in the disease, more so at the elbows and at the knees than distally.

As was mentioned previously, the preceding refers to the typical and classical disease which is described in most of the textbooks. The evolution takes place over many decades, and most patients lead a productive and relatively full life, adapting themselves slowly to their illness. There are, however, two other clinical pictures, which are in my own experience equally common. They have largely been neglected in the more standard texts.

Infantile Facioscapulohumeral Dystrophy

The first and most characteristic is the infantile variety of facioscapulohumeral dystrophy.[2] This is by no means a benign disease and it is noticed within the first two years of life. Curiously, it is seldom noted by the parents in their own children, but the babysitter or another friend comments that the child never smiles, or that the eyes are kept open during sleep. This picture is associated with severe weakness. Not only may there be total paralysis of the face, including the muscles involved in eye closure (Figures 5.15 and 5.16), but severe and crippling weakness of the other muscle groups is seen early. Many of these children are using wheelchairs by the time they are nine or ten years of age. Even their facial weakness produces serious handicap. They are completely unable to smile and are often ostracized at school because of their total lack of emotional response. Many children develop an audible laugh instead of a smile in order to signify amusement. This produces even more difficulty with acquaintances whose casual pleasantries are greeted with a harsh chuckle from a mirthless and impassive face. The patient may make constant sucking noises and use the tongue to try and control the drooling of saliva. Such children are frequently far more depressed than those with other disabling childhood diseases, such as Duchenne's dystrophy.

The inheritance of this severe form of infantile muscular dystrophy is interesting. In all except one of the patients whom we have seen so far with this illness, there are no overt cases of facioscapulohumeral dystrophy in the parents.[3] However, one parent always has mild facial weakness. This may be either the father or mother of the patient, and usually on examination they have the full pouting mouth characteristic of facioscapulohumeral dystrophy. On occasion, such parents have been noted to sleep with their eyes open and have had difficulty with whistling or drinking through a straw, but again this is often not regarded as an abnormality. It is well known that the degree of severity of facioscapulohumeral dystrophy is more variable than that of almost any other illness. In the same family, severe and mild cases may be seen in both the same and different generations. However, the invariable occurrence of the mild, subclinical variety in a parent of a child with the severe infantile type requires more explanation and raises the possibility of a modifying gene, perhaps in the other parent.

Facioscapulohumeral Dystrophy with Late Exacerbation

The third variety of facioscapulohumeral dystrophy is more difficult to document. What follows is tentative, and post mortem confirmation is lacking. There are some patients who have a lifelong mild weakness of the face, perhaps with an inability to blow up balloons or difficulty with whistling. At some stage in their life, they may undergo a sudden and rapid deterioration, such that within a matter of two to three years they have difficulty walking, and even require the use of a wheelchair. Both the hip and shoulder muscles are involved. Although this sudden deterioration may occur at any time, it is more common in middle life. Obviously, the differential diagnosis includes any of the inflammatory myopathics as well as some of the rapid, progressive varieties of limb girdle dystrophy. The lifelong facial weakness which precedes this worsening, however, suggests that it may be a variety of facioscapulohumeral dystrophy. The picture is complicated by the fact that many such patients have inflammatory changes within their muscles. When treated with steroids they do not show the typical response of patients with polymyositis and the muscle biopsy, although it may reveal an inflammatory response, is different.

Laboratory Studies

Laboratory studies in the investigation of facioscapulohumeral dystrophy usually do no more than confirm the diagnosis. The clinical picture is typical enough and although the serum enzymes are often elevated, the EMG "myopathic," and the muscle biopsy substantiates the diagnosis, this adds little (other than reassuring the physician) to the management of the patient. However, it is advisable to biopsy all patients with facioscapulohumeral dystrophy, particularly those with a rapidly progressive form or the infantile type. A number of these patients show quite marked inflammatory responses in the biopsy[4, 5] and, when present, a therapeutic trial on steroids is worthwhile. I have never seen any objective improvement from such treatment, but some patients have a symptomatic improvement and claim to be able to walk with more facility, to arise from the floor more easily, and generally feel improved. It is possible that this is a placebo effect, although it is not an effect that we have noted with a placebo, when this has been substituted for the steroids.

Treatment

Treatment of facioscapulohumeral dystrophy follows the usual and general lines for the treatment of neuromuscular diseases. In addition, the possibility of surgical fixation of the scapula should be considered. If patients are unable to raise their arms above the horizontal level because of the loss of scapular fixation, they may derive some improvement by surgical attachment of the scapula to the posterior thoracic wall. Unfortunately, such operation is not without complications, and one of the more troublesome is that the scapula may break loose again shortly after the procedure. In some cases, the operation can give considerable benefit. We usually recommend surgery on one side only. If it is successful, operation can be considered for the opposite side at some later date. Additionally, useful function of the hand may be restored by providing wrist support when the wrist drop is marked. If a foot drop is noticed, ankle supports, either of the shell type or with a wire spring brace, should be tried. A review of some of the pertinent clinical literature was published by Kazakov and others.[6]

BIBLIOGRAPHY

1. Morton, N. E. and Chung, C. S. Formal genetics of muscular dystrophy. Am. J. Hum. Genet. *11:* 360, 1960.
2. Hanson, P. A. and Rowland, L. P. Moebius syndrome and facioscapulohumeral muscular dystrophy. Arch. Neurol. *24:* 31–39, 1971.

3. Carroll, J. L. and Brooke, M. H. "Infantile facioscapulohumeral dystrophy" in Proceedings of the IV International Conference on Neuromuscular Disease, Marseille. ed. J. Serratrice. In Press.
4. Munsat, T. L., Piper, D., Cancilla, P., and Mednick, J. Inflammatory myopathy with facioscapulohumeral distribution. Neurology *22:* 335–347, 1972.
5. Dubowitz, V., and Brooke, M. H. *Muscle Biopsy: A Modern Approach.* Saunders, London, 1973.
6. Kazakov, V. M., Bogorodinsky, D. K., Znoyko, Z. V., and Skorometz, A. A. The facio-scapulo-limb (or the facioscapulohumeral) type of muscular dystrophy. Eur. Neurol. *11:* 236–260, 1974.

SCAPULOPERONEAL DYSTROPHY

Scapuloperoneal dystrophy is probably a variety of facioscapulohumeral dystrophy. In any one case it may be quite difficult to decide which of the two diagnoses is appropriate. In the scapuloperoneal syndrome, the muscles which are involved early are those of the peroneal and anterior tibial group. Foot drop is among the initial complaints. This is followed shortly by shoulder weakness, which is typically of the type associated with facioscapulohumeral dystrophy (Figures 5.21 and 5.22). In approximately one-half of the patients there is also associated facial weakness and in this instance the differential diagnosis may not only be difficult but irrelevant. The disease is often inherited as an autosomal dominant, but an X-linked recessive pattern has also been described.[1, 2]

The importance in the consideration of this diagnosis lies in the fact that other illnesses may mimic scapuloperoneal dystrophy. Perhaps it would be more appropriate to use the term scapuloperoneal syndrome until a definitive diagnosis is made. Nemaline myopathy may present in the adult in this fashion, and perhaps denervating diseases may also cause such a syndrome. It can be quite difficult to distinguish patients whose weakness is limited to the peroneal and anterior tibial muscles from those with hereditary motor neuropathy. Inspection of the extensor digitorum brevis over the dorsum of the foot may be helpful. The muscle is usually atrophic in chronic peripheral neuropathy but is often hypertrophic in the scapuloperoneal syndrome. This is due to the fact that the patient uses the muscle in a futile attempt to dorsiflex the foot. The toes are then drawn upwards, an action which can be seen when the patient walks.

Treatment of the illness is again symptomatic, and ankle supports may be of great help.

BIBLIOGRAPHY

1. Thomas, P. K., Schott, G. D., and Morgan-Hughes, J. A. Adult onset scapuloperoneal myopathy. J. Neurol. Neurosurg. Psychiatry *38:* 1008–1015, 1975.
2. Thomas, P. K., Calne, D. B., and Elliott, C. F. X-linked scapuloperoneal syndrome. J. Neurol. Neurosurg. Psychiatry *35:* 208–215, 1972.

HEREDITARY DISTAL MYOPATHY

Of the varieties of muscular dystrophy which affect the distal muscles early, only myotonic dystrophy comes readily to mind. Most of the other forms of neuromuscular disease with predominantly distal involvement are due to denervation. An exception is an illness which was first clearly described by Welander.[1] This disease has also been associated with Gowers' name, al-

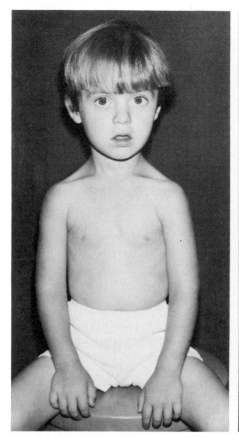 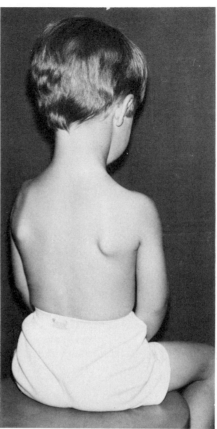

Figures 5.21 (*left*) and 5.22 (*right*). Scapuloperoneal dystrophy. The typical patient with scapuloperoneal dystrophy closely resembles the patient with facioscapulohumeral dystrophy in the appearance of the shoulders. This boy has an abnormal shoulder configuration even though he has little detectable weakness. The clavicles slope downward, the arms are internally rotated with skin creases running upward from the axillae (Figure 5.21). The inferomedial angles of the scapulae are prominent (Figure 5.22). His father had classical scapuloperoneal dystrophy.

though his patients may well have had myotonic dystrophy. Though common in Sweden, it is rarely seen in the rest of the world. Inheritance is as an autosomal dominant with an onset usually between 40 and 60 years of age, when the hand becomes clumsy and fine movements difficult. In a much smaller proportion of patients, the feet are initially involved and a foot drop is noted. Weakness and wasting of the small muscles of the hands and feet, of the extensor muscles of the wrist, and of the foot dorsiflexors may be present. The disease is not only slowly progressive but, in Welander's series, is almost completely limited to these muscles, with less than 10% showing weakness of proximal muscles, wrist flexors, or foot plantar flexors. Although the illness produces some handicap, the typical case does not progress to total incapacity. Among those few whose illness begins with weakness of the feet, either alone or associated with hand weakness, there is more likelihood that the disease will be progressive and that proximal as well as distal muscles will be

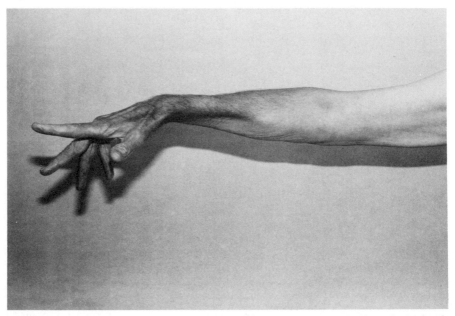

Figure 5.23. The patient is being asked to extend the fingers and wrist as completely as he can. The finger extensors are variably affected and the fingers adopt different postures. The distal wasting of the muscles is also apparent. (Distal myopathy.

involved in this progression. Welander also suggested that there is a homozygous form which commences earlier in life, results in widespread muscle weakness, and has a more rapid course.[2] Reports of the same or a similar entity have appeared from other parts of the world. In general, such reports have stressed that the disease may appear at an earlier age and may produce more generalized weakness even though the distal weakness and late onset pattern remains the more typical presentation.

Examination of the patient shows wasting of the small muscles of the hand, particularly of the thenar eminence. The patient cannot extend the fingers fully, and an attempt to do this produces a posture in which the fingers are held in dissimilar positions (Figure 5.23). There may be a wrist drop, and the wasting of the wrist extensors produces an oblique groove across the posterior surface of the forearm. Wasting of the intrinsic muscles of the feet and of the anterior tibial and peroneal muscles is less common, as mentioned. The deep tendon reflexes are often preserved early in the disease, diminishing particularly at the ankles and wrists as the disease progresses. There is usually no sensory abnormality and, if such is found, the possibility of peripheral neuropathy should be entertained.

Laboratory studies which may be of value include muscle biopsy,[3, 4] which shows changes suggestive of a myopathy with vacuolar changes, and EMG, which demonstrates "myopathic" potentials. Motor end point biopsies fail to show any significant abnormality of the distal innervation.[5] Serum creatine phosphokinase levels may be normal or slightly elevated. Post mortem studies are rare, but those described by Markesbery et al.[3] show involvement of the cardiac musculature as well as the skeletal musculature. Symptoms of cardiomyopathy are rarely described in the reports. The treatment for this illness is again supportive with recommendation for the appropriate bracing.

BIBLIOGRAPHY

1. Welander, L. Myopathia distalis tarda hereditaria. Acta Med. Scand. Suppl. *265:* 1–124, 1951.
2. Welander, L. Homozygous appearance of distal myopathy. Acta Genet. *7:* 321–324, 1957.
3. Markesbery, W. R., Griggs, R. C., Leach, R. P., and Lapham, L. W. Late onset, hereditary distal myopathy. Neurology *24:* 127–134, 1974.
4. Edstrom, L. Histochemical and histopathological changes in skeletal muscle in late onset hereditary distal myopathy (Welander). J. Neurol. Sci. *26:* 147–157, 1975.
5. Sumner, D., Crawfurd, M. d'A., and Harriman, D. G. F. Distal muscular dystrophy in an English family. Brain *94:* 51–60, 1971.

LIMB GIRDLE DYSTROPHY

It is difficult to write of limb girdle dystrophy with much conviction or enthusiasm since the term probably denotes a collection of illnesses with various etiologies. Only the common occurrence of a progressive weakness of the hips and shoulders has resulted in their being considered as a single entity. While it is true that the muscle biopsies from such patients are rather similar, this is at best a tenuous connecting thread. In other respects the patients' illnesses differ widely. There is variety in the mode of inheritance, the age of onset, and the progression of the illness, as well as in the distribution of weakness, which seems to underline the need for reappraisal.

Many cases are sporadic, but an autosomal recessive pattern of inheritance is not unusual. When the disease occurs in a family, the various members of the family seem to have the same type of illness, and even the sporadic cases of the disease may conform to one of several general patterns. Perhaps the commonest of these has its onset during the second or third decade. The illness begins with weakness of the hips, and the symptoms are in no way different from other illnesses causing hip weakness. At about the same time, or shortly thereafter, the patient notices shoulder weakness and the illness progresses so that within twenty years after the onset walking will be difficult, if not impossible. Although the patient is confined to a wheelchair, the skeletal deformities so common in some of the other forms of neuromuscular disease are not frequent. Death may occur from cardiopulmonary complications and terminal pneumonia.

In another version of the disease, the weakness is not noted until the fourth decade or even later, but this late onset does not always mean a good prognosis. In some patients there is a rapid progression of the weakness with an inability to walk within three years of the onset of the disease. The majority of such patients exhibit an autosomal recessive inheritance of the disease. In yet other patients, the disease seems to be predominantly of the hips and thighs or of the shoulders and arms, leading to the term pelvifemoral dystrophy for the one and scapulohumeral dystrophy for the other. These varieties are usually associated with a better prognosis. As in some other neuromuscular diseases, the illness is named for the muscle groups in which the weakness commences. This does not imply that the muscles outside of these groups are uninvolved, and in the terminal stages of the illness the muscles of the lower legs, forearms, and hands are weak, too.

Rarely, families with an autosomal dominant pattern of inheritance have been found and, equally unusually, limb girdle dystrophy may present in the first decade. Occasionally mild weakness of the face is seen; if facial weakness is severe, consideration should be given to the diagnosis of facioscapulohumeral dystrophy. Involvement of the tongue or pharynx is not part of the illness. Sensory symptoms are absent, and other muscular symptoms such as myoglobinuria or muscle pain are also lacking. (Many patients with limb girdle dystrophy suffer from severe and intractable low back pain.) Unless there are associated signs of nerve compression, surgical intervention is usually inadvisable and may indeed exacerbate the pain. The weakness of the lumbar muscles which predisposes to the development of low back pain is not reversed by operation and the instability of the lumbar spine may well be worsened by any surgical maneuver.

Examination of the patient shows the usual abnormalities of gait associated with either hip or shoulder weakness. There may be weakness of the neck muscles, both flexors and extensors. The set of the shoulders may be abnormal. The tips are depressed, giving a webbed appearance to the neck, and the clavicles slope downwards. There is often a crease running from the axilla diagonally toward the neck. This is produced by the shoulders folding forward as scapular fixation is lost; the crease is accentuated by the atrophy of the underlying pectoral muscles. The pattern of weakness is different from that seen in facioscapulohumeral dystrophy (q.v.) since in the latter the strength of the deltoid muscle may be relatively preserved. Similarly, winging of the scapula may be seen, but the tendency of the scapula to ride up over the back and appear as a prominence in the trapezius when viewed from in front is not marked in limb girdle dystrophy. Preferential weakness and atrophy of the biceps is a useful diagnostic sign (Figure 5.24). Although not pathognomonic of limb girdle dystrophy, it is noted frequently in even mild cases. The degree of wasting may be so pronounced that a concavity appears in the upper arm where the biceps should normally be.

The pattern of weakness in the hips is not so characteristic. Both hip flexors and extensors as well as the paravertebral muscles are involved, and the quadriceps and hamstrings share this involvement. Deep tendon reflexes are usually depressed at the elbows and knees early in the illness. Intellectual difficulty is not present and other complications, such as cardiac conduction defects, are rare.

The differential diagnosis includes any of the causes of proximal weakness and it is axiomatic that if the diagnosis of limb girdle dystrophy can be made juvenile spinal muscular atrophy should also be considered. The selective absence of the biceps may be helpful in making the diagnosis of limb girdle dystrophy, whereas the occurrence of more than an occasional fasciculation would suggest spinal muscular atrophy.   .

Laboratory studies that may be helpful include the usual abnormalities of serum creatine phosphokinase and lactic dehydrogenase. The elevation of these enzymes is seldom spectacular, but it may occasionally be increased by a factor of 10. Electromyography reveals the presence of small, short polyphasic potentials. There may be bizarre high frequency discharges, but in general the pattern is a "myopathic" one. Muscle biopsy shows considerable

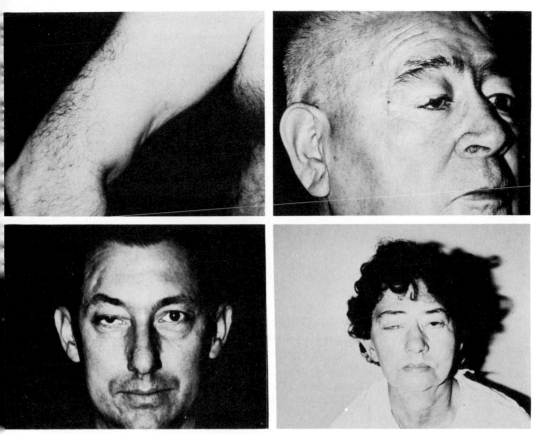

Figure 5.24 (*top left*). Severe wasting of the biceps is not infrequently seen in limb girdle dystrophy. Instead of the normal muscle belly a concavity is noted.

Figures 5.25–5.27. These patients (*top right* and *bottom*) with ocular pharyngeal dystrophy have paralysis of extraocular movement and ptosis. Although the ptosis is bilateral, it is very often asymmetrical as shown here.

variation in the size of fibers, coupled with numerous internal nuclei and fiber splitting. Moth eaten, whorled fibers are usually profuse.

There are probably many conditions causing a proximal myopathy and as more sophisticated methods of evaluation become possible it is likely that we will discover more and more conditions of known etiology which we can split off from the heterogeneous collection called limb girdle dystrophy. A measure of my open hostility to this whole entity can be deduced from the lack of bibliographic references for this particular section.

OCULAR MYOPATHIES

There are three types of neuromuscular disease in which the eye muscles are involved and which share many features in common. These are ocular dystrophy, oculopharyngeal dystrophy, and oculocraniosomatic neuromuscular disease with ragged red fibers. As to the first of these, I have not knowingly seen a case and I shall only parrot what has appeared in the literature. My experience with the second entity involves a number of patients, but since they are probably all derived from a common genetic background in a Spanish-American population in the United States, it may not be readily applicable to other areas. The third entity seems to be the subject of great controversy. It is not that the clinical picture remains unclear, but uncertainty remains as to the name by which the disease should be known. A further description of this last illness is given in the section on metabolic diseases, where it belongs by virtue of the striking abnormalities seen in the mitochondria. Clinically, though, it is often considered in the differential diagnosis of the two preceding illnesses. Although they are called "myopathies," in some instances the proof remains a little shaky. Since the changes of myopathy and denervation are even harder to distinguish in the extraocular muscles than elsewhere, most of the evidence that the ocular diseases are indeed "myopathic" is based on a few post mortem studies showing normal brain stem neurons. In view of these circumstances, this section is undertaken with temerity since it is guaranteed to please no one and irritate many.

Ocular Dystrophy

The existence of a form of dystrophy causing ptosis and weakness of the extraocular muscles has been recognized for many years. Although there are several previous reports, the paper of Kiloh and Nevin was the first of the modern papers delineating this entity.[1] The ptosis usually precedes the weakness of the eye muscles and, although it may occur at any age, the onset is much more common in the first 20 to 30 years of life.[2] The symptoms are caused by drooping of the eyelids which interferes with vision. It is rare for diplopia to be a complaint. The disease is slowly progressive over many years and, although it may be limited to the eye muscles in some stage of the disease, there is always evidence of involvement of other muscle groups later on. Facial weakness is probably most common; a number of patients also have weakness in the limbs. Even those without overt weakness may have areflexia or an abnormal muscle biopsy. An unusual aspect of ocular myopathy is the curare sensitivity reported by Ross[3] and by Matthew, et al.[4] Some patients with ocular myopathy have developed profound ptosis, extraocular palsies, and weakness of the neck and limbs with small doses of curare. This raises a difficult diagnostic problem. Patients with myasthenia who have extraocular weakness also have an extreme sensitivity to curare. If weakness of the eye muscle is the only major expression of the myasthenia, the diagnosis may be quite difficult to prove since the extraocular palsies may not respond to the administration of edrophonium or neostigmine. Ross[3] felt that the entity, ocular myopathy, was nevertheless a real one. It differed from myasthenia since there was a long and slowly progressive history of eye findings which did not wax and wane and which was succeeded by an equally unvarying weakness of the limbs without any of the bulbar signs of myasthenia. Whatever the solution to this diagnostic dilemma, if surgery is to be considered in patients with ocular myopathy, the possibility of abnormal sensitivity to curare should be emphasized.

The disease is often inherited as an autosomal dominant. Occasional sporadic cases and cases with autosomal recessive inheritance have also been described. On examination, the weakness is commonly severe enough to produce a total paralysis of the eye muscles. The marked ptosis causes the patient to retroflex the head. The pupillary responses are normal. Treatment is symptomatic and is aimed at the relief of the ptosis. This may involve surgery or the use of eyelid crutches.

A significant number of the patients who have been diagnosed as having ocular myopathy may complain of dysphagia thus the entity merges with the following one, oculopharyngeal dystrophy. The only case I have seen which could have been classified clinically as a relatively pure ocular myopathy (ptosis, extraocular palsies, and mild facial weakness beginning in the 20's) was in fact a member of a large family with many members suffering from classical oculopharyngeal dystrophy.

Oculopharyngeal Dystrophy

An illness which is perhaps similar but which causes more wide spread abnormalities is oculopharyngeal dystrophy.[5] This illness, which is usually inherited as an autosomal dominant, is rare in most parts of the world but occurs in circumscribed geographical areas. It is quite common in French Canadian families in Quebec, and the disease has been traced to a common ancestor who landed in Quebec from France in 1634.[2, 6] A similar large focus is found among Spanish American families in southern Colorado, northern New Mexico, and Arizona.

The illness begins later than the pure ocular dystrophy, with its onset in the third or fourth decade. The weakness is frequently asymmetrical: a marked ptosis may develop on one side while the other eyelid is only minimally involved (Figures 5.25–5.27). Eventually, however, both lids are extremely ptotic, and all extraocular movement is lost, although pupillary responses remain normal. Usually the dysphagia follows the weakness of the eye muscles although in the French Canadian families difficulty with swallowing occurs at the same time as, or even precedes, weakness of the eyes. Most of the patients have some degree of facial weakness and, as the disease slowly worsens, weakness of the hips and shoulders is common. In one report distal weakness of the limbs was associated with ocular myopathy and dysphagia.[7] With increasing age the dysphagia becomes incapacitating. Saliva pools in the pharynx and it may be impossible for the patient to swallow any solid foods; even liquid foods present some difficulty. In the face of this, there is considerable weight loss and the patient becomes emaciated. In one patient this emaciation did not respond to the administration of a daily diet of 3500 calories by a nasogastric tube over a period of four weeks. The patient still continued to lose weight even though caloric intake should have been sufficient to prevent this.

Examination of the patient will be abnormal, the extent of the abnormality depending upon the stage of the disease. Ptosis, extraocular palsies, and facial weakness are almost always apparent. Weakness and wasting of the masseter muscles may be seen. The tongue may be atrophic, and the pharynx moves poorly. Proximal weakness of the limbs with areflexia is not uncommon. Usually there is no problem in making the diagnosis in view of the strong family history seen in many of these patients. Myotonic dystrophy and myasthenia gravis can give rise to some confusion with this entity, but there are obvious significant differences between oculopharyngeal dystrophy and these two common diseases. Other neuromuscular diseases can present with ptosis and ophthalmoplegia; these vary from myotubular myopathy to oculocraniosomatic neuromuscular disease.

Laboratory studies may be of help. The electromyogram shows small amplitude, polyphasic potentials with short duration. There are none of the associated findings seen in denervation. The serum "muscle" enzymes may be elevated but are seldom more than three to four times normal and more usually are within normal limits. EKG abnormalities have been found and have varied from conduction deficits to changes suggesting old infarction. Since this population is older than the usual group of patients with neuromuscular disease, the findings should be cautiously interpreted. Microscopic abnormalities of the muscle have been described but are not pathognomonic of this illness. Investigation of esophageal motility shows abnormalities throughout the length of the esophagus with decreased peristalsis and incoordinate muscle contraction from the pharynx to the lower part of the esophagus. This implies that smooth muscle is involved as well as striated muscle.[2, 8] Post mortem studies have shown changes in the pharyngeal striated muscle compatible with a dystrophic process, but abnormalities of the smooth muscles could not be demonstrated.[8, 9]

BIBLIOGRAPHY

1. Kiloh, L. G., and Nevin, S. Progressive dystrophy of the external ocular muscles (ocular myopathy). Brain *74:* 115–143, 1951.
2. Bray, G. M., Kaarsoo, N., and Ross, T. Ocular myopathy with dysphagia. Neurology *15:* 678–684, 1965.
3. Ross, R. T. Ocular myopathy sensitive to curare. Brain *86:* 67–76, 1963.
4. Matthew, N. T., Jacob, J. C., and Chandy, J. Familial ocular myopathy with curare sensitivity. Arch. Neurol. *22:* 68–74, 1970.
5. Victor, M., Hayes, R., and Adams, R. D. Oculopharyngeal muscular dystrophy: A familial disease of late life characterized by dysphagia and progressive ptosis of the eyelids. New Engl. J. Med. *267:* 1267–1272, 1962.
6. Barbeau, A. The syndrome of hereditary late onset ptosis and dysphagia in French Canada. In: *Progressive Muskeldystrophie Myotonie Myasthenie,* edited by E. Kuhn. Springer, Berlin, 1966, pp. 102–109.
7. Schotland, D. L., and Rowland, L. P. Muscular dystrophy: Features of ocular myopathy, distal myopathy and myotonic dystrophy. Arch. Neurol. *10:* 433–445, 1964.
8. Roberts, A. H., and Bamforth, J. The pharynx and esophagus in ocular muscular dystrophy. Neurology *18:* 645–652, 1968.
9. Weitzner, S. The histopathology of the pharynx and esophagus in ocularpharyngeal muscular dystrophy: Case report and literature review. Am. J. Gastroenterol. *56:* 378–382, 1971.

6   myotonia

Myotonia is found in several illnesses. In some it plays a dominant part; in others it is overshadowed by other aspects of the disease. Myotonia is a phenomenon in which relaxation of the muscle after contraction is delayed. The period of gradual relaxation may be prolonged over several seconds. Contraction of a myotonic muscle may be produced by mechanical stimulation (e.g. percussion) as well as voluntarily. Electromyography shows repetitive action potentials of the muscle fibers associated with the phase of contraction and relaxation. These trains of potentials may wax and wane in both amplitude and frequency. The phenomenon seems to arise at the sarcolemmal membrane since curare, although obviously preventing the development of myotonia following voluntary activity, does nothing to diminish the myotonia generated by percussion. In addition to human disease, myotonia has also been noted in goats, mice, and horses. Experimentally, myotonia has been produced by the administration of 20, 25-diazacholesterol, by monocarboxylic aromatic acids, such as the insecticide 2,4-D, and by other compounds. In all varieties, there seems to be a rather generalized abnormality of membranes, those of the muscle and red blood cells being the most extensively investigated. Some forms of myotonia have been associated with a decreased chloride conductance through the cell membrane.[1, 2] It has been suggested that in normal muscle following an action potential there is a significant accumulation of potassium in the transverse tubules and the high chloride permeability ordinarily counteracts the depolarization so produced.[3] Decreasing the extracellular chloride concentration experimentally may produce repetitive electrical activity in muscle fibers, and analysis of a mathematical model of the membrane has indicated that this could be a sufficient cause for myotonia.[4]

The exact cause of the decreased permeability to chloride is not known, but it is to be expected that the membrane is at fault. Abnormalities of the fatty acid composition of muscle membrane phospholipids as well as of cholesterol esters have been described.[5] The membranes of both muscle and red blood cells exhibit a decreased ability to phosphorylate protein.[6, 7] An increase in membrane paranitrophenylphosphatase activity of rat microsomes has been found in experimental myotonia.[8] Increase in the activity of sodium potassium ATPase, another enzyme associated with the membrane, has also been found.[9] Detailed discussion of these findings is outside the scope of this book, and more information may be obtained by consulting the reviews quoted above.

The illnesses in which myotonia occurs as a minor component (such as acid maltase deficiency, for example) will be discussed in later sections. The three illnesses which are outlined in this section are myotonic dystrophy, myotonia congenita, and paramyotonia.

BIBLIOGRAPHY

1. Bryant, S. H. Cable properties of external intercostal muscle fibers from myotonic and non-myotonic goats. J. Physiol. *204:* 539–550, 1969.
2. Lipicky, R. J., Bryant, S. H., and Salmon, J. H. Cable parameters: Sodium, potassium, chloride and water content and potassium efflux in isolated external intercostal muscle of the normal volunteers and patients with myotonia congenita. J. Clin. Invest. *50:* 2091–2103, 1971.
3. Adrian, R. H., and Bryant, S. H. On the repetitive discharge in myotonic muscle fibers. J. Physiol. *240:* 505–515, 1974.
4. Barchi, R. L. Myotonia: An evaluation of the chloride hypothesis. Arch. Neurol. *32:* 175–180, 1975.
5. Kuhn, E. Myotonia: A lecture. In: *Clinical Studies in Myology*, edited by B. A. Kakulas. Excerpta Medica, Amsterdam, 1973, pp. 471–480.
6. Roses, A. D., Herbstreith, M. H., and Appel, S. H. Membrane protein kinase alteration in Duchenne muscular dystrophy. Nature *254:* 350–351, 1975.
7. Roses, A. D., and Appel, S. H. Muscle membrane protein kinase in myotonic muscular dystrophy. Nature *250:* 245–247, 1974.
8. Brody, I. A. Myotonia induced by monocarboxylic aromatic acids. Arch. Neurol. *28:* 243–246, 1973.
9. Peter, J. B., Fiehn, W., Nagatomo, T., Andiman, R., Stempel, K., and Bowman, R. Studies of sarcolemma from normal and diseased skeletal muscle. In: *Exploratory Concepts of Muscular Dystrophy, II*, edited by A. T. Milhorat. Excerpta Medica, Amsterdam, 1974, pp. 479–490.

MYOTONIC DYSTROPHY

Clinical Aspects

The adult with advanced myotonic dystrophy has an appearance so characteristic that it is hard to mistake it for any of the other neuromuscular illnesses (Figures 6.1–6.7, 6.11). The face is drawn and lugubrious, with hollowing of the muscles around the temples and jaws. The eyes are hooded, the lower lip droops, and the facial weakness imparts a curious sag to the lower part of the face. The wasting of the neck muscles, particularly the neck flexors, gives a slender appearance, and the patient balances his head precariously rather like trying to balance a cherry on top of its stalk. Descriptive terms such as "hatchet-faced" and "swan-necked" have been given to the myotonic patient. It is perhaps the very typical appearance of the fully developed disease which has caused so many of us to miss the diagnosis in its milder forms. Such diagnostic errors are aided and abetted by the patients themselves, who exhibit an unusual degree of denial towards their illness and towards the existence of the same illness in their families. Indeed, I would suspect that almost half of the patients with myotonic dystrophy present with complaints which have nothing to do with their neuromuscular disease. Neither is it unusual to hear a patient with myotonic dystrophy insist that his disease began only two to three years ago when the hospital charts document the presence of the illness for decades.

Myotonic dystrophy is inherited as an autosomal dominant condition with a prevalence estimated at between 3 and 5 per 100,000. This makes it one of the commoner neuromuscular disorders. Some have suggested genetic heterogeneity of the illness, with one type occurring early and another later in life,[1]

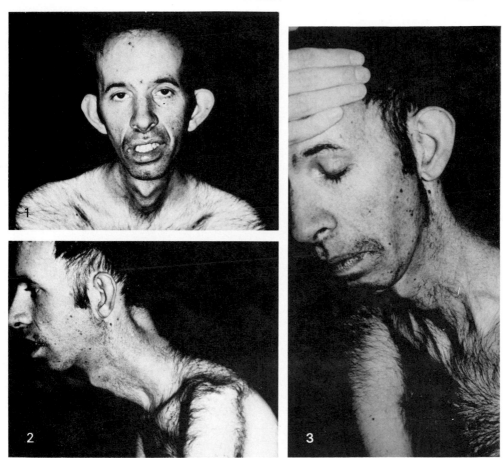

Figures 6.1–6.3. Myotonic dystrophy. The long, thin face with temporal and masseter wasting and frontal balding is characteristic (Figure 6.1). Weakness and wasting of the sternocleidomastoids and other muscles in the neck gives a "swan neck" appearance (Figure 6.2). When the patient attempts to flex his neck against the examiner's hand, atrophy of the sternocleidomastoid is seen (Figure 6.3).

but most of the evidence does not support such a view. Typically, the symptoms of the disease are not noticed until adolescence or early adult life. However, examination of the patient even in the first decade may reveal the presence of myotonia and the characteristic long-faced child with a slightly nasal voice. Although myotonia is noted quite early, it is seldom presented as a complaint by the patient. They may be troubled by some muscle stiffness, cramping pains, or, on occasion, difficulty with relaxing the grasp, but more commonly it is the onset of weakness of the feet and hands which the patient first notices. The weakness increases slowly but steadily and eventually spreads to involve all the muscle groups. Weakness of the flexor muscles of the neck is an early finding, and atrophy of the sternocleidomastoid muscles, which may disappear totally or be present as a thin band, has often been used as a diagnostic clue.

The presence of myotonia upon direct percussion of the muscle is a striking

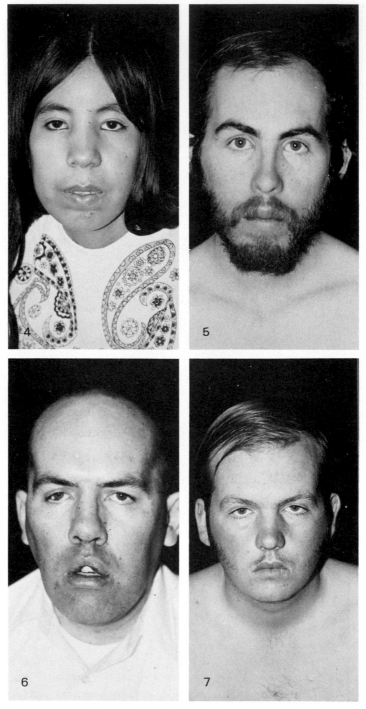

Figures 6.4–6.7. Myotonic dystrophy. Various features are to be noted including the elongated face (Figures 6.4–6.6), the temporal and masseter wasting (Figures 6.5 and 6.6), and the ptosis (Figures 6.4, 6.6, and 6.7). Also notice the shape of the patient's mouth in Figure 6.6 and compare it with Figure 6.8.

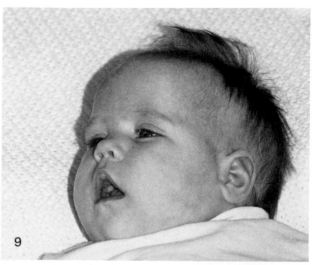

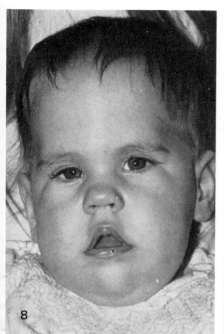

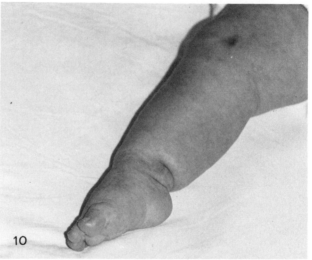

Figures 6.8–6.10. Infantile myotonic dystrophy may present as a facial diplegia with hypotonia at birth. This is associated with an abnormality of the appearance of the mouth in which the upper lid forms an inverted V (Figures 6.8 and 6.9). Skeletal abnormalities such as a club foot (Figure 6.10) are also seen.

finding in more ways than one. In evaluating myotonia, two aspects should be borne in mind. The first is the tendency for the myotonia to disappear as the weakness progresses. Thus, in patients with severe wasting and weakness of the hands it is preferable to search for myotonia in muscles of the forearm or shoulders. Secondly, myotonia should never be confused with the normal contraction response which may be produced by percussion of a muscle. This normal response is usually a brief flickering movement of the muscle but may be pronounced enough to cause the joint to move. The delay in relaxation so characteristic of the myotonic is not seen. Myotonia may be accentuated by cold, but this is less a feature of myotonic dystrophy than in some other forms of myotonia.

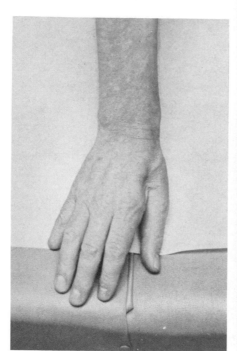
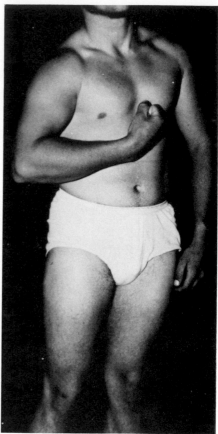

Figure 6.11 (*left*). Myotonic dystrophy often causes wasting of distal musculature, in this case of the small muscles of the hands.

Figure 6.12 (*right*). Myotonia congenita is often, although not always, associated with a well developed musculature.

With the passage of time, the voice becomes increasingly dysarthric and nasal and there may be difficulty in swallowing food. It is interesting that the earlier the illness begins, the more severe is the involvement of the bulbar musculature. With increasing handicap the patient is eventually confined to a wheelchair. Death often occurs during the fifth or sixth decade from cardiorespiratory failure.

In addition to the neuromuscular symptoms, involvement of other organs reflects the fact that myotonic dystrophy seems to be a diffuse disorder. Mild mental retardation is not uncommon and, as already mentioned, there is an odd form of denial in these patients. This is frequently reflected in a suspicious and hostile attitude toward the physician. For example, it is often more difficult to persuade the patient with myotonic dystrophy to accept the use of canes or supportive devices than a patient with other forms of neuromuscular disease. Cataracts are common in myotonic dystrophy. A careful search with the slit lamp will reveal them in almost all cases. The exact form of the cataract varies but, commonly, multi-hued specks are found in the anterior and posterior subscapular zones. Other forms of cataracts are also seen, and surgical extraction may be necessary at some stage. Endocrine abnormalities include disturbances of adrenal, pancreatic and gonadal function. Testicular atrophy is common, with disappearance of the seminiferous tubules. In the female, infertility, habitual abortion, and menstrual irregularities are noted. There may also be difficulty during labor, with a prolonged first stage and hemorrhage with poor uterine contraction during the third stage. It has been suggested that this is secondary to smooth muscle abnormalities in the uterus.[2] Abnormalities of the glucose tolerance test may be a reflection of the muscular atrophy or of obesity as much as of an abnormality of pancreatic function.[3]

Involvement of smooth muscle may be responsible in part for the difficulty with swallowing and perhaps has some association with the increased incidence of gallbladder problems. Although patients frequently complain of chronic constipation and urinary symptoms, these often seem to be rather nonspecific complaints and are less clearly associated with abnormalities of smooth muscle function. Cardiac muscle may also be abnormal, and cardiac conduction defects such as first degree heart block (PR interval greater than 0.2 second) and cardiac arrhythmias are seen in over half the patients.[4] Some patients with myotonic dystrophy may have recurrent dislocations of the jaw.

Terminally, the patient becomes lethargic, develops repeated respiratory infections, and probably suffers from pulmonary hypoventilation. Cyanosis may be pronounced, although there is often no clear evidence of congestive cardiac failure. Perhaps related to this is the increased risk which has been reported with general anesthesia. Patients with myotonic dystrophy may be unduly susceptible to barbiturates and to other medications such as morphine, which may depress the ventilatory drive.[5-8]

In infancy, myotonia presents a different clinical picture. When myotonic dystrophy manifests itself in the neonatal period, it may do so without any evidence of myotonia. Indeed, the only clinical findings may be extreme hypotonia and facial paralysis. These children have an oddly shaped mouth with the upper lip forming an inverted V, an appearance which has been called the shark mouth (Figures 6.8 and 6.9). Club feet are also common in the neonate (Figure 6.10). The pregnancy is often complicated by hydramnios and poor fetal movements. As these children grow older mental retardation is discovered as a prominent part of the picture, more so than in those whose disease commences later. In one series the mean I.Q. of children with neonatal myotonic dystrophy was 66.[9] Frequent respiratory infections are seen at an early age. Myotonia eventually makes its appearance, but may be delayed until the fifth year or later. One of the unusual aspects of this situation is that such children are almost always born to myotonic mothers, rather than inheriting the disease from the father. This has suggested that the severity of the illness may be due to some maternal intrauterine factor. Out of 70 patients with congenital myotonic dystrophy, paternal transmission was shown in only one case.[10] Once the diagnosis of congenital myotonic dystrophy is suspected it is relatively simple to confirm the diagnosis by examination of the child's mother.

The illness may show some "anticipation" when, with each succeeding generation, the illness appears earlier and is more severe. Part of this reflects the inaccuracy of the myotonic's memory. If an adolescent is seen to suffer from the disease, his parent may very often claim that his own illness has lasted but a short while. When this history is taken at face value, then anticipation surely is the rule. However, there is usually evidence for the parent's illness having lasted much longer than he believes, and in my own experience the phenomenon of anticipation has been most uncommon.

Laboratory Studies

The diagnosis of myotonic dystrophy is usually a clinical one and laboratory tests are seldom necessary in the fully advanced case. However, in the early stages when the weakness is still slight it may be comforting to obtain appropriate laboratory studies. Fortunately, in the situation where the patient's disease is mildest, the muscle biopsy is usually the most diagnostic with a combination of internal nuclei and Type 1 fiber atrophy.[11] This is also true in the neonatal disease. The biceps muscle is more prone to this change than other commonly biopsied muscles such as the gastrocnemius and the vastus lateralis.[12] Electromyography demonstrates the classical findings of myotonia, with waxing and waning of the amplitude and frequency. When this activity is heard over a loudspeaker, it has been likened to the sound of a dive-bomber. As World War II recedes, it is more appropriate to compare it to a motor bike being revved up. True myotonia should not be confused with pseudomyotonia or bizarre high frequency potentials in which the amplitude does not wane so markedly and the frequency is more regular, perhaps producing the sound of a motor boat. Associated with the electrical myotonia, small short polyphasic potentials are also found. Although this has often been put forward as evidence for the myogenic origin of myotonic dystrophy, evaluation of the motor units in the illness has suggested that the nerve is also abnormal. Careful measurement of the cutaneous branches of the common peroneal nerve did not reveal any significant morphologic abnormality.[13]

Serum "muscle" enzymes are often abnormal but are of little help in establishing the diagnosis. Abnormal catabolism of IgG and hypogammaglobulinemia are seen in many patients.[14] Bony abnormalities have been described with thickening of the cranial vault and a small pituitary fossa. These changes do not seem to be of any particular significance.

Other findings point to widespread abnormalities in the function and structure of cell membranes. The activity of protein kinase in red blood cells as well as in muscle is abnormally reduced. Using the technique of electron spin resonance spectroscopy, an increased fluidity in the membrane of erythrocytes has been shown.[15] This abnormality was partially corrected by phenytoin. The activity of the NaK pump in the erythrocyte membrane also seems to be abnormal.[16] The Na efflux rate seems to be less and suggests that the stoichiometric ratio indicates an exchange of 2 Na for 2 K, rather than the normal situation in which 3 Na are exchanged for 2K. Such an abnormality of the sodium potassium pump again points to a disorder of membrane function. Platelet aggregation has been found to be abnormally sensitive to adrenalin, perhaps also due to a decrease in phosphorylation of the platelet membrane.[17]

Another enzyme which characterizes the membrane, adenyl cyclase, was found to have reduced activity.[18] An abnormal fatty acid is present in the cholesterol esters of muscle from patients with myotonia dystrophica.[19]

Treatment

The treatment of myotonic dystrophy follows the general principles laid down for other illnesses. Mechanical devices such as ankle supports may be helpful to patients as they develop distal weakness. Breathing exercises and postural drainage should probably be carried out in the advanced stages of the illness. The sensitivity of patients to drugs such as sedatives and narcotics which depress the respiratory center should be borne in mind. Drugs such as quinine, quinidine, dilantin, procainamide, and Diamox have all been recommended for the treatment of patients with myotonic dystrophy. All these drugs are aimed at alleviating the myotonia. Therapy is not universally successful, because the patient with myotonic dystrophy is seldom aware of the myotonia and is more troubled by weakness. A therapeutic trial of one of the medications is worthwhile if the patient's stiffness is a significant part of his complaint. It is difficult to know which of the drugs to recommend for initial therapeutic trial. Procainamide and perhaps quinine prolong the PR interval of the electrocardiogram. Since this interval is abnormally prolonged in many patients with myotonic dystrophy, there are perhaps theoretical reasons for starting with dilantin, a drug which shortens the PR interval.[4] The other side effects of dilantin, however, can be troublesome to the patient, especially since myotonics are occasionally erratic in their dosage schedules. Dantrolene sodium has not been of any help to patients with myotonic dystrophy. As a rule, the patient derives greater benefit from an ankle support than from any of the pills.

Genetic counseling is an important although often unsuccessful part of the management. Since an autosomal dominant gene is involved, any myotonic parent must be warned that there is an even chance of any child developing the disease. Prenatal prediction of affected infants may be possible in certain circumstances. The genes for ABH blood group secretion (which determine whether these ABH substances are secreted into the body fluids, such as saliva) are closely linked to that for myotonic dystrophy. In some families in which the secretor genotype can be evaluated the determination of whether the fetus is a secretor or non-secretor can be used to predict the likelihood of its suffering from myotonic dystrophy.[20, 21]

BIBLIOGRAPHY

1. Bundey, S., and Carter, C. O. Genetic heterogeneity for dystrophia myotonica. J. Med. Genet. *9:* 311–315, 1972.
2. Shore, R. N., and Maclachlan, T. B. Pregnancy with myotonic dystrophy: Course complications and management. Obstet. Gynecol. *38:* 448–454, 1971.
3. Bird, M., and Tzagournis, M. Insulin secretion in myotonic dystrophy. Am. J. Med. Sci. *260:* 351–358, 1970.
4. Griggs, R. C., Davis, R. J., Anderson, D. C., and Dove, J. T. Cardiac conduction in myotonic dystrophy. Am. J. Med. *59:* 37–42, 1975.
5. Ravin, M., Newmark, Z., and Saviello, G. Myotonia dystrophica: An anesthetic hazard: Two case reports. Anesth. Analg. *54:* 216–218, 1975.
6. Dundee, J. W. Thiopentone in dystrophica myotonica. Anesth. Analg. *31:* 257–262, 1952.

7. Kaufman, L. Anesthesia in dystrophia myotonica. Proc. R. Soc. Med. *53:* 183–188, 1960.
8. Bourke, T. D., and Zuck, D. Thiopentone in dystrophia myotonica. Br. J. Anesth. *29:* 35–38, 1957.
9. Harper, P. S. Congenital myotonic dystrophy in Britain. I. Clinical aspects. Arch. Dis. Child. *50:* 505–513, 1975.
10. Harper, P. S. Congenital myotonic dystrophy in Britain. II. Genetic basis. Arch. Dis. Child. *50:* 514–521, 1975.
11. Engel, W. K., and Brooke, M. H. Histochemistry of the myotonic disorders. In: *Progressive Muskeldystrophie, Myotonie, Myasthenie*, edited by E. Kuhn. Springer-Verlag, Berlin, New York, 1966, pp. 203–222.
12. Carroll, J. E., Brooke, M. H., and Kaiser, K. Diagnosis of infantile myotonic dystrophy. Lancet *2:* 608, 1975.
13. Pollock, M., and Dyck, P. J. Peripheral nerve morphometry in myotonic dystrophy. Arch. Neurol. *33:* 33–39, 1976.
14. Wochner, R. D., Drews, G., Strober, W., and Engel, W. K. Accelerated breakdown of immunoglobulin G (IgG) in myotonic dystrophy: A hereditary error of immunoglobulin catabolism. J. Clin. Invest. *45:* 321–329, 1966.
15. Roses, A. D., Butterfield, A., Appel, S. H., and Chestnut, D. B. Phenytoin and membrane fluidity in myotonic dystrophy. Arch. Neurol. *32:* 535–538, 1975.
16. Hull, K. L., and Roses, A. D. Stoichiometry of sodium and potassium transport in erythrocytes from patients with myotonic muscular dystrophy. J. Physiol. *254:* 169–178, 1976.
17. Bousser, M. G., Conard, J., Lecrubier, C., and Samama, M. Increased sensitivity of platelets to adrenalin in human myotonic dystrophy. Lancet *2:* 307–309, 1975.
18. Mawatari, S., Takagi, A., and Rowland, L. P. Adenyl cyclase in normal and pathologic human muscle. Arch. Neurol. *30:* 96–102, 1974.
19. Kuhn, E. Myotonia: A lecture. In: *Clinical Studies in Myology: Proceedings of the 2nd International Congress on Muscle Diseases*, edited by B. A. Kakulas. Excerpta Medica, 1973, pp. 471–479.
20. Schrott, H. G., and Omenn, G. S. Myotonic dystrophy: Opportunities for prenatal prediction. Neurology *25:* 789–791, 1975.
21. Insley, J., Bird, G. W. G., Harper, P. S., and Pearce, G. W. Prenatal prediction of myotonic dystrophy. Lancet *2:* 806, 1976.

MYOTONIA CONGENITA (THOMSEN'S DISEASE)

Clinical Aspects

In myotonia congenita the muscle stiffness is the predominant if not the only complaint from which the patient suffers. There are two varieties: one with an autosomal dominant inheritance, which Dr. Thomsen first recognized in his own family; the second, and probably the commoner form, is an autosomal recessive described by Becker.[1] In the autosomal dominant variety, the myotonia is noticed in earliest childhood, but it may be rather mild and shows no progression. Both sexes are equally affected and there are no associated findings such as the cataracts or testicular atrophy which are found in patients with myotonic dystrophy. In the recessive variety, the disease is said to become noticeable around the age of six and the myotonia is more severe than in the dominant type. Two-thirds of the patients with the recessive variety are male.

The patient describes his condition in a rather stereotyped way. After resting, the muscles are stiff and difficult to move. With continued exercise, the muscles loosen and the patient's movement becomes almost normal. This is seen very typically when the patient arises from a chair. He moves clumsily and starts to walk with a stiff and wooden appearance almost as if he had no joints in his body. As he continues, he can first walk freely and finally can run with ease. A muscle which is stiff from myotonia cannot exert normal power, and this may give a spurious impression of weakness. As the myotonia disappears the strength returns. Exposure to cold makes the symptoms worse and can be used as a provocative test. All the striated muscles of the body seem to share this abnormality and, although it is most noticeable in the limbs, evidence of myotonia can also be found in the face and tongue. The only abnormality which may be seen in addition to the presence of myotonia is muscular hypertrophy (Figure 6.12). This is not always present and seems to be more pronounced in the recessive form than in the autosomal dominant. It is so striking on occasion as to give the appearance of the Farnese Hercules, but the majority of patients, although well muscled, do not demonstrate this degree of hypertrophy and it is certainly not as common as one would anticipate from the various dramatic pictures to be found in the literature.

Laboratory Tests

Electromyography can be helpful in establishing the diagnosis. Well marked myotonia is found with none of the associated dystrophic potentials. The muscle biopsy reveals an absence of Type 2B fibers.[2] This is a subtype of muscle fiber and is characterized by its histochemical properties. Internal nuclei and various other changes may also be seen in the muscle biopsy but these changes are less specific. Evidence for abnormalities of the membrane is also found in myotonia congenita. The abnormalities are different from those present in myotonic dystrophy. The phosphorylation of membrane proteins (protein kinase activity) is normal, chloride conductance is reduced and the membrane resistance is greater than normal. Electron spin resonance shows increased fluidity of the erythrocyte membrane as in myotonic dystrophy although not necessarily from the same cause.[3]

Treatment

Unlike patients with myotonic dystrophy, the patient with myotonia congenita suffers the effects of the myotonia. A therapeutic trial of one of the medications aimed at preventing this is thus always worthwhile. In a double blind comparison of diphenylhydantoin and procainamide, the former drug was found to be more effective.[4] The side effects of procainamide were said to be more troublesome than those of dilantin. Quinine is also well tolerated by patients and seems to be quite effective in the management of myotonia. In my own experience, the beneficial effect of these medications is rather short-lived and tends to disappear after two or three months. For this reason, patients have usually taken such medication at times when they may be particularly under stress, such as in cold weather or when they have an undue amount of activity to undertake. As in myotonic dystrophy, diamox, ACTH, and corticosteroids have also been tried, with varying results.

BIBLIOGRAPHY

1. Becker, P. E. Zur Genetik der Myotonien. In: *Progressive Muskeldystrophie, Myotonie, Myasthenie*, edited by E. Kuhn. Springer-Verlag, Berlin, New York, 1966, pp. 247–255.
2. Crews, J., Kaiser, K. K., and Brooke, M. H. The pathology of myotonia congenita. J. Neurol. Sci. *28:* 449–457, 1976.

3. Butterfield, D. A., Chestnut, D. B., Appel, S. H., and Roses, A. D. Spin label study of erythrocyte membrane fluidity in myotonic and Duchenne muscular dystrophy and congenital myotonia. Nature *263:* 159–161, 1976.
4. Munsat, T. L. Therapy of myotonia. Neurology *17:* 359–367, 1967.

PARAMYOTONIA CONGENITA

Clinical Aspects

Paramyotonia congenita was described by Eulenburg in 1886. It is a rare disorder whose existence has even been denied because of the resemblance that it bears to hyperkalemic periodic paralysis. It is a disease of autosomal dominant inheritance, and the characteristics of the myotonia are slightly different from those in the preceding diseases. The facial muscles and the muscles of the forearms and hands are predominantly involved, and the myotonia shows more sensitivity to cold—may, indeed, be manifest only on exposure to cold.

Myotonia of the face may be noticed by a stiffness of the expression, a narrowing of the palpebral fissures and a dimpling of the chin owing to the contraction of the mentalis muscle. A similar stiffness may be noticed in the tongue. When myotonia occurs in the hand, a peculiar posture is seen with the middle three fingers lightly flexed, particularly at the metacarpophalangeal joint, and the thumb and little finger held abducted. Another unusual aspect of the myotonia is that repetitive activity may make the myotonia worse, rather than better. Finally, the illness differs from the preceding varieties because the patient may experience severe weakness of the muscle following exposure to cold. Exercising a muscle may also provoke weakness as well as myotonia. The disease is manifest from birth and does not improve as the patient gets older.

Laboratory Studies

Laboratory investigation of the disease is directed toward the demonstration of myotonia and to disproving any possible association with the periodic paralyses. Electromyography demonstrates the myotonia and, in addition, reveals an abnormal reduction in the amplitude of the evoked response following stimulation at 25 to 50 Hz.[2] This reduction in amplitude accompanies the increasing weakness and is not corrected by the administration of edrophonium. Its cause is unclear but it is likely to be associated with a membrane defect.

Treatment

Usually no specific treatment of the symptoms is required. Acetazoleamide may, on occasion, make the symptoms worse rather than better. Although this drug is useful in the treatment of hypo- and hyperkalemic periodic paralysis, it should be avoided in paramyotonia congenita.

BIBLIOGRAPHY

1. Thrush, D. C., Morris, C. J., and Salmon, M. V. Paramyotonia congenita: A clinical, histochemical and pathological study. Brain *95:* 537–552, 1972.
2. Burke, D., Skuse, N. F., and Lethlean, A. K. Contractile properties of the abductor digiti minimi muscle in paramyotonia congenita. J. Neurol. Neurosurg. Psychiatry *37:* 894–899, 1974.

OTHER FORMS OF MYOTONIA

An often quoted form of myotonia is that seen in association with dwarfism, diffuse bone disease, and unusual ocular and facial abnormalities.[1] This has also been known as the Schwartz-Jampel Syndrome.[2] Analysis of the electrical activity in this interesting syndrome shows that it really differs from myotonia and is more nearly equivalent to the group of diseases showing abnormal spontaneous activity. Thus, the repetitive activity is of high frequency, does not have the waxing and waning qualities of myotonia, and is also abolished by curare, unlike myotonia.

Myotonia acquistia is another illness which is perhaps mythical. The sudden acquisition of myotonia has been described following trauma, electric shock, and other disasters. However, the usual association is of a sudden traumatic episode which brings to light hitherto undiagnosed myotonic dystrophy or myotonia congenita. Poisoning with 2,4-D or with diazacholesterol may give rise to myotonia and perhaps should be considered as true myotonia acquisita.

BIBLIOGRAPHY

1. Aberfeld, D. C., Hintebuchner, L. P., and Schneider, M. Myotonia dwarfism, diffuse bone disease and unusual ocular and facial abnormalities: A new syndrome. Brain *88:* 313–322, 1965.
2. Taylor, R. G., Layzer, R. B., Davis, H. S., and Fowler, W. M. Continuous muscle fiber activity in the Schwartz-Jampel syndrome. Electroencephalogr. Clin. Neurophysiol. *33:* 497–509, 1972.

7

inflammatory myopathies

POLYMYOSITIS AND DERMATOMYOSITIS

Clinical Aspects

Muscle, no less than other tissues in the body, is at the mercy of various inflammatory processes. The range and diversity of these conditions are impressive: bacterial, viral, and parasitic infections have all been described, as well as the granulomatous conditions due to tuberculosis and sarcoidosis. Yet it is remarkable how seldom one sees any of these diseases and their importance fades, at least in the non-tropical countries, when compared to the prevalence of inflammatory diseases of muscle of unknown cause, often associated with disturbances of the immune system. Dermatomyositis and polymyositis are common diseases in any muscle clinic. The combination of a typical skin rash with the signs and symptoms of muscular weakness makes the diagnosis of dermatomyositis not only probable but, on occasions, inescapable. However, the diagnosis of polymyositis in the absence of the rash may indeed be difficult, and provides a variety of traps for the unwary. There are other illnesses in which inflammatory changes are seen in the muscle; nor does the lack of such pathology exclude the diagnosis of polymyositis. These and other problems in the diagnostic criteria for polymyositis have bedeviled the literature and clouded the evaluation of therapy. It is also hard to know whether to consider polymyositis and dermatomyositis as one entity or whether the two diseases are discrete as to cause, prognosis, and treatment. Before treading this particular clinical morass it would be perhaps better to set down some of the typical features of the illness.

Dermatomyositis is an acquired illness with an acute or subacute course. It may occur at any age, but it is slightly more common in childhood and again in the 5th and 6th decades. It is unusual to see a case between the ages of 15 and 25.[1] Some studies have suggested that women are more prone to the disease than men.[2] As with many other muscle diseases, the true incidence is hard to discover but lies somewhere between 5 and 10 patients per million annually. The disease often begins with a variety of systemic symptoms, including fever, malaise, or mild and nonspecific gastrointestinal symptoms. Sometimes there is a preceding illness or event which causes the patient and even the physician to suspect that it might be related to the onset of the inflammatory myopathy. Such episodes have included upper respiratory infections, immunizations, and drug reactions. Prolonged exposure to sunlight can precede the development of the rash in dermatomyositis. A change in behavior often presages the disease in childhood. Children become fretful and irritable, and a normally good child may become impossible and unruly.

The rash may appear before, after, or concomitant with the weakness and may take several forms. There may be a blotchy flush over the cheekbone which blanches on pressure, with a rather slow return of color when the pressure is released. The eyelids, particularly the upper eyelid, may become discolored and assume a purple color which has been likened to lavender, lilac, or heliotrope. In the black races the rash is neither lavender nor red, but rather a dusky, deep purple shadow on the skin. In severe involvement, the rash is accompanied by marked edema which can cause a puffiness around the eyes. The skin may also break down and present a scaly or weeping appearance. An erythematous rash of the chest and neck often develops in the area that would be exposed by an open shirt or scoop neck dress. The associated telangiectasia makes the rash reminiscent of that associated with irradiation. The skin over the elbows and knees becomes not only discolored but also thickened. Frequently nodules develop which may become necrotic and extrude calcinous material. The rash is equally characteristic on the hands. It varies from a slight puffiness and discoloration around the nail beds to marked edema with telangiectasia. There may be areas of erythema and thickening over the knuckles and the interphalangeal joints. When the skin changes are severe there is a shiny atrophic appearance to the skin over all the fingers and back of the hand. At other times the rash may be diffuse, covering almost the whole body, though there is usually sparing of the skin in the axilla. The end result of such diffuse changes can be disastrous, with the patient's skin reduced to a chitinous, atrophic shell which cracks at every attempted manipulation.

The ancient tenet that inflammation is accompanied by "calor, dolor, turgor, et rubor" is nowhere more misleading than in polymyositis. Fully a third of the patients with the disease have no symptoms of muscle pain whatsoever. The all too often noted comment that a patient could not have polymyositis because of the absence of muscle pain is extremely ill-advised. Not only is its absence no bar to the diagnosis of polymyositis but the majority of patients who do complain of muscle pain have some other illness such as polymyalgia or the ubiquitous "aches, cramps, and pains" syndrome. When pain is present it is usually described as a deep aching within the muscles, a soreness which is helped to some extent by rest and made worse with continued activity. The muscles may be swollen, particularly the proximal muscles of the leg, and palpation of the muscle belly may accentuate the tenderness. In chronic and long standing disease, the muscles may not only become firmly indurated but may be the site of contractures. Rarely, widespread calcification of the soft tissues follows severe poly- or dermatomyositis. Although this calcification is disabling, it is usually found only when the disease itself is inactive.

The symptoms of weakness may begin with surprising suddenness and may render a patient bedfast within several days, but usually the progress of the weakness is measured not in days but in weeks. The symptoms differ in no way from those of patients with other forms of proximal weakness: difficulties in arising from a chair, climbing stairs, and lifting objects onto shelves are common. There is a special predilection for the anterior neck muscles in polymyositis, in which respect it differs from myasthenia gravis where the posterior muscles of the neck are more often involved. Weakness of the facial muscles, although recorded, is unusual and should suggest the possibility of some other diagnosis. Bulbar symptoms are generally unusual, but dysphagia is a common feature of dermato- and polymyositis and may be so severe as to necessitate nasogastric tube feeding. The limb weakness is initially of proximal muscles and spreads to involve more distal muscles as the disease progresses. Whether or not polymyositis is a different disease from dermatomyositis, those patients without the rash have a similar story. They experience the same initial systemic complaints followed by an acute or subacute bout of weakness. It is unusual for a child to have polymyositis (without the rash) so the disease is chiefly seen in adults.

It is difficult to be sure of the natural history of these two diseases although attempts have been made to characterize it.[1-3] Some studies have been plagued by the shifting miasmic quality of the criteria used to diagnose polymyositis. The typical case of dermatomyositis is easy to document, but when cases are adjudged on the basis of the clinical picture alone or of mild inflammatory responses in the muscle biopsy, it is hard to be certain that dystrophies or metabolic myopathies of various types are excluded.[4, 5]

The disease may run a variable course. A patient, particularly a child, may have an acute attack of dermato- or polymyositis with subsequent complete recovery even in the absence of any medical treatment. Other cases suffer a remitting, relapsing illness, usually with imperfect recovery between bouts of myositis. A third variety, and one which may evolve from the previous type, is a chronic indolent form. The best that can be hoped for if this happens (although this is perhaps a physician's viewpoint, not that of a patient) is that the disease burns out before the patient's pulmonary functions are compromised. Death, when it takes place, is usually from inanition, intercurrent infection, or respiratory failure. In one large series about one-third of the patients died in the course of myositis.[3] This study also suggested that the more acute the disease the better the prognosis. Of those patients whose disease had lasted less than 6 months, almost half went into remission, whereas of those whose illness was of longer duration, barely a quarter achieved remission. Perhaps the axiomatic corollary of this should be noted: namely, the longer one suffers a disease the more likely it is to be severe. It is quite probable that the natural history of polymyositis will never be established. We are long into an age when steroid therapy and immunosuppressive drugs have become commonplace, and it is difficult to stand by and watch a patient become enfeebled from polymyositis without at least attempting treatment. Perhaps the only certain statement which can be made is that patients with dermato- and polymyositis do poorly enough in general that some therapy should be sought.

Laboratory Studies

If clinical criteria are difficult and therapeutic response uncertain, how may one essay the diagnosis of poly- or dermatomyositis? Both forms share certain abnormalities. The serum "muscle" enzymes are elevated and in our experience the creatine phosphokinase (CPK) has been the most useful. This has been disputed[2] but there is usually elevation of this enzyme at some stage of the disease and such elevation may on occasion be pronounced. The CPK tends to be higher when the disease is active than when it is inactive, but a normal enzyme level is seen in a number of patients in whom the disease is in exacerbation. The serum CPK should therefore be used only as one of the criteria to judge the progress of the disease. The other muscle enzymes are also elevated and in some patients in whom CPK is normal the lactic dehydrogenase or SGOT can be used to monitor the disease. In others the sedimentation rate may reflect the activity of the illness, but this finding is nonspecific and cannot be used to establish the diagnosis. An EMG can be helpful since a so-called myopathic EMG with short low amplitude polyphasic potentials may be associated with signs of muscle irritability, such as bizarre repetitive discharges, or with fibrillation and positive denervation potentials. The muscle biopsy may be strikingly abnormal and is slightly different in the two forms of the illness. In dermatomyositis there tends to be more perifascicular atrophy, whereas in polymyositis this change is often lacking. Inflammatory changes are obviously part and parcel of the disease but they may be absent in a third of the patients. A novel serological test has been proposed based on the inhibition of a complement fixation reaction between disease serum and thymus extract which is produced by papain digestion of the same polymyositic serum.[6] If confirmation of this test is forthcoming it might be useful diagnostically.

Classification

To have arrived thus far in the discussion of inflammatory myopathies without attempting their classification would be regarded in some circles as a tour de force and in others as a lapse in judgment. The ways in which the various forms of polymyositis may be classified are not yet settled, nor even the question as to whether there really are different forms of myositis. In any group of diseases the advantage of a good system of classification is that it simplifies matters, whereas the disadvantage of a bad one is that it only complicates the subject. Although the classification which has been proposed for the inflammatory myopathies is not based upon the certainty of different etiologies, it does serve as a reminder that the several varieties are not necessarily identical. If this function is to be served it is better to maintain rather wide and general categories. If and when the details are filled in at a later time a new classification will assuredly come into being. For this reason the system suggested by Bohan and Peter,[4, 5] which in itself was adapted from that of Pearson,[2] approaches a reasonable compromise. It is as follows:

Group 1. Primary idiopathic polymyositis.
Group 2. Primary idiopathic dermatomyositis.
Group 3. Dermatomyositis (or polymyositis) associated with neoplasia.
Group 4. Childhood dermatomyositis (or polymyositis) associated with vasculitis.
Group 5. Polymyositis or dermatomyositis associated with collagen vascular disease.

The first two groups are separated on the basis of information which is already available. There is enough difference between polymyositis and dermatomyositis at least to give rise to doubt as to their common identity. Childhood dermatomyositis seems to be a slightly different disease. A category of cases associated with cancer gives tacit recognition to the fact that these patients need to be managed differently, while that associated with collagen vascular disease admits the thin end of a very large wedge to the classification.

It is obvious from the preceding that dermato- and polymyositis may be seen in conjunction with other conditions. In polymyositis and particularly in dermatomyositis there may be associated vascular symptoms. The incidence of Raynaud's phenomenon has been estimated to be as high as 28 per cent, although most of us have encountered this symptom less frequently. Cardiac abnormalities with heart block and pathologically proven involvement of the heart have been noted.[7, 8] Abnormalities of the lung with interstitial fibrosis and pneumonitis may also occur as a rare complication.[9, 10] This type of illness links patients with idiopathic polymyositis whose symptoms chiefly reflect the muscle disease to other patients in whom the muscle disease is clearly complicated by (or perhaps even a complication of) some diffuse collagen vascular disease.

Lupus erythematosus, polyarteritis nodosa, and scleroderma may all have weakness as a facet of the disease complex. The prognosis in such a situation is not as good as with uncomplicated polymyositis, but again this may simply imply that the more widespread a disease the more likely it is to have serious consequences. An exception to this rule is the entity known as mixed connective tissue disease.[11, 12] This is usually a disease of women and clinically resembles a combination of systemic lupus erythematosus, polymyositis, and scleroderma. The diagnostic test is the demonstration of high titers of an extractable nuclear antigen which is very sensitive to digestion with ribonuclease. The antinuclear antibody test shows a speckled positive. Clinically the patients suffer from arthritis, Raynaud's phenomenon, thickened, swollen hands or sclerodermatous skin changes, lymphadenopathy, anemia, leukopenia, fever, disturbances in esophageal motility, hepato- and splenomegaly, and muscle weakness. Kidney disease is very unusual, and the response to steroid treatment is excellent.

There is a special relationship between dermatomyositis (less often polymyositis) and neoplasms. This relationship is chiefly seen in the adult form of dermatomyositis, and the underlying neoplasm is usually a carcinoma. The true incidence of this is difficult to extract from the literature but is probably in the neighborhood of 10 to 20 per cent. Whatever the exact figure, it is high enough that a search for a carcinoma should be undertaken in any adult patient, especially a male of 40 or over, who has either poly- or dermatomyositis. In the not too remote past the incidence of carcinoma was thought to be high enough that repeated evaluation for the possibility of cancer was carried out every 6 months or so. Perhaps a more justifiable approach is to recommend an initial thorough workup for an underlying neoplasm, with simple screening procedures (such as testing for occult blood in the stools, chest x-ray, etc.) at regular intervals throughout the course of the disease. If the patient's symptoms warrant a more complete investigation, this would obviously be advisable. In our own series of patients we have detected only three neoplasms, two of the lung and one of the thyroid, the last being discovered incidentally at post mortem in an unselected series of 62 patients with poly- or dermatomyositis.

Etiology

Much is known about the underlying pathology of the disease, although the precise etiology is still unknown. It has been suggested that the perifascicular distribution of the atrophic muscle fiber indicates vascular insufficiency with selective atrophy of those fibers furthest "downstream."[13] Paulson et al. employed xenon-131 to measure the blood flow in a limb at rest and during hyperemia induced by ischemic exercise and histamine.[14] They showed a decreased muscle blood flow in patients with polymyositis that was present neither in Duchenne's dystrophy nor in limb girdle dystrophy. Morphometric analysis of the skeletal muscle capillaries reveals hypertrophy of the capillary endothelial cells and also basement membrane reduplication, suggesting repeated capillary degeneration as the primary event in the disease.[15] Subtle differences are also found between the changes in polymyositis and in dermatomyositis.

An experimental animal model of myositis has been produced by the injection of muscle extracts in conjunction with complete Freund's adjuvant.[16] Inflammatory lesions were produced, the worst involvement being noted in those animals injected with a myofibrillar fraction.[17] Circulating antibodies to muscle were detected in this animal model. Antimuscle antibodies have also been detected in patients with polymyositis, but the force of this evidence is slightly weakened by their detection in normal controls as well.[18] The possibility of an altered immune state raises the question of whether the damage is produced by humoral factors or by cellular means. In the animal model the disease was transferred to other animals by an infusion of washed lymphocytes from an affected animal.[16] When lymphocytes from patients with polymyositis were incubated with muscle, they released a lymphotoxin which was demonstrated using human fetal muscle as a target organ.[19] The degree of damage to the target cells was evaluated by assaying the incorporation of ^{14}C-labeled amino acids into the cells. The lymphocytes which had been incubated with muscle produced a 50 per cent decrease, which was not quite as complete as the 95 per cent decrease in amino acid incorporation when the lymphocytes were nonspecifically stimulated with phytohemagglutinin. It was nevertheless clearly different from normal. A more direct demonstration of the cytotoxicity was possible by incorporating ^{51}Cr into cultured chick muscle cells.[20] These cells were then incubated with either the serum or lymphocytes of patients with polymyositis and the release of labeled chromium into the supernatant was measured. Only lymphocytes from patients with active disease produced an increased release of chromium into the medium, an indirect indication of damage to the muscle cells. The highest values of chromium release, and therefore the most damage, were seen in the untreated patients or patients being treated with low dose or alternate day steroids. Others have failed to demonstrate any abnormal response of lymphocytes from patients with polymyositis to stimulation by muscle extract or other agents and have concluded that cell mediated immunity does not play a part in the illness.[21]

A humoral mechanism has also been suggested as a cause of polymyositis.[22, 23] A deposition of immunoglobin was noted particularly in children with dermatomyositis. This deposition was more pronounced in small veins than in arteries. These authors felt that, although the lymphocytes in patients with polymyositis were capable of damaging muscle, the cells may have been "turned on" nonspecifically, secondary to the general damage of muscle which occurs in the disease from some other primary cause.

A review of experimental auto allergic myositis and polymyositis[24] concluded that there are indications that there is a relative absence of humoral response in patients with the latter disease. This is indicated by the depressed IgG levels and a decreased response to tetanus toxoid. Whatever the final outcome it is apparent that there is still much to learn about the altered immunity of polymyositis.

Treatment

The treatment of dermato- and polymyositis is simpler to describe than it is to justify. Controlled trials on steroids or other immunosuppressants are few and far between. One large study concluded that the same number of patients achieved remission with no steroids as with a high dose of steroids.[3] A low dose of steroids seemed to be ineffective and only one patient on low dose steroid therapy did well. A hopeful sign for those who believe in the use of these drugs was that twice as many patients were "better" with a high dose of steroids than with no steroids at all. Two seemingly contradictory studies on the results of high dose steroid therapy in polymyositis demonstrated in one series that 7 of 18 patients died and only 3 maintained any improvement.[25] In the other, larger series (118 patients), two-thirds of the patients improved to the point where they had no functional disability.[26] In spite of the dismal state of our knowledge, few of us can observe the worsening of a patient with acute dermato- or polymyositis without prescribing prednisone.

The problem is compounded by the ways in which the drug is used. What follows is a distillation of my own prejudices, based on no firm scientific principles. It seems to me that there are three errors which are prevalent in the treatment of patients with steroids: The first occurs when the medication is started too late, the second is the administration of steroids in doses which are too small, and the third is the termination of the therapy too soon. If steroids have an effect on the disease, they should be used as soon as the diagnosis is made. It seems, in general, that patients who are treated earlier do better.[26, 27] If steroids are to be used they should be used in adequate suppressive doses of between 50 and 80 mg. of prednisone daily (1 to 2 mg. per kilogram of body weight in children). Using smaller doses of prednisone early in the disease in the hope of sparing the patient the untoward side effects is an unhappy compromise at best and may even result in the appearance of side effects in the absence of the possible benefit of suppressive doses. Physicians' insecurity over the value of prednisone also leads to an early withdrawal of the drug, which may sometimes be not only unnecessary but harmful. A typical situation is the patient with moderately severe polymyositis with an elevated CPK whose diagnosis is well substantiated. The patient is placed on suppressive doses of steroids and, instead of the expected immediate improvement, no change in the patient's condition is seen for a week to 10 days. At this point the physician is cither given to doubts about the diagnosis or concludes that steroids are ineffective. Consequently the medication is withdrawn. Very frequently the serum CPK will fall during this first week. The clinical improvement, however, may be quite delayed, a matter of 4 to 6 weeks after the decline in the CPK. The return of the enzymes to more normal levels is not only an encouraging finding but is an indication to persevere with the use of steroids for at least 2 to 3 months before assuming the patient is steroid resistant. The length of time during which patients should be maintained on suppressive doses of steroids is another problem with no proven solution. If the disease is acute and the patient has been started on 80 mg. of prednisone daily, or higher, the dose can be tapered after 2 months or when the enzymes return to normal. This tapering should be gradual; we have usually reduced the total daily dose by 5 mg. every other week. By appropriately reducing the alternate daily dose the patient may be converted to an alternate day regimen of steroids. Some patients do quite well on such a schedule; others do not. As long as the patient is improving, suppressive doses of steroids should be continued. Once the dosage is below 50 mg. every other day the reduction may be even slower, 2.5 mg. at a time. Sometimes an exacerbation of the polymyositis during steroid withdrawal is heralded by a gradual increase in the serum muscle enzyme levels. Such an increase should be treated with great respect and if there is a consistent and progressive elevation of the enzymes an increase in the dose of steroids may be indicated even in the absence of clinical change. Ancillary therapy includes the administration of potassium supplement and an antacid regimen. A high protein, low carbohydrate diet with decreased salt intake is also recommended. During the past 7 years over 50 patients have been treated using this schedule. The commonest side effect has been the occurrence of cataracts. These are usually seen in patients who have been on steroids for 18 months or more and have occurred in about 30 per cent of patients. Several patients also developed cushingoid features but there have been no serious problems with hypertension, diabetes, or gastrointestinal disturbance. Osteoporosis and compression fracture of a thoracic vertebra were seen in one patient. During this time there have been six deaths, all patients with dermatomyositis, three in childhood and three in middle age. Although valid statistics cannot be derived from our results because many patients have been followed only for a brief time, they parallel those of De Vere and Bradley[26] rather than the more ominous outlook seen in the series of Riddoch and Morgan-Hughes.[25]

A different view on the management of juvenile dermatomyositis has been proposed by Dubowitz.[28] Based on the results of steroid therapy in eight cases he suggested using smaller doses of prednisone (1 to 1.5 mg./kg.) and tapering the dosage as soon as clinical improvement begins. Dubowitz also suggested that serum enzyme levels are less reliable than the patient's clinical response.

In addition to steroids, various immunosuppressant agents have been used.[29–35] Patients reported in the literature have responded to methotrexate, azathioprine, and cytoxan. There are good theoretical grounds for trying these medications. My own experience has been limited to azathioprine and, in only two patients, methotrexate. The results obtained were not as good as those in the literature, but it is quite possible that the medications were used too late. Presumably, if they are to be effective, they will be more effective early in the disease. Perhaps the ideal treatment of dermato- and polymyositis would be the immediate use of azathioprine or methotrexate in combination with steroids as soon as the diagnosis is made. Various dosage schedules have been recommended for the various drugs. Methotrexate has been given both intravenously and orally. The least toxic and most effective regimen seems to be to give the drug orally in increasing doses until 0.8 mg. per kilogram of body weight is given per week. The side effects of the medication have been pronounced in some series and relatively absent in others. Among those mentioned were buccal ulcers, hepatitis, pleuritis, and pneumonitis. With methotrexate therapy the maximal response occurred after about 13 weeks of treatment.[34] Azathioprine has been used in doses sufficient to decrease the leukocyte count to around 3,000. Frequent monitoring of the blood is necessary, particularly early in the course of treatment.

It is important to attempt to prevent the joint contractures which may develop during the illness, and a program of "range of motion" passive exercises should be carried out during the acute stages of the disease.

BIBLIOGRAPHY

1. Medsger, T. A., Dawson, W. N., and Masi, A. T. The epidemiology of polymyositis. Am. J. Med. *48:* 715–723, 1970.
2. Pearson, C. M. Polymyositis. Annu. Rev. Med. *17:* 63–82, 1966.
3. Winkelmann, R. K., Mulder, D. W., Lambert, E. H., Howard, F. M., and Diessner, G. R. Dermatomyositis-polymyositis: Comparison of untreated and cortisone treated patients. Mayo Clin. Proc. *43:* 545–556, 1968.
4. Bohan, A., and Peter, J. B. Polymyositis and dermatomyositis. N. Engl. J. Med. *292:* 344–347, 1975.
5. Bohan, A., and Peter, J. B. Polymyositis and dermatomyositis. N. Engl. J. Med. *292:* 403–407, 1975.
6. Reichlin, M., and Mattioli, M. Description of a serological reaction characteristic of polymyositis. Clin. Immunol. Immunopathol. *5:* 12–20, 1976.
7. Schaumburg, H. H., Nielsen, S. L., and Yurchak, P. M. Heartblock in polymyositis: Case with proven involvement of heart. N. Engl. J. Med. *284:* 480–481, 1971.
8. Singsen, B., Goldreyer, B., Stanton, R., and Hanson, V. Childhood polymyositis with cardiac conduction defects. Am. J. Dis. Child. *130:* 72–74, 1976.
9. Duncan, P. E., Griffin, J. P., Garcia, A., and Kaplan, S. B. Fibrosing alveolitis and polymyositis. Am. J. Med. *57:* 621–626, 1974.
10. Schwarz, M. I., Matthay, R. A., Sahn, S. A., et al. Interstitial lung disease in polymyositis and dermatomyositis; analysis of six cases and review of the literature. Medicine *55:* 89–104, 1976.
11. Sharp, G. C., Irvin, W. S., Tan, E. M., Gould, R. G., and Holman, H. R. Mixed connective tissue diseases. Am. J. Med. *52:* 148–159, 1972.
12. Levitin, P. M., Weary, P. E., and Ginliano, V. J. The immunofluorescent "band" test in mixed connective tissue disorders. Ann. Intern. Med. *83:* 53–55, 1975.
13. Banker, B. Q., and Victor, M. Dermatomyositis (systemic angiopathy) of childhood. Medicine *45:* 261, 1966.
14. Paulson, O. F., Engel, A. G., and Gomez, M. R. Muscle blood flow in Duchenne type muscular dystrophy, limb girdle dystrophy, polymyositis and in normal controls. J. Neurol. Neurosurg. Psychiatry *37:* 685–690, 1974.
15. Jerusalem, F., Rakusa, M., Engel, A. G., and MacDonald, R. D. Morphometric analysis of skeletal muscle capillary ultrastructure in inflammatory myopathies. J. Neurol. Sci. *23:* 391–402, 1974.

16. Morgan, G., Peter, J. C., and Newbould, B. B. Experimental allergic myositis in rats. Arthritis Rheum. *14:* 599–609, 1971.
17. Manghani, D., Partridge, T. A., and Sloper, J. C. The role of the myofibrillar fraction of skeletal muscle in the production of experimental polymyositis. J. Neurol. Sci. *23:* 489–503, 1974.
18. Partridge, T. A., Manghani, D., and Sloper, J. C. Antimuscle antibodies in polymyositis. Lancet *1:* 676, 1973.
19. Johnson, R. L., Fink, C. W., and Ziff, M. Lymphotoxin formation by lymphocytes and muscle in polymyositis. J. Clin. Invest. *51:* 2435–2449, 1972.
20. Dawkins, R.L., and Mastaglia, F. L. Cell mediated cytoxicity to muscle in polymyositis. New Engl. J. Med. *288:* 434–438, 1973.
21. Lisak, R. P., and Zweiman, B. Mitogen and muscle extract induced in vitro proliferative responses in myasthenia gravis dermatomyositis and polymyositis. J. Neurol. Neurosurg. Psychiatry *38:* 521–524, 1976.
22. Whitaker, J. N., and Engel, W. K. Mechanisms of muscle injury in idiopathic inflammatory myopathy. N. Engl. J. Med. *289:* 107–108, 1973.
23. Whitaker, J. N., and Engel, W. K. Vascular deposits of immunoglobulin and complement in idiopathic inflammatory myopathy. N. Engl. J. Med. *286:* 333–338, 1972.
24. Dawkins, R. L. Experimental autoallergic myositis, polymyositis and myasthenia gravis. Clin. Exp. Immunol. *21:* 185–201, 1975.
25. Riddoch, D., and Morgan-Hughes, J. A. Prognosis in adult polymyositis. J. Neurol. Sci. *26:* 71–80, 1975.
26. De Vere, R., and Bradley, W. G. Polymyositis: Its presentation morbidity and mortality. Brain *98:* 637–666, 1975.
27. Rose, A. L. Childhood polymyositis. Am. J. Dis. Child. *127:* 518–522, 1974.
28. Dubowitz, V. Treatment of dermatomyositis in childhood. Arch. Dis. Child. *51:* 494–500, 1976.
29. Arnett, F. C., Whelton, J. C., Zizic, T. M., and Stevens, M. B. Methotrexate therapy in polymyositis. Ann. Rheum. Dis. *32:* 536–546, 1973.
30. Benson, M. D., and Aldo, M. A. Azathioprine therapy in polymyositis. Arch. Intern. Med. *132:* 544–551, 1973.
31. Currie, S., and Walton, J. N. Immunosuppressive therapy in polymyositis. J. Neurol. Neurosurg. Psychiatry *34:* 447–452, 1971.
32. Haas, D. C. Treatment of polymyositis with immunosuppressive drugs. Neurology *23:* 55–62, 1973.
33. Metzger, A. L., Bohan, A., Goldberg, L. S., Bluestone, R., and Pearson, C. M. Polymyositis and dermatomyositis: Combined methotrexate and corticoid steroid therapy. Ann. Intern. Med. *81:* 182–189, 1974.
34. Sokoloff, M. C., Goldberg, L. S., and Pearson, C. M. Treatment of corticosteroid-resistant polymyositis with methotrexate. Lancet *1:* 14–16, 1971.
35. Malaviya, A. N., Many, A., and Schwarz, R. S. Treatment of dermatomyositis with methotrexate. Lancet *2:* 485–488, 1968.

POLYMYALGIA RHEUMATICA

There are many illnesses in which muscle pain is a prominent symptom. Sometimes these illnesses are nebulous and the diagnosis difficult to establish. Often the pain seems to be frankly psychosomatic in origin. At other times the physician may take refuge behind a diagnosis such as fibrositis, which often implies no more than a feeling that the disease is organic but an inability to discover any abnormality. One disease, polymyalgia rheumatica, has been gaining increasing acceptance within recent years.[1, 2]

The symptoms of muscle pain and stiffness are so characteristic that different patients will use identical phrases in describing their symptoms. After a period of rest, particularly a prolonged period, the muscles "freeze" or "set like jelly" and any movement of the muscles produces pain or a tearing feeling within the muscle. With continued use and exercise the muscle stiffness and pain may abate. Thus, the discomfort is greatest early in the morning upon arising and, indeed, may be severe enough to prevent the patient from getting out of bed. Usually the shoulder muscles are more involved than any other muscles and in a surprising number, even among the younger patients, there is evidence of cervical arthritis. Women suffer from the illness twice as frequently as men and the disease appears in late life, cases under the age of 55 being quite rare in the literature.

There are often other complaints that go along with muscle stiffness and tenderness. The patient may feel chronically unwell and may run a low grade fever with frequent night sweats. Temporal arteritis with tender, enlarged, and nodular arteries may be associated with the illness. The older patients are particularly afflicted with this complication. It is difficult to determine the true incidence of temporal arteritis, but it may be as high as seventy-five per cent. Some have recommended routine biopsies of the temporal artery to exclude this condition because of the possibility of associated retinal artery occlusion. Our own experience has been somewhat different. We have found pathological evidence of temporal arteritis in less than 20 per cent of patients with classical polymyalgia rheumatica. We do not now routinely biopsy temporal arteries in such patients although any clinical indication of temporal arteritis, no matter how vague, would be an indication for biopsy. Polymyalgia rheumatica may occur with surprising suddenness over a period of a few days. Left without treatment, patients do seem to improve, but this improvement may take place over several years and few are willing to endure the symptoms for that length of time. An association between polymyalgia and neoplasia has been suggested, but this association was not confirmed by one recent study.[3]

Examination of the patient when the symptoms are severe may show the stiffened, cautious walk of a patient in pain. The arms are held close to the side and flexed, protected against any untoward swinging movement, and the legs are moved stiffly and slowly. The muscle is often tender to the touch, although the pain produced with palpation is not as severe as that caused when the patient moves. If the patient can relax, passive movement of the limbs is normal, although often the patient splints the limb against such movement. For the most part, the large joints in the limbs are not abnormal and periarticular tenderness is not generally a part of the disease. If the patient is seen late in the day when his symptoms have abated, he may appear relatively normal. When asked, the patient usually describes his pain as a feeling of stiffness and to illustrate this will often move his arms in a manner reminiscent of a boxer loosening his shoulder muscles.

Laboratory Studies

With one exception, the laboratory studies tend to be normal. The sedimentation rate, however, is elevated, often over 70 mm per hour. For the diagnosis of polymyalgia rheumatica to be made with certainty, the elevated sedimentation rate is an essential parameter. Patients often show a mild hypochromic or normochromic anemia. There is occasional elevation of the alpha globulin, and sometimes positive antinuclear antibodies are found. The muscle biopsy may also show mild abnormalities.[4] There is an increased incidence of HL-A8 antigen in patients with polymyalgia.[5]

Treatment

Little is known of the etiology of this disease, and the only evidence that it belongs in the rheumatoid group of diseases is that it shares some of their clinical characteristics. The description of the disease may be mundane, but response to treatment often approaches the spectacular. The illness not only responds to prednisone but does so with alacrity. The patient is free of symptoms within a week and often within 24 hours of the administration of prednisone. We have usually started patients on between 30 and 50 mg. of prednisone daily and maintain this dosage for two months before decreasing it gradually. These levels of prednisone administration are higher than recommended in the literature, but we have felt that the disease is more effectively suppressed this way and relapses are less common. Maintenance with low doses of steroids, from 10 to 20 mg. daily, may be necessary for a year or more. Withdrawal of the medication below this level may exacerbate the symptoms.

BIBLIOGRAPHY

1. Hunder, G. G., Disney, T. F., and Ward, L. E. Polymyalgia rheumatica. Mayo Clin. Proc. *44:* 849–875, 1969.
2. Andrews, F. M. Polymyalgia rheumatica. Practitioner *205:* 635–640, 1970.
3. von Knorring, J. and Somer, T. Malignancy in association with polymyalgia rheumatica and temporal arteritis. Scand. J. Rheumatol. *3:* 129–135, 1974.
4. Brooke, M. H. and Kaplan, H. Muscle pathology in rheumatoid arthritis, polymyalgia rheumatica, and polymyositis. Arch. Pathol. *94:* 101–118, 1972.
5. Rosenthal, M., Müller, W., Albert, E. D., and Schattenkirchner, M. HL-A Antibodies in polymyalgia rheumatica. N. Engl. J. Med. *292:* 595, 1975.

SARCOID MYOPATHY

In sarcoidosis, the disease may be found in the muscle as in other tissues. The diagnosis of sarcoid myopathy rests upon the clinical demonstration of involvement of other organs as well as the pathological demonstration of noncaseating granulomata in the muscle. It has been suggested that sarcoidosis may affect muscle exclusively. This is not well substantiated and a critical review of the literature reveals that on most occasions, sarcoid myopathy is part of more diffuse disease.[1] The myopathy takes one of several forms, of which the commonest is asymptomatic.[2, 3] As many as half of all patients with sarcoidosis have some involvement of the muscle even in the absence of muscular symptoms. In those patients with overt muscle disease, the majority have a chronic proximal myopathy. Palpable nodules may be found in the muscle, and occasionally a diffuse hypertrophy of the muscle may occur. Women are more commonly affected than men (4:1). Additionally, the age of onset seems to be later in women than in men so that the illness appears predominantly in the postmenopausal woman. A very acute and fulminating myopathy may be seen with marked elevation of creatine phosphokinase, but this is unusual.

Laboratory tests which may substantiate the diagnosis of sarcoidosis include the changes seen in the chest x-ray and the positive skin reaction to the

Kveim-Siltzbach antigen. It is also important to differentiate the granulomatous changes produced by sarcoidosis from those produced by an impressive array of chemical and other agents. These vary from beryllium to cork dust and from fungi to spirochetes.[4] The treatment of sarcoidosis is no more clear than the treatment of polymyositis, probably less so. There is evidence from the literature that the majority of patients are helped by the administration of steroids or ACTH, but controlled studies are lacking. Gardner-Thorpe suggested that, although steroid therapy had been useful in 20 of 26 cases reported in the literature, the hazards of steroid therapy were too great to allow the routine use of the drug.[1] Nevertheless, in a patient whose weakness is secondary to sarcoidosis, the use of prednisone is probably justified at least as a therapeutic trial.

BIBLIOGRAPHY

1. Gardner-Thorpe, C. Muscle weakness due to sarcoid myopathy. Neurology *22:* 917–928, 1972.
2. Silverstein, A. and Siltzbach, L. E. Muscle involvement in sarcoidosis. Arch. Neurol. *21:* 235–241, 1969.
3. Douglas, A. C., Macleod, J. G., and Matthews, J. D. Symptomatic sarcoidosis of skeletal muscle. J. Neurol. Neurosurg. Psychiatry *36:* 1034–1040, 1973.
4. James, D. G. Modern concepts of sarcoidosis (Editorial). Chest *64:* 675–677, 1973.

OTHER INFLAMMATORY CONDITIONS

There are other conditions associated with inflammation of muscle. In some, the etiology is obscure. For example, some patients with an intestinal malabsorption syndrome and IgA deficiency have developed striking muscle weakness with facial and axial muscle involvement.[1] In other patients the inflammatory response is due to direct infection of the muscle by various organisms. Bacterial infections include those seen as part of miliary tuberculosis and with other organisms such as staphylococcus and streptococcus.

In tropical countries pyomyositis is not an uncommon disease. The affecting organism is often *Staphylococcus aureus* and usually the large muscle groups are involved, commonly those of the thigh. The muscle is hot, painful, and swollen, and activity is limited because any movement exacerbates the pain. Systemic signs of bacterial infection with fever and malaise are common. Treatment involves the use of the appropriate antibiotics and surgical drainage of the abscess.[2]

Parasitic infestations of muscle are also well known. The larvae of trichinella may find their way into human muscle after the ingestion of infected pork. General symptoms of malaise and fever are associated with muscle pains and stiffness. There may be periorbital edema. Involvement of the masseter muscles is common, with pain on attempting to open the jaw or on chewing. Skin rashes, petechial hemorrhages, and retinal hemorrhages have been noted. Subclinical infection is probably commoner than is realized, and recent estimates of the prevalence of trichinosis in the population are in the neighborhood of 4 per cent.[3] Laboratory studies, in addition to showing the presence of the parasite in the muscle biopsies may show accompanying evidence of hypersensitivity such as eosinophilia and hypergammaglobulinemia. Heavy infestation with the Trichinella may be fatal. Suggested treatment involves the administration of prednisone in doses of 60 mg. daily together with thiobendazole in doses of 50 mg. per kilogram per day for two weeks.[4]

Cysticercosis may also manifest itself as a disease of muscle. The encysted larvae of the tapeworms may present as a space occupying lesion with central nervous system complaints. Epilepsy is a common symptom. Muscle symptoms, which may be seen in association with neurological deficit or in isolation, include diffuse aches and pains and palpable nodules in the muscle. An unusual form is the pseudohypertrophic variety in which the muscle becomes massively enlarged.[5]

The association between toxoplasma infection and polymyositis has been postulated by some authors.[6, 7] The relationship is at best an indirect one since the organism was not found in the muscle. Serological evidence of a recent toxoplasma infection was more common in patients with a polymyositis like illness than in control groups of patients. Some reduction in the titers of antibodies to the organism followed treatment with pyrimethamine and sulfonamides. The clinical response to such treatment was not very striking.

Viral infections of muscle may be much commoner than is realized. It is possible that the diffuse aches and pains which so often accompany an attack of influenza actually represent viral inflammatory disease of the muscle. Severe muscle symptoms may also be present in viral infections. Acute muscle pains in the legs, especially of the calf muscles, have been associated with influenza B virus. Recovery usually takes place over a period of a week or so.[8] In another report, leg pain was associated with an infection by an echo virus. The muscle biopsy showed vacuolar degeneration and clinical examination showed mild proximal weakness. There was rapid resolution of these symptoms and a presumptive diagnosis of a viral myopathy was made.[9] Infection with coxsackie B virus is well known and may result in severe muscle pain.

An acute myositis bearing some of the hallmarks of a viral infection has been noted in young children, often following an upper respiratory infection. The illness is characterized by the rapid development of muscle pain usually in the leg. The pain is so severe that the child may scream at any attempted movement of the limb. The presence or absence of weakness is difficult to determine because the pain prevents adequate examination. Elevation of the serum CPK to levels of 1,000 to 3,000 IU is not uncommon. The disease abates spontaneously in two to three weeks. Extensive viral studies in 8 such patients showed no evidence of an infection.[10] Viral studies in two similar cases were also negative. In my experience, this illness tends to occur in clusters and when one patient arrives in the muscle clinic it is almost certain that three or four others will follow within two or three weeks.

BIBLIOGRAPHY

1. Carroll, J. E., Silvermann, A., Isobe, Y., Brown, W. R., Kelts, K. A., and Brooke, M. H. Inflammatory myopathy, IgA deficiency and intestinal malabsorption. Pediatrics *89:* 216–219, 1976.
2. Fett,J. D. Staphylococcal pyomyositis. Minn. Med. *56:* 724–725, 1973.
3. Zimmerman, W. J., Steele, J. H., and Kagan, I. G. Trichinosis in the U. S. population, 1966 to 1970. Pub. Health Rep. *88:* 607–623, 1973.
4. Davis, M. J., Cilo, M., Plaitakis, A., and Yahr, M. D. Trichinosis: Severe myopathic involvement with recovery. Neurology *26:* 37–40, 1976.

5. Sawhney, B. B., Chopra, J. S., Banerji, A. K., and Wahi, P. L. Pseudohypertrophic myopathy in cysticercosis. Neurology *26:* 270–272, 1976.

6. Kagen, L. J., Kimball, A. C., and Christian, C. L. Serological evidence of toxoplasmosis among patients with polymyositis. Am. J. Med. *56:* 186–191, 1974.

7. Samuels, B. C., and Rietschel, R. L. Polymyositis and toxoplasmosis. J.A.M.A. *235:* 60–61, 1976.

8. Dietzman, D. E., Schaller, J. G., Ray, C. G., and Reed, M. E. Acute myositis associated with influenza B infection. Pediatrics *57:* 255–258, 1976.

9. Marcus, J. C., and Bill, P. L. A. Acute myopathy in three brothers. Neuropaediatrie *7:* 101–110, 1976.

10. McKinlay, I. A., and Mitchell, I. Transient acute myositis in childhood. Arch. Dis. Child. *51:* 135–137, 1976.

MYOSITIS OSSIFICANS PROGRESSIVA

Ectopic calcification is seen in a variety of conditions. Abnormalities of parathyroid function, the late stages of polymyositis, an excessive intake of Vitamin D, and repeated trauma may all cause abnormal calcification. The disease myositis ossificans progressiva is set apart from these by a clinical picture which is so different as to be almost instantly recognizable. Although traditionally termed myositis, the illness is not truly one of muscle, but an ossification of the fascial planes, tendons, and aponeuroses. It is an extremely rare condition afflicting both sexes and probably inherited as an autosomal dominant with varying penetrance.

The lesions begin with an area of the muscle which becomes acutely hot, swollen, and tender. As this subsides, progressive ossification occurs over the subsequent weeks and the final result is a bony plaque which impedes the action of the muscle and results in a contracture (Figures 7.1 and 7.2). It is not clear why such bone formation occurs, but some events are clearly provocative. Thus, trauma to the muscle or a strain of the muscle is often followed by an area of ossification. One patient developed an extensive plaque of calcification in the area underlying a tuberculin skin test. The disease always commences in the first decade, usually within the first two years of life.

In a survey of a large number of cases,[1, 2] the muscles of the neck were the first affected in a quarter of the patients. The muscles of the paraspinal region, of the face, and of the shoulders and arms were the initial site of involvement in order of decreasing frequency. The hips and legs were not usually the location of early lesions. The muscles of the eyes, larynx, perineum, diaphragm, and tongue are said to be normal, and the heart is also fortunately spared.[3] As the disease progresses, deformities become increasingly severe and bony ankyloses extend across joints locking the limb into immobility. About the best that may be hoped for is that the limb freezes in a position in which it can still be used, but all too often this is not the case and useful function of the arms and legs is lost. Death, which is frequently due to respiratory embarrassment, is postponed until adult life. In the terminal stage the patient is completely immobile. Although this is an extraordinary and dramatic disease, it has not received more than passing attention in the medical literature. Perhaps this is due to its rarity. The first report is usually attributed to Patin, who mentioned in 1692 the case of a woman who became as "hard as wood." No one has had the temerity to cite Lot's wife as another early case.

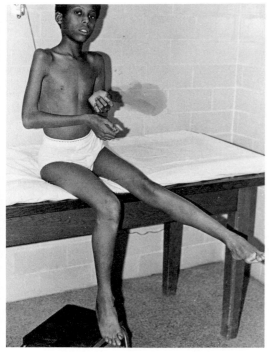 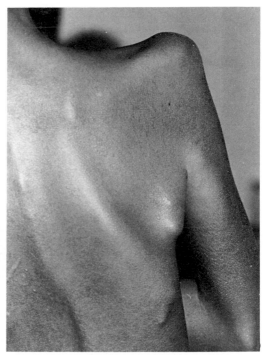

Figures 7.1 (*left*) and 7.2 (*right*). Myositis ossificans. This patient is fixed in the position shown (Figure 7.1) by bony bridges extending across the joints. These deposits of bone are easily palpable and often visible (Figure 7.2). Notice the shortened great toes.

The associated bony abnormalities are common enough to aid the diagnosis. Most of the patients have microdactyly or adactyly, especially of the big toe and thumb. The proximal phalanges may also be shortened. Other abnormalities which have been described are hallux valgus, exostoses, absent ear lobes, and spina bifida. Associated deafness has been reported, perhaps associated with ossification of the muscles of the inner ear.

The pathological changes are best described as centers of ossification occurring between fascicles or in association with tendons and aponeuroses. There are changes in the muscle itself, but these are nonspecific and may be secondary. A muscle biopsy is probably not a wise procedure in patients with myositis ossificans because such trauma to the muscle is almost always followed by ossification. Various medications have been used including steroids, EDTA, sodium citrate, and injections of parathyroid extract. None of these seems to have been of any value. Recently there has been some interest in the use of diphosphonate. This substance is related to pyrophosphate but is resistant to chemical and enzymatic hydrolysis. In experimental situations in animals it has been thought to prevent soft tissue calcification and reduce bone absorption. In higher doses it prevents the mineralization of the bone matrix. Sodium ethane 1-hydroxydiphosphonic acid (EHDP) or sodium etidronate has been used in myositis ossificans in doses of 20 mg. per kilogram of body weight per day. Some reports have suggested that the development of calcification was impeded[4] and have even suggested that some improvement has occurred while on the medication.[5] A more recent study failed to confirm this,[6] but it may be worthwhile trying this medication in a severe or rapidly progressive case.

There may also be a benign entity associated with ossification of a muscle. Four patients were reported in each of whom one area of ossification occurred which did not follow any provocative episodes.[7]

BIBLIOGRAPHY

1. Lutwak, L. Myositis ossificans progressiva. Am. J. Med. *37:* 269–293, 1964.
2. Illingworth, S. Myositis ossificans progressiva (Münchmeyers disease). Arch. Dis. Child. *46:* 264–268, 1971.
3. Simpson, A. J., and Friedman, S. Myositis ossificans progressiva. Mt. Sinai J. Med. N.Y. *38:* 416–422, 1971.
4. Russell, G. G., Smith, R., Bishop, M. C., Price, D. A., and Squire, C. M. Treatment of myositis ossificans progressiva with a diphosphonate. Lancet *1:* 10–12, 1972.
5. Weiss, I. W., Fisher, L., and Phang, J. M. Diphosphonate therapy in a patient with myositis ossificans progressiva. Ann. Intern. Med. *4:* 933–936, 1971.
6. Bland, J. H., Kirshbaum, B., O'Connor, G. T., and Horton, E. Myositis ossificans progressiva. Arch. Intern. Med. *132:* 209–212, 1973.
7. Samuelson, K. M., and Coleman, S. S. Nontraumatic myositis ossificans in healthy individuals. J.A.M.A. *235:* 1132–1133, 1976.

8 metabolic muscle diseases

There are various diseases, some of which are due to endocrine abnormalities and others of which are associated with known or postulated biochemical defects, that are referred to as the metabolic myopathies. Some, such as the endocrine myopathies and acid maltase deficiency, may produce fixed and even progressive muscle weakness. Others in which the energy supply of the muscle is deranged may present with fatigue on exercise, muscle cramps, and myoglobinuria.

GLYCOGEN STORAGE DISEASES

Not all the glycogen storage diseases will be considered in this section, only those in which the muscle involvement is a prominent part of the clinical picture.

Acid Maltase Deficiency (Pompe's Disease, Type 2 Glycogenosis)

Maltase (α-1,4-glucosidase) is an enzyme with widespread distribution in various tissues. Its activity varies with the pH, and this variation is compatible with the existence of two or possibly more forms. One, with a pH optimum of 4.5 to 5, is known as acid maltase. Although the biochemical activity of the enzyme is known, the specific function of maltase in the scheme of carbohydrate metabolism is not clearly understood. It is a lysosomal enzyme and its absence in the disease acid maltase deficiency is associated with the accumulation of glycogen in lysosomes as well as free in the tissue. The infantile variety of acid maltase deficiency was recognized some years ago. The children may be normal for a few weeks after birth but then develop severe hypotonia and enlargement of the heart, tongue, and liver owing to the accumulation of glycogen in these organs. The disease is inherited as an autosomal recessive. There may be some reduction in acid maltase levels in the muscle of the heterozygote carrier.[1] The disease is progressive; the children become intermittently cyanotic and usually die from either cardiac or respiratory failure before one year of age.

Although there is some overlap, a milder form of the illness is seen in patients whose symptoms begin in infancy or early childhood but whose decline is much slower. Many of these patients survive for several years, although not beyond the second decade.[2] A proximal weakness develops, and the muscles may feel firm or rubbery. This makes it difficult to distinguish the disease clinically from Duchenne's muscular dystrophy, a problem which is compounded by a tendency to develop ankle contractures. Some patients may have no enlargement of the tongue, liver, or heart; others show variable involvement of these organs.

The adult variety of acid maltase deficiency begins later and the hereditary basis of the illness is uncertain.[1-3] It may be an autosomal recessive and familial cases have been reported.[4] A proximal weakness is noted, greater in the hips than in the shoulders. The heart and liver are not abnormal, and only one patient has been described with enlargement of the tongue. A clue to the diagnosis may be in the involvement of the respiratory muscles. In general the illness resembles limb girdle dystrophy or polymyositis, but severe respiratory involvement is unusual in these two conditions. Patients may have frankly anoxic symptoms from their respiratory weakness before the hip weakness presents a major problem. Part of this respiratory difficulty may result from an insensitivity of the respiratory center to hypoxic stimulation since we have found a marked decrease in hypoxic ventilatory drive in one patient.[5]

The diagnosis rests with the laboratory studies. There is often mild elevation of the serum "muscle" enzymes. The EMG shows irritable muscles with high frequency repetitive potentials and myotonia. This is more pronounced in the infantile variety. In the adult form, electromyographic changes may be restricted to the paraspinal muscles or other truncal muscles. Clinical myotonia is usually absent. The muscle biopsy shows a striking vacuolar myopathy. With histochemical stains, the vacuoles are acid phosphatase positive and large amounts of glycogen are present. Electron microscopic studies show glycogen in membrane bound packets as well as lying free in the tissue.

The acid maltase activity in muscle is lacking in all the varieties of this disease. Interestingly, there is no difference in the enzyme activity of muscles which are severely affected and those which are relatively spared. Even in those with a normal histologic appearance the enzyme is deficient. An increase of glycogen content accompanies the vauolar changes. The glycogen appears to be of normal structure except in occasional cases where reduction in the length of the outer chain is noted. In the infantile form all muscles show vacuolar changes.

In view of the difference in severity, one might expect some differences in the biochemistry of the three types of illness. Acid maltase is absent in the infantile and childhood varieties. In the adult disease very small amounts of lysosomal enzyme are present.[6] It has been suggested that neutral maltase may be responsible for some of the differences. The latter enzyme is decreased in both liver and muscle of patients with the infantile variety but not in the adult form of the illness. Perhaps its activity compensates in part for that of the absent acid maltase.[7] In the childhood form, neutral maltase is normal in the muscle and in the heart but decreased in the liver.

Acid maltase activity has also been studied in the urine and found to be reduced. Heterozygote carriers also show a reduction in urinary enzyme activity and this fact may be of great importance in genetic counseling.[8] Some reduction of acid maltase activity was noticed in leukocytes. It has also been suggested that a decrease in the ratio of acid maltase to neutral maltase may be helpful in the diagnosis of adult acid maltase deficiency. This is one of the few illnesses in which the enzyme defect has been reproduced in tissue culture, suggesting that it is a true primary myopathy.[9]

EKG studies are abnormal in the infantile variety; there is a depression of the ST segment with inversion of the T-waves. There may be giant QRS complexes, and the PR interval is usually shortened.

In an illness marked by accumulation of glycogen and in which the usual degradative pathways are preserved, attempts to mobilize tissue glycogen with epinephrine injections and to limit the intake of dietary carbohydrates are worthwhile. Unfortunately, the results obtained with this treatment over a period of years were something less than dramatic, although possible benefit was obtained in two adults.[2]

BIBLIOGRAPHY

1. Engel, A. G., and Gomez, M. R. Acid maltase levels in heterozygous acid maltase deficiency and in non-weak and neuromuscular disease controls. J. Neurol. Neurosurg. Psychiatry *33:* 801–804, 1970.
2. Engel, A. G., Gomez, M. R, Seybold, M. E., and Lambert, E. H. The spectrum and diagnosis of acid maltase deficiency. Neurology *23:* 95–106, 1073.
3. Hudgson, P., and Fulthorpe, J. J. The pathology of type II skeletal muscle glycogenosis. J. Pathol. *116:* 139–147, 1975.
4. Martin, J. J., deBarsy, T., and den Tandt, W. R. Acid maltase deficiency in non-identical twins; a morphological and biochemical study. J. Neurol. *213:* 105–118, 1976.
5. Carroll, J., and Brooke, M. H. Unpublished observations.
6. Mehler, M., and Di Mauro, S. Residual acid maltase activity in late onset acid maltase deficiency. Neurology *27:* 178–184, 1977
7. Angelini, C., and Engel, A. G. Comparative study of acid maltase deficiency: Biochemical difference between childhood and adult types. Arch. Neurol. *26:* 344–349, 1972.
8. Mehler, J., and Di Mauro, S. Late onset acid maltase deficiency. Arch. Neurol. *33:* 692–695, 1976.
9. Askanas, V., Engel, W. K., Di Mauro, S., Brooks, B. R., and Mehler, M. Adult-onset acid maltase deficiency. New Engl. J. Med. *294:* 573–578, 1976.

Amylo-1,6-glucosidase Deficiency (Debrancher Deficiency, Type 3 Glycogenosis)

An autosomal recessively inherited deficiency of this enzyme is associated with hepatomegaly and a failure to thrive in the first year of life. Frequently, the children are floppy and have poor head control.[1] They are mentally unimpaired. The enzyme deficit is associated with the deposition of glycogen in liver, striated muscle, and, to a lesser extent, cardiac muscle. Although in the majority the enzyme is lacking in all tissues, it is occasionally detected in muscle or in both liver and muscle of a few patients. The patient may slowly improve and the liver may return to normal size by adolescence, but the enzymatic abnormality persists. Why the disease should improve when the enzyme deficit remains unchanged is not known. There are scattered reports of patients with Type 3 glycogenosis who develop muscular weakness. One man presented with an eight month history of distal weakness and wasting beginning at the age of 43.[2] There was a preceding story of muscle fatigue and weakness associated with pain, but this was insubstantial. On clinical examination the disorder resembled a motor neuron disease. A slightly different clinical picture was seen in an 18 year old patient whose muscle symptoms were those of fatigue, stiffness, and weakness of the leg muscles, a picture compounded by a history of gouty arthritis.[3] Other laboratory tests may also be of value. A diabetic glucose tolerance curve, fasting hypoglycemia, and a lack of response of the serum glucose to epinephrine or glucagon are to be expected. The glycogen content of tissues is increased, and the glycogen has an abnormal structure with short outer chains. There may be no increase in serum lactate levels after ischemic exercise. Serum "muscle" enzymes are often abnormal, which is not surprising in view of the great distortion of the muscle architecture. The fibers are disrupted by a large number of glycogen filled vacuoles.

EMG findings in this disease show changes similar to those seen in acid maltase deficiency. There are high frequency repetitive discharges resembling myotonia.

BIBLIOGRAPHY

1. Swaiman, K. F., and Wright, F. S. *The Practice of Pediatric Neurology*. C. V. Mosby, St. Louis, 1975.
2. Brunberg, J. A., McCormick, W. F., and Schochet, S. S. Type III glycogenosis: an adult with diffuse weakness and muscle wasting. Arch. Neurol. *25:* 171–178, 1971.
3. Murase, T., Ikada, H., Muro, T., Nakao, K., and Sugita, H. Myopathy associated with Type 3 glycogenosis. J. Neurol. Sci. *20:* 287–295, 1973.

Amylo-1,4- to -1,6-transglucosidase Deficiency (Brancher Enzyme Deficiency, Type 4 Glycogenosis)

This illness generally causes a failure to thrive, hepatosplenomegaly, and liver failure. Inheritance is as an autosomal recessive. Respiratory muscle and skeletal muscles are affected, but only rarely are muscular symptoms a prominent part of the picture. In one case a child with this illness was thought to have Werdnig-Hoffmann disease on clinical grounds.[1] She was born with hip dislocations, had a poor sucking response, hypotonia, and severe atrophy. Her muscles were scarcely able to move the limbs against gravity, and reflexes were absent. Serum creatine phosphokinase was normal. Hepatosplenomegaly and ascites developed, and the child died in the 2nd year from cardiorespiratory failure. Widespread deposits of amylopectin were found at post mortem.

The enzyme is absent not only in the muscle but also in the peripheral white blood cells. Cultured fibroblasts are also deficient in the enzyme in the patients and in their parents.

BIBLIOGRAPHY

1. Zellweger, H., Mueller, S., Ionasescu, V., Schochet, S. S., and McCormick, W. F. Glycogenosis IV: A new cause of infantile hypotonia. J. Pediatr. *80:* 842–844, 1972.

Myophosphorylase Deficiency (McArdle's Disease, Type 5 Glycogenosis)

The patient with this illness suffers from an inability to break down glycogen, owing to a defect in myophosphorylase.[1-3] Because of this the patient is unable to utilize glycogen as a source of energy when it becomes necessary for heavy work loads or in conditions of ischemia. The illness is inherited as an autosomal recessive or rarely as an autosomal dominant.[4] It is commoner in the male than female. Usually before the child is ten years old, he starts to complain of fatigue and an inability to keep up with others of his age. There may be mild aching in the legs, but this symptom is often noted for the first time in early adolescence. It then becomes increasingly severe and may be provoked by anything more than the mildest exertion.

Often at some stage in teen-age life, a particularly heavy bout of exercise will be accompanied by painful cramps in the muscles which have been used. These pains will last for several hours, even overnight, and the patient may notice that his urine becomes the color of a Burgundy because of the attendant myoglobinuria. At a stage when muscle pain becomes severe, the patient's activity may be severely curtailed and walking the length of a city block is arduous. A muscle that is exercised hard enough to produce a cramp becomes shortened and cannot be stretched passively without producing severe pain. As the years progress, with repeated bouts of muscle pain, a permanent weakness of the proximal muscles may be found. An unusual presentation with neither fatigue, cramps, nor myoglobinuria but merely a gradual progressive proximal weakness beginning in adult life has also been described.[5]

Quite early in the disease, patients notice their exercise tolerance may increase enormously if they slow down immediately upon the initial sensation of muscle fatigue. When they then resume exercise at a slow rate, they experience a "second wind" as does a long distance runner. Many patients with McArdle's disease are able to tell exactly when this occurs and can exercise for long periods of time at a rate which would have totally disabled them if attempted initially. One patient referred to this as a "barrier" and said that initial exercise was accompanied by a sense of laboring and tightness in the muscle, but once the barrier was broken, he had a sense of ease and relaxation and could exercise for as long as he wished. Patients may also notice a rapid acceleration of heart rate and of breathing with the beginning of exercise. In spite of the tachycardia there is only rarely evidence of cardiac abnormality.[6] Since the absence of the enzyme is limited to muscle, no other organs suffer from the primary effects of the disease. Secondary involvement of the kidney and even acute renal failure may be seen after myoglobinuria.[7, 8] Most patients are aware of the amount of exercise which can produce this degree of damage and assiduously avoid situations which might demand it.

Initial examination of the patient reveals little untoward. There is no apparent wasting; indeed, some patients are unusually muscular. Weakness is detected only in the older patients, and the reflexes are all normal. The ischemic exercise test is markedly abnormal. It is to be emphasized that ischemic tests in patients with McArdle's disease and some of the other abnormalities of glycolysis are not benign tests. The contracture and the pain that are produced are indicative of muscle damage, and occasionally frank myoglobinuria may be produced. Although it is vital to employ this test in the diagnosis, it should not be used in frivolous demonstrations. When the forearm muscles are exercised ischemically they fatigue rapidly, within one or two minutes; the pattern of this fatigue is quite abnormal. In the average person, such fatigue ensues after five or six minutes and, if exercise is continued until the hand is paralyzed, the muscles of the forearm are completely limp. The wrist and fingers can be moved passively without any resistance. In the patient with McArdle's disease, as the paralysis occurs, the muscles become increasingly tight and the wrist becomes fixed in flexion with the fingers gripped firmly around the dynamometer or whatever object is being used in the exercise. The wrist and fingers cannot then be passively straightened but remain locked in an iron grip. This is a true contracture, since placement of an EMG needle in the tightened muscles reveals no electrical activity whatsoever.

The chemical accompaniment of this is the absence of rise in lactate levels in the venous blood from the exercised forearm. Ordinarily, the breakdown of glycogen which is provoked under ischemic conditions results in the production of lactate. Since it is impossible for the patient to break down glycogen, no lactate is produced. With a little planning it is possible to carry out a single ischemic exercise test and combine the clinical, electrical, and biochemical studies (and perhaps even grand rounds!). This avoids the necessity of repeated ischemic tests.

Munsat[9] has suggested a standardized forearm ischemic exercise test which has proved useful. A catheter is placed in a superficial vein and a cuff around the upper arm is inflated to a level above systolic pressure. The patient is then asked to grip an ergometer or dynamometer repetitively at about 60 strokes per minute sufficient to produce a work load of four to seven kilograms per meter. The test was found to be reliable as long as work exceeded four kilograms per meter. After one minute the exercise is stopped and the cuff is deflated. In addition to a resting sample obtained before the test, the venous blood is collected at 1, 3, 5, 10, and 20 minute intervals after the cessation of work. The peak lactate level occurs in normals at about 3 minutes and should be 3 to 5 times normal. In patients with McArdle's disease, as with some of the other enzyme deficiencies mentioned below, there is no rise in the lactate level.

The exact diagnosis depends on the estimation of phosphorylase activity in the muscle. This can be accomplished either histochemically or, more reliably, biochemically. Other laboratory studies which may be abnormal are the serum "muscle" enzymes, which, as in any disease which damages muscles, can be quite elevated. Myoglobin may be found in the urine. The muscle biopsy shows subsarcolemmal glycogen and scattered necrotic fibers.

Experimental investigations in patients with McArdle's disease have therapeutic implications. The marked tachycardia which is found on exercise is not an indication of cardiac damage but of the response of the cardiovascular system to unusual changes in the vascular bed or other abnormal vasoregulatory responses. In one patient, if exercise were sufficient to increase oxygen uptake to greater than 60% of the maximal value, the heart rate became maximal after two minutes. The administration of glucose tended to lessen this abnormality.[10] The "second wind" phenomenon occurred only if the initial blood flow on resuming exercise was more than thrice the normal resting level.

An early investigation into the second wind phenomenon suggested that it was associated with a change in the free fatty acid supply to the muscle. This would be logical, since the only alternate source of energy for the muscle other than carbohydrate is derived from fat.[11] Other investigators, while noting the mobilization of free fatty acids which is associated with the "second wind", suggested that the phenomenon was more closely associated with change in the blood flow to the muscle.[12] While they found that the "second wind" was usually associated with a rise in free fatty acids and that the tolerance to exercise was reduced by nicotinic acid (a drug that blocks the release of free fatty acids and glycerol from fat) and increased by isoproterenol and norepinephrine (which increase the free fatty acid levels), they noted an unusual effect with forearm exercise. With hand exercise a local "second wind" occurred only in the muscles being exercised. If the "second wind" is truly associated with the arterial level of free fatty acids it would be a general phenomenon and not one localized to the exercised muscle.

The exercise tolerance of patients has been augmented by the intravenous infusion of glucose and the oral administration of fructose. The sublingual administration of isoproterenol has also been recommended. None of these measures seems to be of universal therapeutic value. Although occasional patients are helped by sublingual isoproterenol, most find the side effects more troublesome than the disease. Honey, which is rich in fructose, has been given to patients but, again, without notable success.

Initially the statement was made that the disease is due to a defect in the enzyme myophosphorylase. It is fitting to conclude the section by pointing out how inexact our knowledge of this is. Phosphorylase exists in two forms, the active form, phosphorylase *a* which is a dimer, and the inactive tetramer phosphorylase *b*.[13] The conversion of phosphorylase *b* to *a* takes place under the influence of phosphorylase kinase. This enzyme is itself activated by a protein kinase, and the protein kinase is activated by cyclic AMP which is produced under the influence of adenyl cyclase. There is thus a cascading series of reactions, and a defect in any one of these might result in an absence of phosphorylase activity. One therefore cannot assume that absence of the activity implies an absence of the enzyme. In this regard, patients have been described without detectable phosphorylase activity who yet had a protein in the muscle which cross-reacted with antibody to normal phosphorylase, suggesting an inactive enzyme.[8] Similar evidence was presented in another case, although a small amount of enzymatic activity was detected.[7] Two different molecular etiologies for the same disease are also suggested by the finding of some patients with McArdle's disease in whom a protein was detectable resembling the phosphorylase protein but without enzyme activity. In other patients, no such protein was detected.[14] It is also possible that the enzyme is inactive because of some inhibitory factor. Muscle fibers cultured from a patient with McArdle's disease were found to demonstrate phosphorylase activity in culture conditions even though the patient from whom they were derived had no detectable activity.[15]

The cause of the contracture which occurs in McArdle's disease is not known. It was suggested that calcium uptake by sarcoplasm reticulum might be impaired leading to prolonged contractures.[16] Other studies have shown no abnormality in such function.[17]

BIBLIOGRAPHY

1. McArdle, B. Myopathy due to a defect in muscle glycogen breakdown. Clin. Sci. *10:* 13–33, 1951.
2. Schmid, R., and Mahler, R. Chronic progressive myopathy with myoglobinuria; demonstration of a glycogenolytic defect in the muscle. J. Clin. Invest. *38:* 2044–2058, 1959.
3. Mommaerts, W. F. H. M., Illingworth, B., Peason, C. M., Geuillory, P. J., and Seraydar-

ian, K. A functional disorder associated with the absence of phosphorylase. Proc. Nat. Acad. Sci. *45:* 791–797, 1959.

4. Chui, L. A., and Munsat, T. L. Dominant inheritance of McArdle syndrome. Arch. Neurol. *33:* 636–641, 1976.

5. Engel, W. K., Eyerman, E. L., and Williams, H. E. Late onset type of skeletal msucle phosphorylase deficiency. N. Engl. J. Med. *268:* 135–141, 1963.

6. Ratinov, G., Baker, W. P., and Swaimam, K. F. McArdle's syndrome with previously unreported electrocardiographic and serum enzyme abnormalities. Ann. Intern. Med. *62:* 328–334, 1965.

7. Grunfeld, J. P., Ganeval, D., Chanard, J., Fardeau, M., and Dreyfus, J. C. Acute renal failure in McArdle's disease. N. Engl. J. Med. *286:* 1237–1241, 1972.

8. Bank, W. J., DiMauro, S., Rowland, L. P., and Milestone, R. Heterozygotes in muscle phosphorylase deficiency. Trans. Am. Neurol. Assoc. *97:* 179–181, 1972.

9. Munsat, T. L. A standardized forearm ischemic exercise test. Neurology *20:* 1171–1178, 1970.

10. Andersen, K. L., Lund-Johansen, B., and Clausen, G. Metabolic and circulatory responses to muscular exercise in a subject with glycogen storage disease (McArdle's disease). Scan. J. Clin. Lab. Invest. *24:* 105–113, 1969.

11. Porte, D., Crawford, D. W., Jennings, D. B., Aber, C., and McIlroy, M. B. Cardiovascular and metabolic responses to exercise in a patient with McArdle's syndrome. N. Engl. J. Med. *275:* 406–412, 1966.

12. Pernow, B. B., Havel, R. J., and Jennings, D. B The second wind phenomenon in McArdle's syndrome. Acta Med. Scand. Suppl. *472:* 294–307, 1967.

13. Howell, R. R. The glycogen storage diseases. In: *The Metabolic Basis of Inherited Disease*, 3rd edition, edited by J. B. Stanbury, J. B. Wyngaarden, and D. S. Fredrickson. McGraw-Hill, New York, 1972, pp. 149–173.

14. Feit, H., and Brooke, M. H. Myophosphorylase deficiency: Two different molecular etiologies. Neurology, *26:* 963–967, 1976.

15. Roelofs, R. L., Engel, W. K., and Shauvin, P. B. Histochemical phosphorylase activity in regenerating muscle fibers from myophosphorylase deficiency patients. Science 177: 795–797, 1972.

16. Gruener, R., McArdle, B., Ryman, B. E., and Weller, R. D. Contracture of phosphorylase deficient muscle. J. Neurol. Neurosurg. Psychiatry *31:* 268, 1968.

17. Brody, I. A., Gerber, C. T., and Sidbury, J. B. Relaxing factor in McArdle's disease: calcium uptake by sarcoplasmic reticulum. Neurology *20:* 555–558, 1970.

Phosphofructokinase Deficiency (Type 7 Glycogenosis)

The enzyme phosphofructokinase (PFK) is responsible for the phosphorylation of fructose 6-phosphate to fructose 1:6-diphosphate, a reaction which is essential in the glycolytic process. It is one of the rate limiting steps, and the control of glycolysis by aerobic metabolism may be brought about by regulating the activity of PFK. The absence of this enzyme is associated with an illness which closely resembles phosphorylase deficiency for the obvious reason that the defect is in the same chain of metabolic reactions. The patients have almost identical symptoms, with early onset of fatigue and aching pains in the muscles. With more strenuous exertion, severe pains, contractures of the muscles and myoglobinuria occur. Most patients experience occasional episodes of nausea and vomiting, an attack which is not common with McArdle's disease.[1–3] The pattern of inheritance, as with many of the glycogenoses, is autosomal recessive.

The laboratory investigations show changes similar to those found in phosphorylase deficiency. There is no rise in lactate production with ischemic exercise, the creatine phosphokinase may be abnormal, and the muscle biopsy may show subsarcolemmal "blebs" which contain glycogen. The histochemical reaction for phosphorylase is preserved, but the phosphofructoki-nase reaction is absent.[4] Immunological studies failed to show a muscle protein which cross-reacted with normal PFK, failing to support the hypothesis that the deficiency of enzyme activity might be due to an inert protein.[2] In addition to the absence of muscle PFK, the enzyme is deficient in erythrocytes, which contain only about half the normal quantities. PFK is composed of subunits which combine to form an active tetramer. Muscle phosphofructokinase is composed of identical (M) subunits, whereas that of the erythrocyte contains two dissimilar kinds of subunits, M, which is identical to that in muscle, and R. The latter subunits are intact, explaining the residual amount of activity in the erythrocytes of patients with phosphofructokinase deficiency.

BIBLIOGRAPHY

1. Tarui, S., Okuno, G., and Ikura, Y. Phosphofructokinase deficiency in skeletal muscle; a new type of glycogenosis. Biochem. Biophys. Res. Commun. *19:* 517–523, 1965.
2. Layzer, R. B., Rowland, L. P., and Ranney, H. M. Muscle phosphofructokinase deficiency. Arch. Neurol. *17:* 512–523, 1967.
3. Tobin, W. E., Huijing, F., Porro, R. S., and Salzman, R. T. Muscle phosphofructokinase deficiency. Arch. Neurol. *28:* 128–130, 1973.
4. Bonilla E., and Schotland, D. L. Histochemical diagnosis of muscle phosphofructokinase deficiency. Arch. Neurol. *22:* 8–12, 1970.

Other Abnormalities of Carbohydrate Metabolism

Satoyoshi and Kowa[1] described a family, members of which had muscle pains and stiffness which were generally more troublesome in adult life than in childhood. The symptoms were provoked by exercise and especially prominent during rest or sleep. There were no abnormalities on examination other than tenderness and stiffness of the muscles after exercise. With the ischemic exercise test no contractures were seen although the normal elevation of lactate in such a test was absent. The authors postulated a defect of phos-phohexoisomerase, although when this enzyme was assayed it was found to be normal. The phosphofructokinase activity was reduced to about half. A beneficial effect was thought to be seen with the oral administration of fructose.[1]

BIBLIOGRAPHY

1. Satoyoshi, E., and Kowa, H. A myopathy due to glycolytic abnormality. Arch. Neurol. *17:* 248–256, 1967.

DISORDERS OF LIPID METABOLISM

At rest and during prolonged exercise, free fatty acids provide a major portion of the energy supply to muscle. Fatty acids are characterized by the length of the chains in the carbon "skeleton". Long chain fatty acids such as palmitic and oleic are predominantly released from stored fat, particularly in the fasting state. Thus, during a fast or during prolonged exercise, the mobilization of free fatty acids and their oxidation in muscle is a vital part of the energy supply. Such oxidation takes place within the mitochondria, but the fatty acids are unable to pass across the mitochondrial membrane unless they are first coupled to carnitine, which acts as a shuttle. Carnitine palmityl transferase is the enzyme which effects the combination. There are actually two such enzymes: Type I, which is situated on the outer surface of the inner mitochondrial membrane, and Type II, which is on the inner surface. This is represented in diagrammatic form in Figure 8.1. Carnitine seems to be present in insufficient quantities in the normal diet to provide the body's needs. It is synthesized in the liver from other precursors and then transported to the muscle. There are two known defects in lipid metabolism which cause neuromuscular disease, and probably several others which will come to light in the near future.

Carnitine Palmityl Transferase Deficiency

Two brothers were described with recurrent bouts of myoglobinuria which commenced in their teens.[1] In one there was a history of muscle cramps associated with fatigue; the other was without pain although he did have some stiffness of exercised muscles. Both had episodes of renal failure presumably due to myoglobinuria. The patients were especially likely to experience symptoms if they had been without food for some time and then undertook some prolonged exercise. Physical examination showed no weakness or other neuromuscular changes, and ischemic contractures, such as are noted in phosphorylase deficiency, were not found. Neither had to limit his activities

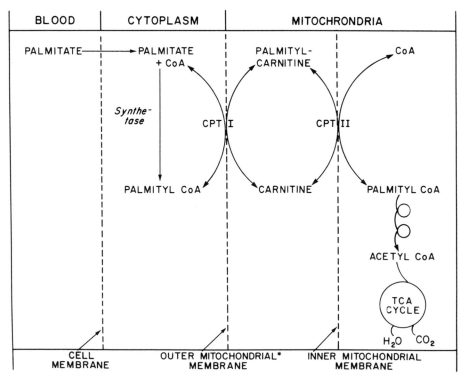

Figure 8.1. Oxidation of palmitate in muscle. (Reproduced by kind permission of Dr. D. DeVivo.)

* Recent work suggests that CPT I is located on the outer surface of the inner mitochondrial membrane.

because of the symptoms of fatigue, and both were of normal athletic ability. The major abnormality in the serum was an elevation of cholesterol and of triglycerides, with an increase of the β and pre-β lipoproteins. The serum muscle enzymes were normal unless provocative tests such as prolonged fasting were performed, when there was a rise in creatine phosphokinase associated with myoglobin in the urine. Urinary ketone bodies were only barely detectable by the third day of the fast although these compounds appeared in the plasma on the third day of fasting. Muscle biopsy showed no abnormality under the light microscope with either routine or histochemical reactions. The electron microscope revealed minor abnormalities with some non-membrane bound material of low electron density. Biochemically the muscle had normal levels of glycogen and of phosphorylase and phosphofructokinase activity. The amount of carnitine in the muscle was more than usual but carnitine palmityl transferase was markedly diminished in both patients. The ischemic exercise test caused a normal rise in lactate levels. There was a prompt rise in plasma acetoacetate after triglycerides containing medium chain (8 to 10 carbon) fatty acids were administered, suggesting that medium chain and short chain fatty acids could be be metabolized. The persistently elevated triglycerides and an anomalous response in which a dramatic increase of triglycerides occurred after fasting were thought to be secondary to the impaired ability of muscle to metabolize the fatty acids. Thus, during fasting, the fatty acids were mobilized normally but instead of being used appropriately by muscle, the plasma surplus was disposed of by the liver with the consequent formation of triglycerides.

BIBLIOGRAPHY

1. Bank, W. J., DiMauro, S., Bonilla, E., Capuzzi, D. M., and Rowland, L. P. A disorder of muscle lipid metabolism and myoglobinuria: Absence of carnitine palmityl transferase. N. Engl. J. Med. *292:* 443–448, 1975.

Carnitine Deficiency

There have been several recent reports of an illness in which muscle carnitine is absent or diminished. The number of cases described has been too few to draw any firm conclusions, but in general the disease seems to be marked by a slowly progressive weakness, superimposed upon which are sudden exacerbations.[1,2] Thus Engel and Siekert described a 24 year old woman who had never been able to sit up from the supine position without using her hands and who slept with her eyes slightly open. At the age of 18 she had a sudden exacerbation and was confined to bed by her weakness. At the same time she developed a nasal voice and in addition to the proximal weakness of shoulders and hips had weakness of her face, palate, and neck and poor esophageal motility.[1] Another example was a young boy who had always been somewhat clumsy with a "floppy" head.[3] At the age of 11 his weakness progressed so that within months he was no longer able to walk to school. Most of the patients have noted some symptoms in childhood. The single exception was a 61 year old woman afflicted since the age of 38 with progressive weakness of the legs and arms, both proximal and distal.[4] In general, the weakness is of the limb girdle more than of distal muscles and there is greater involvement of facial and jaw muscles than in many of the other varieties of proximal muscle disease. A common symptom is weakness of the neck with loss of proper head control.[1, 3, 5, 6] The head may bob around in an unsupported fashion while the patient walks. Also noted in the history are convulsions or syncope which may be associated with evidence of abnormalities in liver function[1, 7] and which in one patient was tentatively diagnosed as Reye's syndrome.[3] In one there was additional evidence of CNS abnormality with deafness, basal ganglia calcification, elevated spinal fluid protein, and a mildly abnormal EEG.[7] Mental retardation has not been a prominent part of the picture. Only one patient had some difficulties at school and was given remedial training.[3] His formal I.Q. was 99.

Physical examination shows the weakness and wasting in the distribution mentioned. Atrophy of the temporal and masseter muscles has been described. The deep tendon reflexes are usually decreased to absent. The patients may be frail and small for their age. Two patients have had palpably enlarged liver,[3, 7] and in another the liver was tender to palpation. Laboratory studies may include either normal or slightly elevated levels of creatine phosphokinase. The EMG is "myopathic" or demonstrates hyperirritability. In one patient conduction velocity was decreased in the peroneal nerve, which was thought to represent evidence of a neuropathic component. This patient also had diabetes and was rather atypical, if atypical is the right word to use in such a small series of patients.[4]

The disease may have a hereditary basis, since reduced carnitine levels were found in the muscles of both parents of one patient, although abnormalities in the muscle biopsy of these parents were not seen.[5] EKG abnormalities have also been described in one patient.[5] The muscle biopsy may give a clue to the diagnosis since it is markedly abnormal, with myriads of lipid droplets scattered throughout the fibers. This change affects Type 1 fibers more than Type 2 but is not exclusive. Other evidence of abnormalities in lipid metabolism is rather scanty. The serum free fatty acids were markedly elevated in one patient; plasma cholesterol, triglycerides, and carnitine may be present in normal qualtities,[5] although decreased levels of serum carnitine have been recorded. Unlike the findings in other varieties of lipid abnormalities, ketone bodies were present after a 16-hour fast.[5] In the muscle, the level of carnitine is markedly reduced to around one-tenth of the normal value. Metabolic studies of the forearm[3] showed that long chain fatty acids were not utilized by the muscle, although there was excessive glucose uptake. Treatment of patients with prednisone has been associated with improvement, and in recent reports[3, 6, 7] the administration of carnitine caused quite marked improvement even though the levels of muscle carnitine were not changed in one patient. The disease may involve more than just the muscle. There is evidence that the liver suffers the effects of carnitine deficiency in some but not all patients. Vacuoles have been described in the leukocytes and Schwann cells of the patient with the onset in later life.

BIBLIOGRAPHY

1. Engel, A. G, and Siekert, F. G. Lipid storage myopathy response to prednisone. Arch. Neurol. *27:* 174–181, 1972.

2. Engel, A. G., and Angelini, C. Carnitine deficiency of human skeletal muscle with associated lipid storage myopathy: A new syndrome. Science *173:* 899–902, 1973.

3. Karpati, G., Carpenter, S., Engel, A. G., Watters, G., Allen, J., Rothmann, S., Klassen, G., and Mamer, O. A. The syndrome of systemic carnitine deficiency. Neurology *25:* 16–24, 1975.

4. Markesbery, W. R., McQuillen, M. P., Procopis, E. G., Harrison, A. R., and Engel, A. G. Muscle carnitine deficiency, association with lipid myopathy, vacuolar neuropathy and vacuolated leukocytes. Arch. Neurol. *31:* 320–324, 1974.

5. Van Dyke, D. H., Griggs, R. C., Markesbery, W., and DiMauro, S. Hereditary carnitine deficiency of muscle. Neurology *25:* 154–159, 1975.

6. Angelini, C. Carnitine deficiency. Lancet *2:* 1151, 1975.

7. Smyth, D. P. L., Lake, B. D., MacDermot, J., and Wilson, J. Inborn error of carnitine metabolism (carnitine deficiency) in man. Lancet *1:* 1198–1199, 1975.

Other Abnormalities of Lipid Metabolism

Another illness characterized by the deposition of lipid in muscle fibers was described by Engel et al.[1] Eighteen year old identical twin girls had aching of the muscles with cramps since childhood. These were occasionally severe and sometimes associated with myoglobinuria. The pains could come on at any time of the day or night and were often related to some preceding exercise hours before. The discomfort lasted for several hours to several days. Neither weakness nor wasting was noticed, and no other abnormality was found. Ischemic exercise tests showed a normal rise in lactate. The symptoms were made worse by a 60 hour fast, during which time the serum creatine phosphokinase (CPK) and other "muscle" enzymes became abnormal. Additionally, the patients failed to produce ketone bodies in the urine during this fast, in contrast to normal controls in whom the production of ketone bodies occurred within 36 hours of fasting. The plasma cholesterol was normal and the triglycerides were at the lower limits of normal. The lipoprotein pattern was also unchanged. When the patients were fed triglycerides containing medium chain fatty acids, there was not only some amelioration of the symptoms but ketone bodies were readily produced. The possible relationship of this illness to one of the preceding is not settled. Clinically, these girls resemble the patient with carnitine palmityl transferase (CPT) deficiency but the normal triglycerides, free fatty acids, and lipoprotein pattern suggest that the etiology is somehow different. There were also increased deposits of lipid in the muscle as opposed to the relatively normal biopsy seen in CPT deficiency. The history is somewhat different from those patients with carnitine deficiency, and ketone bodies were present in patients with carnitine deficiency after 16 hours of fasting.[2] Undoubtedly, however, the defect in this illness must lie somewhere along the pathway of lipid metabolism.

That lipid storage myopathy can occur with normal carnitine palmityl transferase and carnitine is suggested by a case reported by Jerusalem et al.[3] They describe a 28 year old woman with periods of weakness and easy fatigability from infancy. There were some feeding difficulties during the first year of her life, with possible retardation of growth. She had no muscle pains but on examination had slight muscle weakness of the neck and of the proximal muscles of the arms and legs. She used her hands for support in getting up from a sitting position. Deep tendon reflexes were decreased. There was no enlargement of the liver, and blood tests were normal including serum CPK. Some deposition of lipid was noted in the muscle fibers although, to judge from the photographs, this was much less than in other cases. Carnitine and carnitine palmityl transferase values were within normal limits.

Other patients have also been described with deposition of lipid in the muscle fibers. A selective proximal weakness was seen in a 23 year old woman. This seemed to have an episodic course, and there was spontaneous improvement of an attack without any specific therapy. The first attack lasted a few weeks and the second, which began a year later, lasted about two and a half years. She failed to respond to prednisone during one attack. The amount of triglyceride in the muscle was three times the normal level.[4]

Johnson et al.[5] described a 38 year old man with fatigue and proximal weakness who also had weakness of his neck muscles. He was originally thought to have polymyositis. The EMG showed myopathic potentials. The deep tendon reflexes were diminished. Chemical evaluation showed increased cholesterol and slightly elevated levels of triglycerides. Lipoprotein electrophoresis showed an increase in the β-lipoprotein. The patient did well with steroids. Neither carnitine nor carnitine-palmityl transferase was assayed.[5]

BIBLIOGRAPHY

1. Engel, W. K., Vick, N. A., Glueck, C. J., and Levy, R. I. A skeletal muscle disorder associated with intermittent symptoms and a possible defect of lipid metabolism. N. Engl. J. Med. *282:* 697–704, 1970.
2. Van Dyke, D. H., Griggs, R. C., Markesbery, W., and DiMauro, S. Hereditary carnitine deficiency of muscle. Neurology *25:* 154–159, 1975.
3. Jerusalem, F., Spiess, H., and Baumgartner, G. Lipid storage myopathy with normal carnitine levels. J. Neurol. Sci. *24:* 273–282, 1975.
4. Bradley, W. G., Jenkison, M., Park, D., Hudgson, P., Gardner-Medwin, D., Pennington, R. J. T., and Walton, J. N. A myopathy associated with lipid storage. J. Neurol. Sci. *16:* 137–154, 1972.
5. Johnson, M. A., Fulthorpe, J. J., and Hudgson, P. Lipid storage myopathy, a recognizable clinical, pathological entity. Acta Neuropathol. *24:* 97–106, 1973.

MITOCHONDRIAL DISEASES

Some years ago it appeared that we were to be inundated with diseases in which structural abnormalities of the mitochondria were associated with particular clinical entities. "Pleoconial" and "megaconial" myopathies vied with other myopathies with atypical mitochondria , and the result was a series of remarkable pictures of ultrastructural changes that could have graced the walls of the Museum of Modern Art. The belief that each would characterize a particular clinical entity has turned out to be no more than a pious hope and the only survivors of the group, or at least the only ones commonly discussed, are those presented in the succeeding section, oculocraniosomatic neuromuscular disease with ragged red fibers, and Luft's syndrome.

Oculocraniosomatic Neuromuscular Disease with Ragged Red Fibers (Kearns and Sayres Ophthalmoplegia; Kearns-Shy Syndrome; Ophthalmoplegia Plus)

Progressive weakness of the extraocular muscles may occur as part of a complex and varied picture of dysfunction (Figs. 8.2–8.4).[1–3] It may be associated with neurological, cardiac, and other deficits. Recently, many of these different syndromes have seemed to coalesce into one entity, the hallmark of which is the pathological change in muscle biopsy which is known as the ragged red fiber and which is indicative of mitochondrial abnormality (Fig. 8.5).[4]

Most cases are sporadic rather than familial. The symptoms may appear at any time in life, but most often appear during childhood or adolescence. In some patients there may be a history of a flu-like illness sometimes associated with drowsiness, although no definite encephalitic episode has been documented. An early sign may be the development of weakness of the extraocular muscles and ptosis. Muscle fatigue during exercise is also a common symptom. In two patients in our clinic, the fatigue has been severe enough that the patients were unable to walk for a period of time. The illness is progressive, and there may be any or all of the following abnormalities: pigmentary degeneration of the retina, sensorineural deafness, pyramidal tract disease, cerebellar incoordination, endocrine abnormalities (such as amenorrhea), cardiac conduction defects, and, when the illness begins early in life, mental and growth retardation. There is also a defect in ventilatory drive, the patient's respiration responding poorly to increasing hypoxia or hypercapnia.[5] This may have been the cause of an episode of confusion and lethargy which one patient experienced when traveling at an altitude of 10,000 feet. It is also important to bear such respiratory abnormality in mind if anesthesia is being contemplated, since patients may be abnormally sensitive to drugs which are respiratory depressants.

Although the diagnosis can be suspected from the clinical picture, laboratory tests are necessary before it is conclusively proved. Almost all patients with the disease have a moderate increase in cerebrospinal fluid protein. One report indicated that the IgA and IgG fractions were all increased but that the albumin was normal.[6] These authors suggested that the increased CSF immunoglobulins and other proteins were due to an alteration of the blood-CSF barrier. Serum creatine phosphokinase (CPK) is often mildly elevated, but the marked elevation seen in florid myopathies is not to be expected. EMG is not usually helpful in substantiating the diagnosis, although there may be some "myopathic" changes.

The muscle biopsy shows a striking and peculiar change. Even in those biopsies in which general abnormalities (variation of fiber size, internal nuclei, etc.) are not striking, there are scattered fibers with a heavy granular network pattern. Since these stain red or purplish red with the modified trichrome, they have been called "ragged red" fibers. With the more conventional H and E stain this network stains blue. Under the electron microscope, the mitochondria are not only increased in number, but have other abnormalities as well. Crystalloid structures may be present within them, often comprising four sets of parallel lines (quadrilemmal bodies).[7] Abnormal mitochondria are nt limited to the muscle. Systemic involvement is evidenced by abnormal mitochondria in the cerebellum,[8] the liver,[9] and also in the sweat glands.[6] In addition to the abnormal mitochondria there may be a heavy deposition of glycogen and/or lipid in the muscle fibers.[6, 10] The mitochondrial changes are not specific for this illness and may be seen in many different diseases. However, in the oculocraniosomatic neuromuscular disorder they present as the principal abnormality.

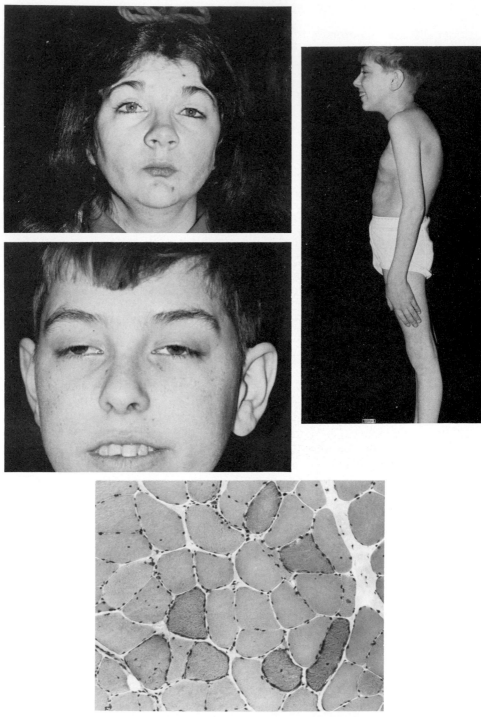

Figures 8.2–8.5. Oculo-cranio-somatic neuromuscular disease with ragged red fibers. Ptosis and extra-ocular palsies are a prominent part of this syndrome (Fig. 8.2, *top, left*, and Fig. 8.3, *center, left*). Minor degrees of axial muscle weakness are found and occasionally a mild kyphosis is noted (Fig. 8.4, *right*). The muscle biopsy shows a large number of "ragged red" fibers, these are fibers with an abnormal granular appearance and a bright red stain with modified trichrome stains (Fig. 8.5, *bottom*). The red staining material is frequently around the periphery fibers and is due to large numbers of abnormal mitochondria.

In this and other diseases marked by structural abnormalities of mitochondria there are associated chemical abnormalities although the exact defect remains unclear.[11, 12] Oxidative phosphorylation, which ordinarily produces the high energy phosphates necessary for the energy supply in muscle, may become uncoupled and control of respiratory function by the changes in the levels of the high energy phosphate compounds may be lost. The mitochondria are in a sense spinning their wheels. High resting lactate and pyruvate levels have been described in some patients with typical oculocraniosomatic neuromuscular disease[2, 13] as well as in others with less typical disease.[14] In one patient the response to exercise was also abnormal. The pyruvate and lactate levels were much higher than normal, as was the lactate to pyruvate ratio. There was also an abnormal change in the hydroxybutyrate to acetoacetate ratio following exercise, which suggested that there was relative hypoxia.[13] A block in carbohydrate utilization was postulated to explain this.

The morphological change may be produced experimentally by the administration of compounds which are known to uncouple oxidative phosphorylation. Thus 2,4-dinitrophenol (DNP) produces ragged red fibers when administered experimentally.[15] Experimental thiamine deficiency has also been associated with the same mitochondrial abnormalities.[16] In spite of these tempting leads, there is as yet no treatment for this illness other than the usual supportive measures. The EKG should be monitored; the conduction defect may become severe enough on occasions that implantation of a pacemaker becomes necessary.

BIBLIOGRAPHY

1. Kearns, T. P. External ophthalmoplegia, pigmentary degeneration of the retina and cardiomyopathy: A newly recognized syndrome. Trans. Am. Ophthalmol. Soc. *63:* 559–625, 1965.
2. Shy, G. M., Silberberg, A. H., Appel, S. H., Mishkin, M. M., and Godfrey, E. H. A generalized disorder of nervous system, skeletal muscle and heart resembling Refsum's disease and Hurler's syndrome, Part I. Am. J. Med. 42: 163–178, 1967.
3. Drachman, D. A. Ophthalmoplegia plus. Arch. Neurol. *18:* 654–674, 1968.
4. Olson, W., Engel, W. K., Walsh, G. O., and Einaugler, R. Oculocraniosomatic neuromuscular disease with ragged red fibers. Arch. Neurol. *26:* 193–211, 1972.
5. Carroll, J. E., Zwillich, C., Weil, J. V., and Brooke, M. H. Depressed ventilatory response in oculocraniosomatic neuromuscular disease. Neurology *26:* 140–146, 1976.
6. Karpati, G., Carpenter, S., Larbrisseau, A., and Lafontaine, R. The Kearns-Shy syndrome: A multi-system disease with mitochondrial abnormality demonstrated in skeletal muscle and skin. J. Neurol. Sci. *19:* 133–151, 1973.
7. Price, H. M., Gordon, G. B., Munsat, T. L., and Pearson, C. M. Myopathy with atypical mitochondria in Type 1 skeletal muscle fibers. J. Neuropathol. Exp. Neurol. *26:* 475–497, 1967.
8. Schneck, L., Adachi, M., Brite, P., Wolintz, A., and Volk, B. W. Ophthalmoplegia plus with morphological and chemical studies of cerebellar and muscle tissue. J. Neurol. Sci. *19:* 37–44, 1973.
9. Okamura, K., Santa, T., Nagae, K., and Omae, T. Congenital oculoskeletal myopathy with abnormal muscle and liver mitochondria. J. Neurol. Sci. *27:* 79–91, 1976.
10. DiMauro, S., Schotland, D. L., Bonilla, E., Lee, C. P., Gambetti, P., and Rowland, L. P. Progressive ophthalmoplegia, glycogen storage and abnormal mitochondria. Arch. Neurol. *29:* 170–179, 1973.
11. DiMauro, S., Schotland, D. L., Bonilla, E., Lee, C. P., DiMauro, P. M. M., and Scarpa, A. Mitochondrial myopathies; which and how many? In: *Exploratory Concepts in Muscular Dystrophy, II*, edited by A. T. Milhorat. Excerpta Medica, New York, 1974, pp. 506–515.
12. Worsford, M., Park, D. C., and Pennington, R. J. Familial mitochondrial myopathy; a

myopathy associated with disordered oxidative metabolism in muscle fibers. Part II. Biochemical findings. J. Neurol. Sci. *19:* 261–274, 1973.

13. Sulaiman, W. R., Doyle, D., Johnson, R. H., and Jennett, S. Myopathy with mitochondrial inclusion bodies; histological and metabolic studies. J. Neurol. Neurosurg. Psychiatry *37:* 1236–1246, 1974.

14. Shapira, Y., Cederbaum, S. D., Cancilla, P. A., Neilsen, D., and Lippe, B. M. Familial poliodystrophy, mitochondrial myopathy, and lactate acidemia. Neurology *25:* 614–621, 1975.

15. Melmed, C. Karpati, G., and Carpenter, S. Experimental mitochondrial myopathy produced by in vivo uncoupling of oxidative phosphorylation. J. Neurol. Sci. *26:* 305–318, 1975.

16. Kark, R. A. P., Brown, W. J., Edgerton, V. R., Reynolds, S. F., and Gibson, G. Experimental thiamine deficiency. Arch. Neurol. *32:* 818–825, 1975.

Luft's Disease

Luft's disease is regularly mentioned in the neuromuscular literature, even though there are only two known cases and the muscular symptoms are minor. Both patients were women suffering from a disorder of hypermetabolism.[1, 2] The patients experienced fever, profuse sweating, and heat intolerance. One preferred to spend her time in a cold room at 4°C. Thirst and appetite were excessive; polyuria was also noted. The general physical examination showed a tachycardia with rapid respirations, profuse sweating, and warm, flushed skin. Blotchy erythematous changes of the skin over the legs were seen. The basal metabolic rate was elevated, but thyroid studies were entirely normal. Some degree of muscle weakness was noted in both patients, although this was mild and generalized. The electromyogram showed a pattern "consistent with a myopathy," with short polyphasic potentials.[3] Serum muscle enzymes were within normal limits. There was no family history of any similar illness. In contrast to the rather mild clinical involvement of muscle, morphological studies showed a striking change. Typical ragged red fibers were seen with the histochemical reactions. Ultrastructural studies revealed the mitochondria to be more numerous than usual, and many were enlarged. They contained tightly packed cristae with paracrystalline and round osmiophilic inclusions.

Biochemically, the disease was characterized by defective respiratory control, indicating relative uncoupling of oxidative phosphorylation. In the second patient, although the uptake of calcium by the mitochondria was normal, it could not be retained by the mitochondria.[4] Thus, respiratory activity, instead of being coupled to the formation of energy rich phosphates, was merely used in a futile attempt to retain calcium within the mitochondria. The constant and uncontrolled mitochondrial respiratory activity resulted in heat production and was probably the basis of the rest of the patient's symptoms and signs. There is no treatment for the illness, although the administration of chloramphenicol, which depresses mitochondrial respiration, was associated with clinical benefit in the second patient.

BIBLIOGRAPHY

1. Luft, R., Ikkos, D., Palmieri, G., Urnster, L., and Afselius, B. A case of severe hypermetabolism of nonthyroid origin with a defect in the maintenance of mitochondrial respiratory control; a correlated clinical, biochemical and morphological study. J. Clin. Invest. *21:* 1776–1804, 1962.

2. Haydar, N. A., Conn, H. L., Afifi, A., Wakid, N., Ballas, S., and Fawaz, K. Severe hypermetabolism with primary abnormality of skeletal muscle mitochondria: Functional and therapeutic effects of chloramphenicol treatment. Ann. Intern. Med. *74:* 548–558, 1971.
3. deJesus, P. V. Neuromuscular physiology in Luft's syndrome. Electromyogr. Clin. Neurophysiol. *14:* 17–27, 1974.
4. DiMauro, S., Bonilla, E., Lee, C. P., Schotland, D., Scarpa, A., Conn, H., and Chance, B. Luft's disease; further biochemical and ultrastructural studies of skeletal muscle in the second case. J. Neurol. Sci. *27:* 217–232, 1976.

MYOGLOBINURIA

Myoglobin is a respiratory pigment with a molecular weight of about 17,000. Its function, although not known precisely, is related to the transport of oxygen. When there is acute damage to muscle fibers, myoglobin may be released into the serum and thence into the urine. The renal threshold is quite low, in the neighborhood of 0.5 mg. per 100 ml. Under extreme circumstances the release of myoglobin is sufficient to cause the urine to become dark, reddish brown, and the accumulation of pigment casts in the renal tubules may be associated with tubular necrosis and renal failure.

Clinical Aspects

Myoglobin may be released from "normal" muscle under the stress of excessive exercise. Forty per cent of naval recruits demonstrated increased quantities of myoglobin in the serum during the first six days of training camp,[1] and an unusually strenuous exercise program was associated with six cases of overt myoglobinuria in a Marine camp.[2]

Muscle is susceptible to damage in situations other than excessive exercise. Sometimes the stress is an external one, such as a crush injury. At other times, a metabolic anomaly is responsible. Various classifications have been proposed; one of the most useful differentiates the hereditary myoglobinurias from the sporadic.[3] The hereditary causes of myoglobinuria are probably all associated with metabolic defects, and there are some which are already known. Thus, phosphorylase deficiency, phosphofructokinase deficiency, and carnitine-palmityl transferase deficiency all belong in the category of hereditary myoglobinurias. Since the enzyme defect is known they have been described separately.

Malignant hyperthermia probably belongs to the category of familiar myoglobinuria, but this is also discussed in a separate section.

Another illness which has been partially characterized gives rise to fatigue, pain, and myoglobinuria with exercise.[4, 5] It is inherited as an autosomal recessive; in childhood the affected members have a limited ability to exercise. There may be periods of exacerbation when only a few steps will provoke muscle pain and fatigue and further exercise is not tolerated. Exercise also gives rise to an abnormal tachycardia and dyspnea. If exercise is forced on the patient during such times, myoglobinuria may result. Some of these patients have fixed weakness, while others are normally strong when the muscle is tested with brief contractions. Occasionally, hypertrophy of the calf muscles is noted, but the examination is not otherwise abnormal. Although the illness is reminiscent of McArdle's disease, elevation of lactate levels and more especially of pyruvate levels is noted following exercise. The authors suggest that the predominant feature is a hyperkinetic circulatory state, perhaps due to a reflex effect following the accumulation of abnormal metabolites in the muscle.

In another report,[6] a patient suffering from exertional myoglobinuria was described in whom an abnormally high lactate production was noted following exercise. The patient's tolerance for exercise was also reduced because of aching and fatigue of the muscles which developed after a few minutes on a treadmill. The picture was complicated by a history of high alcoholic intake, at least at the beginning of the studies. The authors suggested that oxidative phosphorylation may have been uncoupled and the dependence upon anaerobic metabolism resulted in the excessive lactate production.

The sporadic occurrence of myoglobinuria is often seen with unusual or forced exercise. Various picturesque names, such as "squat jump" myoglobinuria, have been coined to indicate the provocative exercise. Myoglobinuria may also be seen in the muscle damage sustained during severe electric shock or after convulsions. Crush injuries such as those caused by falling masonry may also be associated with myoglobinuria, hardly a surprising finding in view of the enormous damage which may occur. Others have suffered from crush injuries from the weight of the body lying on an arm. In this case, a combination of factors is probably responsible. Ordinarily a person will turn over even during deep sleep; otherwise the discomfort will lead to awakening. This type of crush injury is therefore more readily seen in comatose patients, particularly when the coma is due to heroin or alcohol, drugs which may themselves be toxic to muscle.

Interruption of the blood supply to a muscle causes infarction and widespread muscle destruction. For this reason embolism of a major artery is sometimes associated with myoglobinuria. Many drugs are associated with disturbances of oxidative metabolism and may place an additional strain on the necessary energy supplies to muscle. Carbon monoxide, various narcotics, and barbiturates have all been responsible for myoglobinuric episodes, as have other metabolic derangements such as diabetic acidosis and non-ketotic hyperglycemic hyperosmolar coma. Toxins, such as plasmocid, damage the muscle directly and may cause widespread necrosis. Other toxic causes of myoglobinuria vary from the mundane, such as alcohol, to the exotic, such as a bite from the Malaysian sea snake. Heroin, licorice, succinylcholine, ϵ-amino caproic acid, and amphotericin B are also agents which have been associated with muscle breakdown. Contamination of fish with industrial toxins was thought to cause myoglobinuria in the outbreak of the illness known as Haff disease. Other precipitating events include hypokalemia, heat stroke, and high fever. Rarely, an acute muscle illness such as polymyositis may be accompanied by myoglobinuria.

The symptoms of exercise-provoked myoglobinuria are rather stereotyped. The patient has a sense of aching and fatigue in the muscles while exercising. Often this exercise is forced, either because the patient is in a situation, such as the military, where the exercise is compulsory or because the activity has to be continued for the patient's safety, as in mountain climbing. With the continuation of exercise, the muscles become weaker and the patient feels generally unwell with headache, nausea, and, not infrequently, vomiting.

Exercise while fasting is particularly liable to provoke attacks in susceptible individuals. The patient may collapse and be admitted to the hospital in coma. The combination of coma and anuria due to the attendant renal damage may mask the underlying muscle destruction unless an accurate history can be obtained. In less severe cases, the muscle pain and weakness are followed by pigmenturia, which may occur up to 24 hours afterwards. The relationship of the symptoms to exercise is illustrated by a case of a 22 year old girl who attempted a difficult hike up a mountain. Half way to the summit her legs became fatigued and painful, but she had no symptoms in her arms. Her companion carried her on his back much of the rest of the way, and she had to use her arms for support. Thereupon fatigue and pain developed in her arms, so that by the time she arrived at the top of the mountain she was totally incapacitated. The muscles most often affected are the large muscles of the limbs. The cranial musculature and the respiratory muscles are seldom involved in this illness, perhaps because they are never subject to the forceful contractions that are demanded of the limb muscles under conditions of unusual exertion.

Patients who have myoglobinuria which is unrelated to exercise may not notice the onset of the muscular symptoms, perhaps because so many of the provocative causes are associated with a disturbance of consciousness.

Upon examination of a patient during an acute bout of myoglobinuria the muscles are painful, swollen, and indurated. Weakness is always present in such muscles and may amount to a total paralysis. In general the degree of weakness parallels the pain and swelling.

Laboratory Studies

The identification of myoglobin in the urine is necessary in order to make the diagnosis. The urine should be freshly voided and neutralized to prevent the breakdown of myoglobin. Myoglobinuria can be confused both with hemoglobinuria and with the urine seen in porphyria. Myoglobin and hemoglobin react with the benzidine test for heme pigment, a reaction which is not seen in porphyria. In hemoglobinuria, red cells may be detected in the urine. If they are not seen it would imply that the destruction of red blood cells must have taken place in the circulation, in which case the serum should be pink. In myoglobinuria the serum is not tinted. The most reliable identification of myoglobin depends upon electrophoresis and immunoprecipitation by an antibody prepared against purified myoglobin.

Supporting evidence for myoglobinuria is an extreme elevation of the levels of serum "muscle" enzymes. These are high initially, with creatine phosphokinase levels of several thousand, and then decline over a period of days. Renal failure is the most serious complication of myoglobinuria. The patient's survival depends upon the early recognition of this and the appropriate treatment with dialysis. Even in those patients without overt clinical evidence of renal failure there is often a decrease of renal function. Thus, creatinine clearance may be abnormal and increased levels of blood urea may be found.

After an acute attack, the patient's muscle function returns to normal within one to three weeks. Renal function may be impaired much longer, and it may take up to six or seven weeks before creatinine clearance returns to normal values. Some degree of hyperkalemia is also seen in myoglobinuria; it may be severe.

The treatment of the acute attack of myoglobinuria is largely supportive. It seems sensible to keep the patient at rest to prevent further stress on the muscles. Renal function should be closely monitored and dialysis carried out where appropriate. The administration of mannitol to promote diuresis has been recommended in those patients whose renal function is relatively well preserved.

BIBLIOGRAPHY

1. Olerud, J. E., Homer, L. D., and Carroll, H. W. Serum myoglobin levels predicted from serum enzyme values. N. Engl. J. Med. *293:* 483–485, 1975.
2. Demos, M. A. and Gitin, E. L. Acute exertional rhabdomyolysis. Arch. Intern. Med. *133:* 233–239, 1974.
3. Rowland, L. P. and Penn, A. S. Myoglobinuria. Med. Clin. North Am. *56:* 1233–1256, 1972.
4. Larsson, L. E., Linderholm, H., Muller, R., Ringqvist, T., and Sornas, R. Hereditary metabolic myopathy with paroxysmal myoglobinuria due to abnormal glycolysis. J. Neurol. Neurosurg. Psychiatry *27:* 361–380, 1964.
5. Linderholm, H., Muller, R., Ringqvist, T., and Sornas, R. Hereditary abnormal muscle metabolism with hyperkinetic circulation during exercise. Acta Med. Scand. *185:* 153–166, 1969.
6. Kontos, H. A., Harley, E. L., Wasserman, A. J., Kelly, J. J., and Magee, J. H. Exertional idiopathic paroxysmal myoglobinuria; evidence for a defect in skeletal muscle metabolism. Am. J. Med. *35:* 283–292, 1963.

MALIGNANT HYPERPYREXIA (MALIGNANT HYPERTHERMIA)

Clinical Aspects

Man shares with the pig an unusual illness in which an explosive rise in temperature is associated with muscular rigidity and necrosis. The onset is provoked by anesthesia, especially by the administration of halothane and succinylcholine, and it usually occurs in a patient whose prior history gives no clue to the existence of the illness. Following the infusion of succinylcholine the muscles may fasciculate, and tone in the muscles may be increased. This is particularly true of the masseter muscles, and a clenched jaw during the induction of anesthesia is an ominous sign. A short time thereafter there commences an extraordinary rise in body temperature, which may climb at a rate of 2°C per hour. An intense rigidity appears in all muscle groups, and a progressive metabolic acidosis develops. Untreated patients usually die. Convulsions are common shortly before death.

Although the development of malignant hyperpyrexia is unusual (between one in fourteen thousand and one in seventy-five thousand anesthesias),[1] its severity has prompted attempts to define the susceptible population. In many cases the disease is inherited as an autosomal dominant. At times overt signs and symptoms of muscle disease have been found. Thus, hypertrophy of thigh muscles, atrophy of the distal part of the thighs, lumbar lordosis, mild hip weakness, and diminished deep tendon reflexes have all been observed. Myotonia has been noted on several occasions. The lack of specificity of these signs reduces their diagnostic value unless the family history indicates that the patient is at risk.

Laboratory Studies

Persistently high values of serum creatine phosphokinase (CPK) have been recorded in some patients, and if a patient about to undergo surgery has a family history of malignant hyperpyrexia, CPK testing is mandatory. Unfortunately there may be susceptible patients who have normal levels of CPK.

Ellis et al.[1] suggested that patients prone to malignant hyperthermia could be detected by the action of halothane, with or without the addition of succinylcholine, on an excised strip of muscle. Ordinarily this would not cause any contracture in the muscle, but these authors found that in patients with malignant hyperthermia the muscle underwent contracture. This finding has been disputed by others, although their experimental conditions were slightly different.[2]

The abnormal muscle exhibits several interesting pharmacological anomalies. The first is an abnormal sensitivity to caffeine. When this drug is applied locally to normal muscle a contracture occurs. This is associated with an increase in the concentration of calcium in the sarcoplasm either because caffeine promotes the release of calcium from the sarcoplasmic reticulum or because it impedes its uptake. This muscle contracture is markedly potentiated by halothane, a phenomenon which occurs in both normal individuals and patients with hyperpyrexia. The concentration of caffeine necessary to produce this contracture is much lower in patients with malignant hyperpyrexia than in the normal. This applies both with and without halothane.[2] The ability of the sarcoplasmic reticulum to take up calcium is also decreased when compared to normal controls. Halothane has a paradoxical effect on this accumulation of calcium. Ordinarily the effect of halothane is slight and it increases the uptake of calcium by normal sarcoplasmic reticulum. In patients with malignant hyperpyrexia the opposite effect was reported, with a reduction in the uptake of calcium by the sarcoplasmic reticulum. Isaacs and Heffron[3] were unable to duplicate this paradoxical effect of halothane, although they also found the calcium uptake in the sarcoplasmic reticulum of patients with malignant hyperthermia was 28 per cent less than in normal.

The remarkable production of heat which is the hallmark of malignant hyperpyrexia is due to a metabolic aberration, but the nature of this is not clear. In pigs, a progressive loss of ATP and accumulation of phosphate in the blood have been described.[4] There is also an increased "cycling" of fructose 6-phosphate to fructose 1,6-diphosphate and back. With each turn of this cycle, ATP is hydrolyzed and heat is generated. Halothane increases the rate of cycling. There are, however, differences between the human disease and that of the pig, and the etiology may be quite different.

Treatment

The treatment of the illness depends upon its early recognition, and the development of hyperpyrexia and muscle stiffness during anesthesia is an indication to discontinue the surgical procedure. It is also possible that the treatment of this illness will change radically in the next few years since it has been shown that dantrolene sodium reverses the disease in swine. After the intravenous injection of 7 to 10 mg. of dantrolene per kilogram, the rigidity disappears, the temperature returns towards normal, and the metabolic acidosis is controlled. Studies on humans will undoubtedly follow shortly and, if they are as successful as the experiments with pigs would indicate, death from malignant hyperthermia may be a thing of the past.[5] Treatment of the illness up to the present time has followed a regimen similar to that outlined by Maisel et al.[6] As soon as the diagnosis is suspected, all anesthetic agents are discontinued and 100% oxygen is given by endotracheal tube. The patient is cooled by all possible means and the metabolic acidosis is controlled with bicarbonate. Procaine may be given intravenously, with a loading dose of 15 to 20 mg. per kilogram followed by 0.2 mg. per kilogram per minute, with an EKG monitor to detect any ventricular arrhythmia. Steroids such as dexamethazone may be given, and thorazine may also be administered to aid in the cooling process. A patient who recovers from the illness should be watched for renal failure, since an acute attack may be associated with massive myoglobinuria.

BIBLIOGRAPHY

1. Ellis, F. R., Keane, N. P., Harriman, D. G. F., Sumner, D. W., Kyei-Mensah, K., Tyrrell, J. H., Hargreaves, J. B., Parikh, R. K., and Mulrooney, P. L. Screening for malignant hyperpyrexia. Br. Med. J. *3:* 559–561, 1972.
2. Britt, B. A., Kalow, W., Gordon, A., Humphrey, J. G., and Rewcastle, N. B. Malignant hyperthermia; an investigation of five patients. Can. Anaesth. Soc. J. *20:* 431–467, 1973.
3. Isaacs, H. and Heffron, J. J. A. Morphological and biochemical defects in muscles of human carriers of the malignant hyperthermia syndrome. Br. J. Anaesth. *47:* 475–481, 1975.
4. Clark, M. G., Williams, C. H., Pfeifer, W. F., Bloxham, D. P., Holland, P. C., Taylor, C. A., and Lardy, H. A. Accelerated substrate cycling of fructose 6 phosphate in the muscle of malignant hyperthermic pigs. Nature *245:* 99–101, 1973.
5. Harrison, G. G. Control of malignant hyperpyrexia syndrome in swine by dantrolene sodium. Br. J. Anaesth. *47:* 62–65, 1975.
6. Maisel, R. H., Sessions, D. G., and Miller, R. N. Malignant hyperpyrexia during general anesthesia. Successful management of a case. Ann. Otol. Rhinol. Laryngol. *85:* 729–733, 1973.

"ENDOCRINE" MYOPATHIES

Hyperthyroidism

Disorders of thyroid function cause a multitude of different symptoms, and muscle involvement is often minor and overlooked by the patient. On rare occasions the neuromuscular symptoms predominate, but even then other signs of thyroid disorder are usually to be found. Patients with thyrotoxicosis may develop proximal weakness with some muscular wasting. The shoulders are often more affected than the hips. The reflexes may be preserved. The majority of patients with thyrotoxicosis probably have some muscle involvement.[1] Although this usually occurs in the adult, it may also be seen in children.[2] The older literature describes the spontaneous occurrence of muscle twitching, the so-called "fasciculating myopathy of thyrotoxicosis." However, this entity may be largely mythical since electromyography does not typically reveal fasciculations. In one case in which obvious twitching was noted, myokymia was found to be the cause.[3] Neither the muscle biopsy nor the EMG give any further clues as to the underlying etiology; although abnormalities are seen in both studies, these are nonspecific. The serum creatine phosphokinase may be normal. Treatment of the thyrotoxicosis usually alleviates the muscle symptoms. Biochemical studies of mitochondrial function have been carried out, but again fail to give precise information on the way in which the disease occurs.[4]

A common complication of thyrotoxicosis is exophthalmic ophthalmoplegia with associated abnormalities in the extraocular muscles. Standard texts should be consulted for further description of this illness.

Hypothyroidism

Patients with hypothyroidism also have signs of muscular abnormality. The best known is a peculiar change in contractility of the muscles. When a deep tendon reflex is elicited, instead of prompt relaxation after the initial contraction, the relaxation phase is slowed. Thus, when an ankle jerk is obtained, the prompt return of the foot to its resting position is replaced by a slow drift. In patients whose muscular symptoms are marked, not only may there be delay in relaxation but stiffness and cramps may be found and the muscle may hypertrophy. Myedema is found, but percussion myotonia is not part of the picture. Electromyography may demonstrate increased insertional activity with trains of repetitive activity, but true myotonia is not found.

In children, the disease is associated with an impressive hypertrophy and seems to occur more often in boys than in girls (Kocher-Debre-Semelaigne syndrome).[5] Some authors have been impressed by the fact that these children are unusually strong.[6] The development of the illness may be related to the duration and the severity of the hypothyroid state; after treatment the muscle bulk returns to normal, although the strength does not change. In adults, the symptoms are similar although the occurrence of painful cramps is more noticeable. Again, the disease usually responds to appropriate treatment of the hypothyroid condition. Proximal weakness may occur in hypothyroidism and is associated with elevation of creatine phosphokinase.

Associated Disorders

Thyroid dysfunction has as adverse an effect on the strength of patients with muscle disease as on that of normal patients. It is not surprising that patients with various forms of weakness may become worse if their thyroid function is abnormal. There are two diseases which are more commonly associated with thyroid disturbance than can be explained purely by chance. Exacerbations of myasthenia gravis are sometimes associated with the onset of dysthyroid states, and the onset of the one should be sufficient grounds to consider the possibility of the other.

Hypokalemic periodic paralysis may also be seen with thyrotoxicosis. Males suffer from the illness more than females and almost 85 per cent of the cases occur in the third and fourth decades. Ninety-five per cent of cases are sporadic, and the vacuolar myopathy which is often noted in the other varieties is uncommon in thyrotoxic periodic paralysis. Pharmacologically the disease has a different reaction to intra-arterial epinephrine. In familial periodic paralysis the intra-arterial injection of minute amounts of epinephrine causes a prompt paralysis of the arm, even in the absence of attacks, whereas in thyrotoxic periodic paralysis, patients tolerate epinephrine without such paralysis.[7]

Parathyroid Dysfunction

Tetany is the only neuromuscular complication of hypoparathyroidism, but neuromuscular symptoms in hyperparathyroidism have been described frequently.[8-10] Cystic bone disease, kidney stones, renal failure, peptic ulceration, pancreatitis, and mental disturbances are most often thought of as the presenting complaints of patients with hyperparathyroidism, but a significant number of patients also have muscular weakness. The incidence of this weakness in hyperparathyroidism is difficult to ascertain, but it may be as high as 75 to 80 per cent, although it may be overshadowed by the more dramatic effects of the disease. Patients experience fatigue as well as aching in the muscles and may have overt weakness and wasting of the proximal muscles. The hips are usually more involved than the shoulders. The deep tendon reflexes are not only preserved but may be hyperactive. At least two reports stress that the illness may simulate a primary neuromuscular disorder.[8, 10] Some patients have bulbar findings, with hoarseness, fasciculations of the tongue, and dysarthria. These when combined with axial weakness, hyperreflexia, and, in some patients, extensor plantar responses simulate motor neuron disease. In some patients these symptoms respond to correction of the hyperparathyroidism. The possibility that the patients actually had motor neuron disease as well as hyperparathyroidism is not totally excluded. In addition to primary hyperparathyroidism, patients with other forms of osteomalacia may experience similar weakness. The administration of vitamin D seems to help such patients considerably. The severity of the disease does not seem to be correlated with the calcium or phosphate levels in the blood, and the exact mechanism whereby weakness occurs is again unknown. The most helpful laboratory tests are those designed to uncover the hyperparathyroid abnormalities. Changes seen on the muscle biopsy suggest some denervation, but Type 2 atrophy is prominent.

Adrenal and Pituitary Dysfunction

Muscle weakness is part of the clinical picture of acromegaly and Cushing's syndrome. It is also present in Addison's disease and is seen with the administration of steroids, particularly the halogenated compounds. All of these situations are associated with a rather nonspecific muscle weakness which is usually proximal and which responds to the correction of the underlying abnormality. The muscle biopsy in these conditions usually reveals Type 2 fiber atrophy, another nonspecific change.[11]

BIBLIOGRAPHY

1. Ramsay, I. D. Muscle dysfunction in hyperthyroidism. Lancet 2: 931–934, 1966.
2. Johnston, D. M. Thyrotoxic myopathy. Arch. Dis. Child. 49: 968–969, 1974.
3. Harman, J. B. and Richardson, A. T. Generalized myokymia in thyrotoxicosis. Lancet 2: 473–474, 1954.
4. Peter, J. B. In "Hyperthyroidism," Solomon, D. H. (moderator). Ann. Intern. Med. 69: 1015–1035, 1968.
5. Najjar, S. S. Muscular hypertrophy in hypothyroid children; the Kocher-Debré – Semelaigne syndrome. J. Pediatr. 85: 236–239, 1974.
6. Hopwood, N. J., Lockhart, L. H., and Bryan, G. T. Acquired hypothyroidism with muscular hypertrophy and precocious testicular enlargement. J. Pediatr. 85: 233–236, 1974.

7. Engel, A. G. Neuromuscular manifestations of Graves' disease. Mayo Clin. Proc. *47:* 919–925, 1972.

8. Smith, R. and Stern, G. Myopathy osteomalacia and hyperparathyroidism. Brain *90:* 593–602, 1967.

9. Cholod, D. J., Haust, M. D., Hudson, A. J., and Lewis, F. N. Myopathy in primary familial hyperparathyrodism. Am. J. Med. *48:* 700–707, 1970.

10. Patten, B. M., Bilezikian, J. P., Mallette, L. E., Prince, A., Engel, W. K., and Aurbach, G. D. Neuromuscular disease in primary hyperparathyroidism. Ann. Intern. Med. *80:* 182–193, 1974.

11. Pleasure, D. E., Walsh, G. O., and Engel, W. K. Atrophy of skeletal muscle in patients with Cushing's syndrome. Arch. Neurol. *22:* 118–125, 1970.

NUTRITIONAL AND TOXIC MYOPATHIES

Man is spared some of the muscle diseases which affect other animals as a result of nutritional deficiencies. Thus the presence or absence of Vitamin E, selenium, and other compounds is not recognized as a clinical problem. There are, of course, nutritional deficiencies such as are seen with protein deprivation and starvation, but these are not selectively muscle diseases. The nutritional myopathies of man seem to be a result not so much of what is missing from the diet as of what is added. Alcohol remains one of the commonest, and alcoholic myopathy is now well recognized and well described.[1, 2] The typical illness takes one of two forms: either an acute attack of muscle pain, swelling, and weakness after "binge" drinking or a more chronic, rather slowly progressive proximal weakness in alcoholics who maintain a steady intake. In some patients there is evidence of muscle destruction resulting in elevation of serum creatine phosphokinase levels without any overt signs or symptoms.

In the acute alcoholic myopathy, after a bout of enthusiastic drinking the patient may experience the sudden onset of pain and swelling in the muscles. This usually affects the thigh muscles, but other large muscle groups may be involved. The muscle is tense, swollen, and exquisitely tender. Weakness can be profound and there may be associated myoglobinuria. Renal failure may ensue, and the disease should be treated the same way as any acute myoglobinuria. Such an attack may resolve completely, or there may be residual weakness.

In patients with chronic alcoholic myopathy, the weakness is usually of the legs, although occasionally additional weakness of the shoulders is seen. This picture is sometimes superimposed on a preceding history of acute alcoholic myopathy, although it may be difficult to obtain such a story from the patient. In some chronic alcoholics whose acute myopathy has been documented, a later visit to the clinic with the chronic syndrome has revealed no memory of the acute attacks. In addition to the rather typical clinical picture, the muscle biopsy may show a variety of changes, all of them unfortunately nonspecific. There may be muscle breakdown in the same fashion as in other patients with myoglobinuria, and there may be more peculiar alterations such as the tubular aggregates described by Chui et al.[3] An unexplained chemical abnormality is the failure to develop a normal rise of lactate with ischemic exercise and a deficiency in the activity of phosphorylase in the muscle.

Other chemicals have been associated with muscle breakdown. Chloroquine and vincristine may be associated with a myopathy. The myotonia associated with the administration of diazacholesterol is known in both experimental and therapeutic situations. Clofibrate may produce muscle cramps, although the mechanism is not known, and toxins such as plasmocid are also associated with muscle breakdown. Such patients, however, rarely present to a muscle clinic and usually the etiology is obvious.

BIBLIOGRAPHY

1. Ekbom, K., Hed, R., Kirstein, L., and Astrom, K. E. Muscular affections in chronic alcoholism. Arch. Neurol. *10:* 449–458, 1964.
2. Perkoff, G. T. Alcoholic myopathy. Ann. Rev. Med. *22:* 125–132, 1971.
3. Chui, L. A., Neustein, H., and Munsat, T. L. Tubular aggregates in subclinical alcoholic myopathy. Neurology *25:* 405–412, 1975.

PERIODIC PARALYSES

Episodic bouts of weakness which occur with varying severity and frequency are common to all the periodic paralyses. Such paralyses are classified according to whether the serum potassium is increased, decreased, or unchanged during an attack. Hence, there are three major categories: hypokalemic, hyperkalemic, and normokalemic. The distinction into separate categories based on the age of onset, the severity and duration of the attack, and the nature of the provocative factors seems quite clear as one reads the literature. Unfortunately these lines of distinction become blurred by a number of features which all three varieties share in common, and the clarity of the textbook definition may disappear entirely at the bedside. There are enough similarities in each of the three groups to make one suspect that the change in potassium is merely an epiphenomenon which may be of more hindrance than help in the classification of these diseases. Nevertheless, inadequate though the criterion may be, it is the only one available and we shall follow the traditional path, presenting the three types of disease in sequence.

Hypokalemic Periodic Paralysis

Familial Hypokalemic Periodic Paralysis

Clinical Aspects. This illness occurs as an autosomal dominant, but it is often not expressed in the female and may appear to be an autosomal recessive if an asymptomatic mother has affected children. Similarly, there are three times as many men with the illness as there are women. Although the disease may begin at any time, it commonly does so in the second decade, when the patient complains of episodes of severe weakness. The weakness often starts in the legs with a feeling of heaviness and aching in the back and thighs and gradually, over a period of an hour or so, spreads to other muscle groups. Muscles of the shoulders and hips are usually more affected than distal muscles. The attack may be severe enough to paralyze the patient's arms and legs completely and prevent him from raising his head from the pillow. Weakness of the eye muscles occurs rarely, if at all, and the facial muscles are seldom involved. Mild disturbance of breathing may be seen in a severe attack, but respiratory paralysis of a severity to threaten the patient's life is very rare. At the height of the weakness, the muscle is electrically and mechanically inexcitable and the reflexes are lost. The muscles feel swollen, and an increased circumference of the limb has been noted.[1] Usually an attack will last from half a day to a day. The patient's strength will return as suddenly as it disappeared; the last muscles to become weak are usually the first to recover. Even after recovery from an attack, there may be residual weakness for 2 to 3 days before completely normal strength returns.

The frequency of these attacks varies from several times a week to isolated attacks separated by intervals of years. The severity of the attack ranges from mild focal weakness of a few muscles to a total flaccid paralysis of all limbs. During and preceding an attack there is often an increased thirst and, not uncommonly, oliguria. The reverse is seen after an attack, when diuresis and diaphoresis may occur. The patient may also differentiate between "light" and "heavy" attacks. The latter is an episode of paralysis, and the former, a transient sense of weakness lasting for an hour or two.

Provocative factors are fairly stereotyped. Heavy exercise (or exercise to which a patient is not accustomed) followed by a period of sleep or rest, a heavy meal, particularly one rich in carbohydrates and salt, emotional stress, alcohol, trauma, and cold may all precipitate the weakness. Thus, the man who mows the lawn in the afternoon prior to playing a game of touch football, later going out with the team to slake a ravenous appetite with beer, pizza, and popcorn, and arrives back home late enough to become embroiled in a domestic argument may wake up with considerable weakness the next morning.

Although an attack commonly develops in the early hours of the morning, it may occur at other times during the day. It may be warded off by gentle exercise in the early stages, although less commonly than in the hyperkalemic variety. Some drugs, such as epinephrine, norepinephrine, and corticosteroids, may have a provocative effect on the disease. In patients who have frequent attacks, particularly if these attacks are severe, a permanent weakness may develop which is usually proximal and which involves the hips more than the shoulders.[2-4] Eyelid myotonia, originally described in hyperkalemic periodic paralysis, may be prominent in the hypokalemic disease.[5] The disease is usually at its worst during the third and fourth decades and may improve spontaneously thereafter.

Laboratory Studies. Studies during an attack are essential to make the diagnosis. There is a fall in the serum potassium. Serum potassium may be as low as 1.5 meq. per liter during the height of an attack, but the patient's weakness may commence with levels of 3 meq. and become quite marked by the time it has dropped to 2 to 2.5 meq., levels which are better tolerated by the normal person. There are concomitant electrocardiographic changes. Bradycardia is often seen, the T waves are flattened, and there are prominent U waves with prolongation of the PR and QT interval. The heart size has been observed to increase during an attack. Since patients do not always present themselves conveniently at the height of an attack, it is necessary on occasion to use provocative measures so that the change in potassium can be monitored while the paralysis is present. In patients with hypokalemic periodic paralysis, the usual method is to administer glucose and insulin. One hundred grams of glucose can be given orally in conjunction with 20 units of insulin subcutaneously. Alternatively a liter of 10 per cent dextrose containing 20 units of insulin can be given intravenously. The EKG should be monitored throughout the procedure and potassium levels drawn at regular intervals (15 to 30 minutes). A clinical attack of weakness can occur at any time, but it may be delayed for as long as six to seven hours after the administration of glucose. A clear cut attack of paralysis is indicative of hypokalemic periodic paralysis. If no weakness develops it is important to make sure the serum potassium level has fallen to at least 2.5 meq. per liter. Even then it may be difficult to interpret a negative test. The serum creatine phosphokinase may be elevated during or after an attack.

Treatment. The treatment of the disease is not always easy. A clear cut episode of paralysis is best treated by oral potassium, between 5 and 10 gm. being an average dose. This may be repeated in one hour if no response is seen. It is, of course, important to evaluate renal function before administering potassium to a patient. The long term treatment of the disease to prevent attacks may be less successful. The prophylactic administration of potassium chloride has been recommended. Spironolactone has also been found effective, but there are some disturbing side effects such as gynecomastia. The use of a carbonic anhydrase inhibitor such as acetazolamide (Diamox)[6] or dichlorphenamide[7] has been the subject of some enthusiastic reports. These compounds are diuretics and, since they further the loss of potassium, the effect seems paradoxical, but it is probable that the benefit pertains more to changes in membrane function than to changes in the potassium content of the body. Experimentally acetazolamide reduces the movement of potassium into red blood cells. It also diminishes the hypokalemic effect of glucose insulin provocation in patients with periodic paralysis, and possibly part of its effect is mediated through the production of metabolic acidosis.[8] Acetazolamide works well for some patients, but there are others for whom the drug is of no value.

A disease in which the pathophysiology is associated with fluxes in electrolytes must surely be amenable to investigative research. Unhappily the basic defect is still elusive. That the inexcitability of the muscle during an attack was not due to the contractile mechanism but was due to dysfunction of the membrane was shown by Engel and Lambert.[9] The muscle from patients during the paralytic phase of the disease is inexcitable either upon stimulation or when calcium is applied locally to the intact muscle. If the sarcolemmal membrane is stripped from the muscle, the fiber regains its contractile response to the local application of calcium.

During the early stages of the acute attack there is a movement of potassium into muscle cells. This is probably associated with a similar movement of water and sodium ions. The reason for this flux is not known and various theories such as changes in the membrane permeability, the accumulation of abnormal negatively charged intermediates of carbohydrate metabolism, and the abnormal production of aldosterone have all been proposed as underlying mechanisms; however, all have received rather substantial challenges.

Hofmann and Smith[10] studied single muscle fibers in vitro and found that the fibers were not able to withstand the isolation procedure as well as those from normal individuals. There was a significant degree of depolarization regardless of the patient's clinical condition at the time of biopsy (none of the patients was studied during the time of an attack, although one had weakness). There was also an anomalous response to insulin, which caused repolarization of fibers when the external potassium levels were markedly reduced.

Structural alterations within the fibers have also pointed to abnormalities of membranous components. With the light microscope little may be seen, but on occasion some atrophic fibers are present and vacuoles may be found in the central part of muscle fibers. These vacuoles may be numerous and are often reactive with the PAS stains for glycogen. Collections of tubular structures (tubular aggregates), although more common in hyperkalemic paralysis, are also to be found. Such structural changes are not the invariable accompaniment to an acute attack. They may be florid in the interictal period and absent during the attack itself. Electron microscopic studies show that the vacuoles arise from local dilatation of the T tubules and sarcoplasmic reticular vesicles,[11] but whether these changes are associated with the primary abnormality or whether they represent a secondary change is not yet certain.

Secondary Hypokalemic Paralysis

Probably the best known form of this is the periodic paralysis associated with thyrotoxicosis. There is a high incidence in the oriental population. The reason for this close association is unknown. Usually the disease is sporadic and affects men more commonly than women. It is seldom seen before the second decade, and the illness disappears when the thyroid function returns to normal. The attacks are usually not as disabling as in the familial variety, and residual weakness is unusual.

Episodic weakness is also seen in many of the illnesses in which potassium is depleted. Attacks of weakness may occur in hyperaldosteronism, with chronic diarrhea or vomiting, as well as in the chronic administration of potassium depleting diuretics. An interesting, although rare example occurs after the chronic ingestion of licorice.[12] The compound responsible is glycyrrhizate, which is a potent mineralocorticoid.

BIBLIOGRAPHY

1. McArdle, B. Metabolic myopathies. Am. J. Med. *35:* 661–672, 1963.
2. Engel, A. G., Lambert, E. H., Rosevear, J. W., and Tauxe, M. N. Clinical and electromyographic studies in a patient with primary hypokalemia periodic paralysis. Am. J. Med. *38:* 626, 1965.
3. Pearson, C. M. The periodic paralyses; differential features and pathological observations in permanent myopathic weakness. Brain *87:* 341, 1963.
4. Dyken, M., Zeman, W., and Rusch, T. Hypokalemic periodic paralysis. Neurology *19:* 691–699, 1969.
5. Resnick, J. S. and Engel, W. K. Myotonic lid lag in hypokalemic periodic paralysis. J. Neurol. Neurosurg. Psychiatry *30:* 47–51, 1967.
6. Griggs, R. C., Engel, W. K., and Resnick, J. S. Acetazolamide treatment of hypokalemic periodic paralysis. Ann. Intern. Med. *73:* 39–48, 1970.
7. McArdle, B. Metabolic and endocrine myopathies. In: *Disorders of Voluntary Muscle,* edited by J. N. Walton. Churchill-Livingstone, London, 1974.
8. Vroom, F. Q., Jarrell, M. A., and Maren, T. H. Acetazolamide treatment of hypokalemic periodic paralysis. Arch. Neurol. *32:* 385–392, 1975.
9. Engel, A. G. and Lambert, E. H. Calcium activation of electrically inexcitable muscle fibers in primary hypokalemic periodic paralysis. Neurology *19:* 851–858, 1969.
10. Hofmann, W. W. and Smith, R. A. Hypokalemic periodic paralysis studied in vitro. Brain *93:* 445–474, 1970.

11. Engel, A. G. Evolution and content of vacuoles in primary hypokalemic periodic paralysis. Mayo Clin. Proc. *45:* 774–814, 1970.

12. Conn, J. W., Rovner, D. R., and Cohen, E. L. Licorice induced pseudoaldosteronism. JAMA *205:* 492–496, 1968.

Hyperkalemic Periodic Paralysis (Adynamia Episodica Hereditaria[1])

If in one variety of periodic paralysis the serum potassium was always abnormally reduced and in the other abnormally increased, it would be a good deal easier to write about hyperkalemic periodic paralysis. However, the matter is not so straight forward, and perhaps it is safer merely to state that the electrolyte changes are different from those seen in hypokalemic paralysis.

Clinical Aspects. Clinically, the disease is inherited as an autosomal dominant with strong penetrance and an equal involvement of the two sexes. The disease begins early in childhood and often in infancy. Such children have spells during which they become unusually floppy and more poorly. In some, the sound of the child's crying changes. The parents may notice a staring appearance which the child develops either spontaneously or on exposure to cold. This is probably due to the eyelid myotonia which exposes the sclera on downward gaze.

The attacks are usually provoked by rest after exercise but, unlike the hypokalemic form, the weakness develops in a shorter time interval. In one patient, sitting in a chair after carrying out her household chores would cause a feeling of tiredness in the back and legs and within 30 minutes it would be difficult for her to get up out of the chair. The onset of the weakness while sitting at a desk at school or while sitting in the theater has been described. The patient may be able to "walk off" the symptoms early in an attack. This postponement of an attack seems to be only temporary, and the maneuver is sometimes associated with the development of painful "knots" in the muscles.[2] Many patients also prefer to allow an attack to develop because it will be followed by a period of relative freedom from weakness. At times, eating candy or taking a light meal postpones an attack.

There may be odd sensory complaints that vary from a full, heavy feeling in the legs to the occurrence of a "musty" odor preceding an attack.[3] The wife of one patient commented that her husband's skin had a peculiar taste just before an attack. Others have noted that patients smell of ketone bodies during induced paralysis.[4] The duration of the paralysis is said to be much briefer than in the hypokalemic form, and it usually lasts less than an hour. However, more prolonged attacks have also been described which are clinically indistinguishable from those in hypokalemic periodic paralysis. In my experience patients complain of two types of attack, "light" and "heavy." It is not uncommon for mild weakness to be present several days after an episode of paralysis. The frequency varies from two or three mild attacks a day to attacks which are separated by intervals of months.

Although it has been emphasized that hyperkalemic periodic paralysis is the milder form, the literature does not always bear this out. Fixed, permanent weakness is often found; it affects the abdominal muscles, the hip flexors, and then spreads to the other muscles of the legs and shoulders. In some this has been severe enough to keep the patient confined to a wheelchair. Some patients tell the story of a very slow but steady progress in weakness upon which are superimposed briefer and more dramatic attacks of paralysis. In addition to rest after exercise, other provocative factors include exposure to cold, anesthesia, and sleep. The illness may also worsen during pregnancy.

The association of a form of myotonia with hyperkalemic paralysis is well recognized. Symptomatic myotonia suggests the diagnosis of hyperkalemic paralysis, but it is not exclusive to this disease and has been noted in hypokalemic paralysis. The myotonia often involves the muscles of the face, eyes, and tongue as well as the hands. In order to demonstrate eyelid myotonia, the patient is asked to gaze upward for a short period of time and then to look swiftly downwards. The eyelids "hang up" exposing the sclera and then slowly descend to their proper level as the myotonia relaxes. The myotonia is made worse by cold, and immersion of a limb in cool water can be used as a provocative test not only for the production of myotonia but also for exacerbation of the paralysis. For the demonstration of eyelid myotonia it is helpful to lay a towel soaked in cold water across the eyes for a few minutes before carrying out the test. The same phenomenon may be responsible for the tongue stiffening when the patient attempts to eat ice cream. Symptomatically the patient may feel his face stiffen when he walks out in cold weather and the ocular myotonia may make it difficult to look from side to side. The similarity between this myotonia and that seen in paramyotonia congenita together with the episodic weakness, which patients with paramyotonia congenita experience upon exposure to cold, has led some to suggest that paramyotonia and hyperkalemic paralysis are merely two aspects of the same disease. Families in which both types of illness are found lend credence to this view.[5]

When a patient is examined during an attack, the muscles are inexcitable as in the hypokalemic form. Some evidence of nerve hyperexcitability may be seen in the presence of a Chvostek sign.[1] This probably represents the minority of cases, and it is important to differentiate the myotonic response on percussion from this sign.

Laboratory Studies. The diagnosis may be established in hyperkalemic periodic paralysis by finding an elevated serum potassium during an attack of weakness. As in the hypokalemic form, patients become paralyzed with levels of serum potassium which would not be sufficient to affect the normal individual. Attacks are associated with the exit of potassium from muscle into the serum. This may be a local phenomenon and limited to the blood supply from paralyzed muscles, perhaps explaining why some patients with leg weakness may have a normal serum potassium when blood is drawn from the arm.[3] It is not a complete explanation, however, since there are undoubtedly some who suffer from the disease with a normal potassium level in the face of generalized weakness. Pearson found that 80 per cent of a patient's attacks were associated with increased potassium, in 15 per cent there was no change, and in 5 per cent the potassium was actually decreased in the serum.[6]

The EKG may show the changes of hyperkalemia. The creatine phosphokinase may also be elevated during an attack or in the interictal period. Physiological studies during an attack show slight depolarization of the muscle fibers.[3, 7, 8] Decreased potassium levels in the muscle and an increase in the sodium, water, and chloride contents have been reported.

Treatment. Treatment of an acute attack is seldom necessary since many of them are mild and brief. In the event of a more severe attack of weakness, intravenous calcium gluconate has been recommended. Intravenous sodium chloride may rarely abort an attack. Maintenance therapy on acetazolamide (Diamox) or chlorthiazide is helpful in decreasing the frequency of attacks. Acetazolamide has been shown to lessen the changes in serum potassium following provocative maneuvers.[4] The combination of chlorthiazide with potassium may be even more effective although the reason is unclear. Since acetazolamide is a sulfonamide, it should not be used in combination with other sulfonamides because of the dangers of renal damage. Dichlorphenamide, another carbonic anhydrase inhibitor, has been used in daily doses of 50 to 100 mg.[9] Bendrofluazide, 5 mg daily, is also reported to be beneficial. None of these medicines improves the permanent fixed weakness which may develop.

In this regard I would like to mention four patients who are of some historical interest. In 1951 Tyler et al.[10] described a large kindred with a variety of periodic paralysis which differed from the previously recognized hypokalemic variety not only in the clinical picture but also in the response to provocative stimulation with glucose and insulin. It was noted that the potassium in the serum was not reduced during the attacks. The administration of potassium, although it did not cause an attack, was unpopular with the patients, who felt worse on receiving this medication. The provocative effect of rest after exercise was noted, as well as the ability of the patients to "fight off" an attack by continued activity. The initial attacks occurred during the first year of life and were easily recognized by affected parents. The comment was made that the episodes were more frequent during childhood and then decreased in severity with advancing age. The presence or absence of myotonia was not commented on, but no symptoms of myotonia were elicited. Although some have quoted this article as an example of hyperkalemic periodic paralysis,[2] others have suggested it represented the normokalemic variety.[3]

In the last two years we have seen four new members of this kindred. These were a father and son and a mother and son from two separate branches of the family. Interestingly, neither knew of the others' existence although they were both aware that the illness ran in the family. All four had symptoms of myotonia and periodic bouts of weakness. The attacks of paralysis were associated with elevation of potassium, and the administration of potassium to one patient produced unequivocal weakness. Electrical myotonia was present at rest and was exacerbated on exposure to cold. The oldest patient was confined to a wheelchair, whereas the youngest one merely had slight difficulty arising from the floor. The disease appears to be the hyperkalemic variety although the poor response to treatment exhibited by one patient is noteworthy. Their histories are appended at the end of this chapter (Appendix A).

Secondary Hyperkalemic Paralysis

Retention of potassium in the body is associated with many different symptoms, one of which is weakness. This weakness is seen only with extremely high levels of potassium, and usually cardiac abnormalities take precedence over weakness. Causes include renal failure (when the associated uremia may mask the symptoms of hyperkalemia), adrenal failure, or the administration of potassium retaining diuretics. Possibly due to the potassium abnormality or to the associated metabolic abnormalities, muscle twitching and facial myokymia are not uncommon. The muscle is also unduly irritable to percussion.

BIBLIOGRAPHY

1. Gamstorp, I. Adynamia episodica hereditaria. Acta Paediatr. Scand. 45, Suppl. *108:* 1–126, 1956.
2. McArdle, B. Adynamia episodica hereditaria and its treatment. Brain *85:* 121–148, 1962.
3. Bradley, W. G. Adynamia episodica hereditaria; clinical, pathological and electrophysiological studies in an affected family. Brain: *92:* 345–378, 1969.
4. Hoskins, B. and Vroom, F. Q. Hyperkalemic periodic paralysis; effects of potassium, exercise, glucose and acetazolamide on blood chemistry. Arch. Neurol. **32:** 519–523, 1975.
5. Layzer, R. B., Lovelace, R. E., and Rowland, L. P. Hyperkalemic periodic paralysis. Arch. Neurol. *16:* 455–472, 1967.
6. Pearson, C. M. Periodic paralysis; differential features and pathological observations in permanent myopathic weakness. Brain *87:* 341–353, 1964.
7. Creutzfeldt, O. D., Abbott, B. C., Fowler, W. M., and Pearson, C. M. Muscle membrane potentials in episodic adynamia. Electroencephalogr. Clin. Neurophysiol. *15:* 508–519, 1963.
8. Brooks, J. E. Hyperkalemic periodic paralysis; intracellular electromyographic studies. Arch. Neurol. *20:* 13–18, 1969.
9. McArdle, B. Metabolic and endocrine myopathies. In: *Disorders of Voluntary Muscle,* edited by J. N. Walton. Churchill-Livingstone, London, 1974.
10. Tyler, F. H., Stephens, F. E., Gunn, F. D., and Perkoff, G. T. Studies in disorders of muscle. VII. Clinical manifestations and inheritance of a type of periodic paralysis without hypopotassemia. J. Clin. Invest. *30:* 492–502, 1951.

Normokalemic Periodic Paralysis

It is difficult to know whether this is an entity in its own right or whether the reports cited are of slightly atypical varieties of hyperkalemic paralysis, a disease to which it bears a suspicious resemblance. At all events, it must be a rare disease as there have been very few reports following the description by Poskanzer and Kerr of a type of episodic paralysis which had its onset in childhood, was associated with normal serum levels of potassium, and responded to treatment with 9-fluorohydrocortisone and acetazolamide.[1] The weakness was exacerbated by potassium and relieved by sodium chloride. Another report detailed the occurrence of episodic weakness in a mother and son.[2] Serum potassium levels were normal and the muscle biopsy showed tubular aggregates. The authors commented on the similarity between their patients and those in the report of Tyler et al. which was discussed in the section on hyperkalemic paralysis.

BIBLIOGRAPHY

1. Poskanzer, D. C., and Kerr, D. N. S. A third type of periodic paralysis, with normokalemia and a favourable response to sodium chloride. Am. J. Med. *31:* 328–342, 1961.
2. Meyers, K. R., Gilden, D. H., Rinaldi, C. F., and Hansen, J. L. Periodic muscle weakness, normokalemia and tubular aggregates. Neurology *22:* 269–279, 1972.

APPENDIX A

(1) P.K. is a thirty-five year old man (patient VI 30 of Tyler et al.[10]). He was referred to the Muscle Clinic because of an exacerbation of lifelong weakness. In early childhood he had attacks of paralysis of the arms and legs and would be limp during these periods. These spells recurred every week or so and lasted for a few hours, at the end of which time his strength returned spontaneously. Sometimes he had as many as two or three attacks a week. As an adult, he took a job farming and noticed that his weakness often began when he relaxed after heavy exercise. He could then abort an attack by gentle exercise. While his symptoms were inconvenient they did not interfere with his life, and in fact he took no medications. When questioned he commented that he had noticed some stiffness of his hands and face in cold weather but could not think of any other factors that either exacerbated or relieved his symptoms. In his late twenties he developed hip weakness and started to have difficulty climbing stairs. In the year prior to his visit to the Muscle Clinic he had found it difficult to get out of a chair. In order to stand for any period of time, he said he had to "lock his knees backwards." He ascribed the onset of this to being placed on hydrochlorothiazide for treatment of mild hypertension. He had suffered no other medical illnesses. In addition to many other family members, his own son also suffered from the illness.

On examination, he had a moderate degree of weakness of all muscles. The proximal muscles were worse than the distal muscles and the legs were worse than the arms. The gastrocnemii were bulky but there was no shortening of the heel cords. Clinical myotonia was not demonstrated on admission although with cold provocation he developed myotonia of both the eyelids and the hands.

Muscle biopsies were obtained from the biceps and the quadriceps. In the biceps, which was the stronger muscle, many of the fibers contained tubular aggregates (figs. 8.6 and 8.7). There was also variation in the size of fibers, internal nuclei, fibrosis, and fiber splitting. The muscle biopsy from the vastus showed even more dramatic changes, with many vacuoles, gross distortions of the architecture of muscle fibers, moth eaten, whorled fibers, fibrosis, and internal nuclei (Figs. 8.8–8.11). EMG showed abnormal insertional activity with high frequency repetitive discharges and typical myotonia. The myotonia was increased after immersion of the hand in cold water.

He was given 80 meq. of potassium and, five hours later, had an exacerbation of weakness. The EKG showed markedly peaked T waves and the serum potassium was 5.7 meq. per liter. This was not felt to be a clear cut response

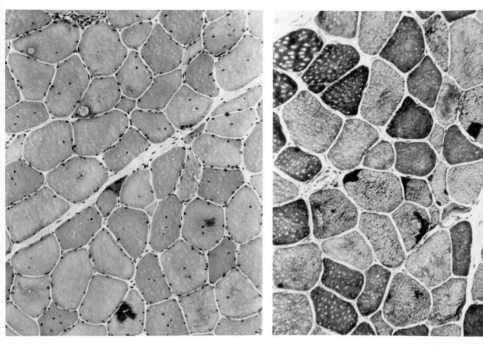

Figure 8.6. (*Left*) *Patient P. K*. Biceps muscle. There is a marked variation in the size of fibers with increased fibrosis and many internal nuclei. The darkly staining areas in the muscle fibers are tubular aggregates (H & E ×138).

Figure 8.7. (*Right*) *Patient P. K*. Biceps muscle. This histochemical reaction highlights the tubular aggregates. These appear as intensely dark areas in the muscle fibers. The small holes in the fibers are artifact, due to ice crystal formation (NADH-Tetrazolium Reductase ×138).

but because of the changes on the EKG it was felt inadvisable to administer higher doses of potassium.

Over the next year he was successively treated with acetazolamide, hydrochlorothiazide, prednisone, and dichlorphenamide. In spite of this he became progressively weaker, although the periodic bouts of weakness were lessened. The serum potassium was within normal values during this time. This gave rise to some doubt as to the diagnosis, and for a period of time he was maintained on potassium supplement alone. This was associated with the return of bouts of paralysis. One year after his original examination he was using a wheelchair and could stand on his own only with great difficulty.

(2) R.K., the eleven year old son of the previous patient was noticed to be abnormal during the first three months of life, when he had spells of floppiness. His mother noted that his cry was weak during these attacks. The symptoms lasted anywhere from minutes to hours and subsided spontaneously. During the attacks the arms and legs would hang limply by his side. In the intervening years he continued to have attacks usually brought on by exercise or anxiety. His mother stated that if he exercised when the attack began, he could usually lessen the degree of weakness. Occasionally he woke at night with an attack of severe weakness. The symptoms began in the legs but the arms were also involved. The boy complained of difficulty with

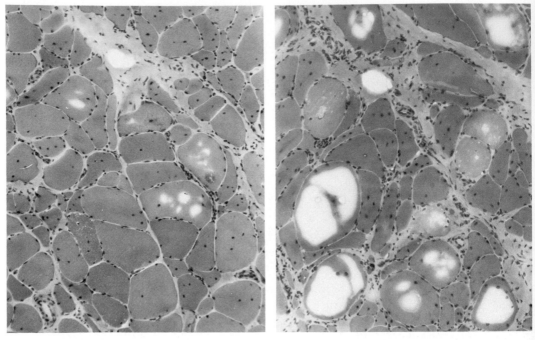

Figure 8.8. (*Left*) *Patient P. K.* Quadriceps. This muscle, which is more severely affected than the biceps, shows variation in the size of fibers, fibrosis and internal nuclei. Vacuoles are obvious in three of the fibers (H & E ×138).

Figure 8.9. (*Right*) *Patient P. K.* Quadricepts. Another area from the same biopsy shows even more severe vacuolar change (H & E ×138).

moving his tongue and swallowing. He was started on acetazolamide and the frequency of the attacks was markedly reduced. At the time of his visit to the clinic he was having only one attack a month. On examination he had mild fixed proximal weakness such that when he arose from the floor he used one hand to support his knee. The muscle biopsy revealed tubular aggregates in some of the muscle fibers together with an occasional central vacuole. There were also atrophic fibers and some internal nuclei (Fig. 8.12).

(3)   P.P. was a twenty-four year old woman, a distant cousin of P.K., who was seen in the clinic because she had been falling frequently. She is a member of generation VII in Tyler's paper, although it is not clear whether she appears on the published pedigree or not. Her weakness was first noticed at the age of six months when she became limp and was unable to move her limbs. She had recurrent episodes of such paralysis usually associated with rest after exercise. If she continued to use certain muscles during the early phase of the weakness, those muscles remained strong while the other muscles became very weak. At times she had several episodes a day and over the preceding few years had at least one episode daily. She could provoke an attack by drinking orange juice. When the weather was cold, both her face and eye movements were hampered because of stiffness. During both of her pregnancies she had noted difficulty in releasing her grasp.

On examination there was mild weakness of the hip. She had a slight "hip dip" when using the right leg. She arose from a chair with the assistance of her

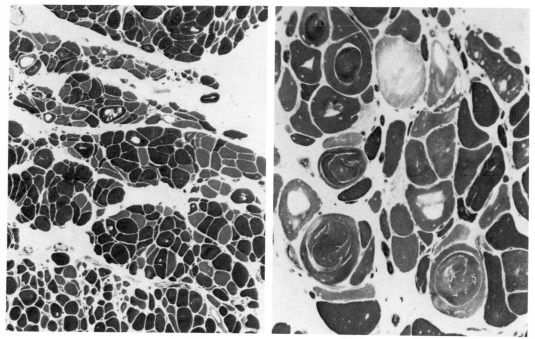

Figure 8.10. (*Left*) *Patient P. K.* Quadriceps. There is marked variation in the size of fibers and vacuoles (ATPase × 55).

Figure 8.11. (*Right*) *Patient P. K.* Quadriceps. Another area of the biopsy shows bizarre distortions in the muscle fibers in addition to the vacuoles. (ATPase ×138).

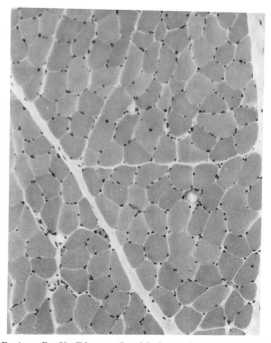

Figure 8.12. *Patient R. K.* Biceps. In this boy, the 11 year old son of P. K., the changes are very mild. One fiber is undergoing vacuolar degeneration and in the lower right corner, a small angulated fiber can be seen. Several other small fibers are scattered in the biopsy. (H & E stain ×138).

hands and was unable to do a situp. Eyelid myotonia and myotonia of the hand could be provoked by cooling. The administration of 40 meq. of potassium was associated with pronounced weakness at a time when the serum potassium was 5.9 meq. per litre. An EMG was not done. Her muscle biopsy was mildly abnormal with numerous internal nuclei, variability in the size of the fibers, and increased fibrosis. The administration of Diamox, 250 mg. t.i.d., was associated with relief of her attacks of paralysis although her fixed weakness was unchanged.

(4)   W.P. was the three year old son of the previous patient. His motor milestones were slightly delayed. He sat at the age of seven months and rolled over at eleven months. At about one year of age his mother noticed occasional episodes of weakness which almost always followed his nap. At this time, the mother would hear a weak cry from the bedroom and would find him to be flaccid. She had not noted any other symptoms. The only abnormality on examination was of mild hip weakness so that he used one hand to assist himself in standing. Provocative studies were not carried out in this child. A muscle biopsy showed only occasional internal nuclei.

9 abnormal muscle activity

Abnormal and repetitive muscle activity occurs as part of many different diseases. Myokymia is not infrequently seen in abnormal metabolic states. Carpopedal spasms are a part of calcium deficiency, and myotonia may occur in acid maltase deficiency. There are two clinical syndromes in which abnormal activity in the muscle is the dominant part of the illness. The first of these has come to be known as the stiff man syndrome, and the second as continuous muscle fiber activity. In both of these conditions there is sustained repetitive activity of muscle fibers.

STIFF MAN SYNDROME

A muscle cramp is a not uncommon experience in normal people. The physiology of this phenomenon is unclear, but it seems to be associated with an unduly powerful, voluntary contraction of a muscle, especially when it is held in a shortened position. The muscle then sustains an excruciatingly painful contraction of its own volition. Fortunately for most of us the threshold to produce such an unpleasant phenomenon is high. In the stiff man syndrome it is as if this threshold were lowered and extraordinary and disabling cramps are produced in many muscle groups under slight, or even no, provocation. It is not known whether the normal physiological cramp and the abnormal muscle activity in the stiff man syndrome have the same origin, but it is perhaps a useful way to remember the clinical stigmata of the disease.

Clinical Aspects

The illnes was first described by Moersch and Woltman.[1] Since then, many reports have appeared in the literature, and a review of these has presented a composite and rather typical picture[2, 3] The disease is usually one of adult life and affects both men and women. There may be some preceding aching and tightness of the back and chest muscles before the full manifestation of the illness. Firm and uncontrollable contractions of the muscles particularly of the hips, thighs, and shoulders then ensue, and these may spread to all the muscles of the body. Facial grimacing, difficulty with swallowing, and difficulty with breathing may be noted. The contractions themselves are unlike any produced voluntarily. The limbs are held rigid and immobile, the bellies of the muscles stand out in sharp relief and feel as if carved out from wood. The limb is usually held in a distorted position since the most powerful muscles in the limb overcome the antagonistic action of other muscles. The foot, for example, is often held in a position of inversion and plantar flexion since the slender muscles in the anterior compartment are no match for the bulky gastrocnemius and soleus group.

The spasms are extremely painful and may cause the patient to cry out aloud. During the worst of them, voluntary movements are not possible and the patient is totally immobilized. Some idea of the force which the contracting muscle exerts is illustrated by the fact that fractures of the long bones have occurred during such spasms. Stiffness disappears entirely during sleep and during general anesthesia but reoccurs following many different stimuli. These include voluntary movement, passive movement of the limb, emotional stress, and even the sudden appearance of visitors in the room. Although the symptoms disappear during sleep, the patient may wake frequently during the night, and when he does so the spasms return promptly.

The physical examination reveals no neurological abnormalities other than occasional increase in the reflexes and, rarely, extensor plantar responses. The latter should not be accepted automatically as part of the syndrome and may indicate other pathology.

A condition in which the abnormalities resemble the cramps which the patient can produce by voluntary movement, which disappear during sleep, and which are associated with a normal EMG pattern may make the examiner suspect that hysteria is the basis for this disease. It is unlikely, however, that the hysteric would have the fortitude to produce contractions strong enough to break long bones, and these titanic contractions take the disease out of the realm of the more gentle symptoms which the average hysteric manifests. Another intriguing question which is not yet answered about this illness is whether it exists in a sub-clinical form. Many patients who have aches, cramps, and pains of their limbs also have some degree of stiffness. Although there has been a tendency in the past to dismiss these patients as having functional disease, it is possible that they represent subclinical variety of the stiff man syndrome. It is wise to remember that strychnine and tetanus may also produce abnormal muscle spasms.

Laboratory Studies

Electromyographic examination shows a sustained interference pattern that persists in spite of all attempts to relax the muscle. Electroencephalographic investigation has shown an abnormality in the sleep pattern with less REM sleep than usual. These patients rarely attain stage three or stage four sleep.[4]

The spasms are easily abolished by curarization, block of the peripheral nerve with local anesthetic, or spinal anesthesia. In some patients, excretion of an abnormal metabolite perhaps derived from norepinephrine has been reported.[5] The origin of the disease is not clear. It has been ascribed to an overactivity of the gamma efferent system. A selective block of the gamma system by xylocaine, which was not sufficient to cause paralysis of the limb, abolished the spasms. This possible abnormality of gamma motor neurons was said to be due to a persistent drive from suprasegmental areas. The block of the gamma efferent system produced by xylocaine would remove the tonic "driving" of the intrafusal fibers and might be expected to decrease the reflex evoked activity of the alpha motor neurons. Others have felt that the disease is caused by some loss of the inhibitory influence from interneurons or by a deficiency in Renshaw cell function preventing the normal inhibitory feedback on anterior horn cells. An imbalance between a catecholaminergic and a GABA system has also been proposed.[4] Defective activity of the interneuronal inhibitory pool might impair the release of GABA and cause overactivity of the catecholaminergic neurons.

Treatment

This is one neuromuscular disease for which an effective form of treatment is known. The use of high doses of valium is recommended.[6] The dose of valium necessary to give relief of the symptoms may be 300 mg. a day or even higher. For some patients the side effects of this dose are too great to allow the drug to be used. Others tolerate enormous doses of valium without any side effects. As in many conditions in which valium is effective, the drug takes some days before it exerts its maximum effect.

BIBLIOGRAPHY

1. Moersch, F. P., and Woltman, H. W.: Progressive fluctuating muscular rigidity and spasm (stiff man syndrome). Proc. Staff Meet. Mayo Clin. *31:* 421–427, 1956.
2. Gordon, E. E., Januszko, D. M., and Kaufman, L. A critical survey of the stiff man syndrome. Am. J. Med. *42:*582–599, 1967.
3. Franck, G., Cornett, M., Grisar, T., Moonen, G., and Gerebtzoff, M. A. Le syndrome de l'homme raide. Acta Neurol. Belg. *74:* 221–240, 1974.
4. Guilleminault, C., Sigwald, J., and Castaigne, E. Sleep studies and therapeutic trial with L-dopa in a case of stiff man syndrome. Eur. Neurol. *10:* 89–96, 1973.
5. Schmidt, R. T., Stahl, S. M., and Spehlmann, R. A pharmacologic study of the stiff-man syndrome. Neurology *25:* 622–626, 1975.
6. Howard, F. M. A new and effective drug in the treatment of stiff man syndrome. Mayo Clin. Proc. *38:* 203–212, 1963.

CONTINUOUS MUSCLE FIBER ACTIVITY (NEUROMYOTONIA)

Another condition in which the motor unit has a tendency to discharge spontaneously is known as continuous muscle fiber activity.[1, 2] This entity has been known under many different names and may be present with varying degrees of severity. Perhaps in the same way that the stiff man syndrome may be thought of as an extension of the sometimes normal phenomenon of muscle cramping, continuous muscle fiber activity may be an extension of the normal phenomenon of fasciculations or at least an extension of the tendency of the motor unit to discharge spontaneously. In its mildest forms, it occurs as myokymia. This is a brief contraction of parts of the muscle a phenomenon which is difficult to distinguish from fasciculations, and indeed the words in the past have been used interchangeably. There is, however, an important point of distinction when electrical studies are carried out. A fasciculation is an isolated motor unit discharge and, although it may be repetitive, the interval between individual fasciculations of the same motor unit are quite prolonged. In myokymia, one or more motor units discharge in rapid sequence. Thus, short bursts of action potentials are seen on the EMG and are associated with brief tetanic contractions of the muscle fibers. The frequency of these trains of motor units varies from roughly ten to a hundred Hz. The length of the trains also varies from doublets and triplets to sustained bursts lasting several seconds. The appearance of the muscle during these times is of a quivering, undulating "bag of worms." When the myokymic trains are prolonged, they are easy to differentiate from fasciculations because the strip of muscle that is contracting does so over a long period of time and does not resemble the brief twitch of a fasciculation. On the other hand, brief myokymic trains are impossible to distinguish with the naked eye from the contraction seen with a fasciculation.

Clinical Aspects

In the mild form of the disease the patient suffers no particular handicap. The movements may be disturbing since the patient is aware of them and they may keep him awake at night. The myokymia does not disappear during sleep. There may be difficulty relaxing the muscle after a voluntary contraction. In the most severe form, stiffness is present at rest and impedes movement. When walking, the patient may give the impression of wading through a sea of molasses. The disease occurs at any age, even during the neonatal period.[3] There is usually no precipitating cause and most of the cases occur sporadically.

The symptoms often start gradually with a period of increasing stiffness, frequently in the legs. In one or two cases muscle pains have been noted.[4] The patient notices the twitching movements in the legs and may also complain of excessive sweating. This is perhaps related to the necessary dissipation of heat generated by the constant muscle activity, but its exact cause is unclear. With increasing symptoms, the body becomes stiff and the wrists are flexed with the fingers extended. The feet turn into an equinus position. The patient may have a stooped posture because of the rigidity. When the patient tries to move, the stiffness is quite variable. Initially it may increase and then decrease again, waxing and waning throughout the course of movement. Laryngeal stridor has been noted in one patient.[5]

The abnormal tone and myokymia do not disappear during sleep. The fact that they are not altered during spinal block, during pentothal anesthesia, or by proximal nerve block suggests that the defect lies in the distal part of the motor unit. A motor point infiltration with xylocaine reduces the activity although it does not abolish it completely. Curarization is associated with abolition of the spontaneous activity. Sometimes the muscle fiber activity is also absent for a few seconds after voluntary contraction. In several patients, peripheral wasting has been noted, perhaps further evidence of a neuropathic problem in this illness.

Laboratory Studies

The EMG abnormalities are characteristic and have already been described. The pathology is obscure, but most of the cases have shown not only physiological evidence of damage to the peripheral nerves but pathological evidence with signs of denervation and reinnervation in the muscle as well as anatomical changes in the peripheral verve. In two cases, abnormal chemicals have been incriminated. In a severe case in an infant, a derivative of DDT was found in the serum and in another case[4] exposure to the herbicide 2,4-D was noted. These two cases may closely resemble myotonia which can be produced experimentally by 2,4-D.

Treatment

The treatment of the disease with diphenylhydantoin has been remarkably successful and in patients with myokymia alone as well as those with the fully developed syndrome, the administration of diphenylhydantoin has removed the symptoms. Carbamazepine (Tegretol) has also been reported to help the illness.[6]

BIBLIOGRAPHY

1. Isaacs, H. A syndrome of continuous muscle fiber activity. J. Neurol. Neurosurg. Psychiatry *24:* 319–325, 1961.
2. Mertens, H. G., and Zschocke, S. Neuromyotonie. Klin. Wochenschr. *17:* 917–925, 1965.
3. Black, J. T., Garcia-Mullin, R., Good, R., and Brown, S. Muscle rigidity in a newborn due to continuous peripheral nerve hyperactivity. Arch. Neurol. *27:* 413–425, 1972.
4. Wallis, W. E., Van Poznak, A., and Plum, F. Generalized muscular stiffness, fasciculations and myokymia of peripheral nerve origin. Arch. Neurol. *22:* 430–439, 1970.
5. Levinson, S., Canalis, R. F., and Kaplan, H. J. Laryngeal spasm complicating pseudomyotonia. Arch. Otolaryngol. *102:* 185–187, 1976.
6. Isaacs, H., and Heffron, J. J. A. The syndrome of "continuous muscle fiber activity" cured: further studies. J. Neurol. Neurosurg. Psychiatry *37:* 1231–1235, 1974.

10 congenital (more or less) muscle diseases

The ungainly title to the chapter is a measure of the uncertainty associated with the diseases described herein. Originally the chapter was to be entitled, "Congenital Nonprogressive Myopathies," but although most are congenital many are in fact progressive, and the evidence that these illnesses are primarily of the muscle itself is shaky. "Morphologically Distinct Myopathies" was equally inexact since the morphology by which they are distinguished may, in fact, represent epiphenomena in the muscle rather than any fundamental part of the disease. The ideal solution, a chapter entitled "Other," seemed somehow escapist. In some of these illnesses, such as the congenital hypotonias, the pathology is uncertain although the clinical picture is better described. In others, the abnormalities in the muscle are so striking that they are embodied in the name of the disease, and in yet others, such as the congenital dystrophies, we are certain of neither the clinical picture nor the pathological changes. The first section will deal with floppy infants, excluding children, such as those with infantile spinal muscular atrophy, whose diseases have been described in preceding chapters. This will be followed by discussion of the various illnesses characterized by peculiar structural alterations, such as central core disease and nemaline myopathy.

CONGENITAL HYPOTONIA

Observation of the way in which a baby moves and the postures adopted by its limbs, together with an evaluation of the passive tone, are the most useful tests of muscle function in the newborn period. Poverty of movement, the assumption of abnormal postures, and a reduction in the baby's tone are the characteristics of the floppy infant. Such infants may have respiratory difficulties at birth and shortly afterwards are noted to be lying with the limbs externally rotated and abducted, the so-called "frog leg" position. The hypotonia is expressed in various ways. When the child is pulled by his hands from the supine position the head falls backwards in extreme retroflexion. When supported under the abdomen and lifted from the bed (ventral suspension) the hypotonia causes the child to droop in an inverted "U." A more precise description is given elsewhere.[1] Hypotonia may be due to causes other than abnormalities of the neuromuscular system, mental retardation and other forms of cerebral damage being among the commonest. Usually in such circumstances the floppiness is an incidental part of the picture and the diagnosis is readily apparent. In upper motor neuron disease or with cerebral palsy, the initial hypotonia may give way to increased tone and spasticity. In the patient with mental retardation, such as is seen in Down's syndrome, the floppiness improves as the child grows older. In other children there is weakness of the muscles in addition to the disturbance of tone; these children either have been discussed in preceding chapters or will be considered later in this chapter. A substantial number of babies have no clear weakness, and these fall into three main groups: benign congenital hypotonia, the Prader-Willi syndrome, and congenital hypotonia associated with Type 1 fiber predominance.

Benign Congenital Hypotonia

The concept of benign congenital hypotonia is a very useful one and if stringent criteria are applied to its diagnosis the prognosis is always good. Benign congenital hypotonia refers to those children whose physical examination reveals only abnormal tone. The deep tendon reflexes are normal. There is neither weakness nor wasting. Occasionally strabismus is noted, but this may be merely incidental rather than part of the illness. The laboratory tests, including the serum "muscle" enzymes, electromyography, and, even more importantly, muscle biopsy, are all normal. Children in this group have a uniformly good prognosis and the parents can be reassured that eventually the child will develop normally. It is possible that some children with additional findings such as a decrease in deep tendon reflexes or with mild abnormalities of muscle histochemistry may do equally well. However, if the category of benign congenital hypotonia is broadened to include these patients, a small percentage will be shown later to have some other illness and an excellent prognosis cannot be given with such certainty.

Congenital Hypotonia With Type 1 Fiber Predominance

Muscle fibers can be differentiated into two basic types using the appropriate histochemical reactions. These have been termed Type 1 and Type 2; in normal muscle the Type 2 fibers usually outnumber the Type 1 fibers by about 2:1. Type 1 fiber predominance refers to a change in which the Type 1 fibers comprise more than 60% of the fibers in the biopsy.

Type 1 fiber predominance is a common connecting link that joins many of the illnesses to be described in this chapter. It is, perhaps, not surprising that in some instances it is the only change to be found. Such may be the case in children who present with congenital hypotonia (Figures 10.1 and 10.2). There may be some decrease in the deep tendon reflexes and a higher incidence of skeletal anomalies such as flat feet or pes cavus, congenital hip dislocation, and, very rarely, kyphoscoliosis. Mild weakness of the limbs may persist into adult life, but most of these children improve. They may remain ungainly and somewhat clumsy, but a normal life is possible. Type 1 fiber predominance is the only abnormality in the biopsy and the presence of fibrosis, internal nuclei, phagocytosis and necrosis, or variability in the size of fibers is probably a reason to exclude the diagnosis.

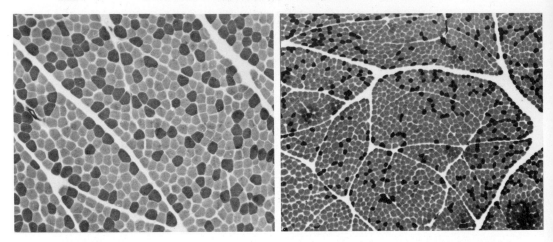

Figure 10.1 (*left*). In an eighteen month old boy who had a history of congenital hypotonia and some delay in the attainment of motor milestones, the muscle biopsy from the biceps showed the majority of fibers to be Type 1 (light). This is an example of congenital hypotonia with Type 1 fiber predominance (ATPase pH 9.4).

Figure 10.2 (*right*). A similar patient with congenital hypotonia, in whom there was mild weakness of the legs and decreased reflexes, showed Type 1 fiber predominance in a biopsy from the biceps muscle (ATPase pH 9.4).

Prader-Willi Syndrome

A cause of hypotonia which is not uncommon in a muscle clinic is the Prader-Willi syndrome.[2] These children are floppy at birth. Very frequently they have a low birth weight and experience considerable feeding difficulties in the neonatal period, with a poor suck response and some difficulty swallowing. The cause for the hypotonia often goes undiagnosed until about the age of three years, when they gain weight in a striking and characteristic fashion. These children become enormously obese and their appetite is legendary. It is not uncommon for the parents to have to padlock the refrigerator or for the children to be found rummaging in the garbage cans of their neighbors in search of food. The face is rather characteristic although difficult to describe (Figures 10.3 and 10.4). Boys are more often affected with the illness than girls. Hypogonadism with a small penis and undescended testicles is characteristic.

The symptoms all point towards a defect in hypothalamic function, but none has yet been found. An abnormality in growth hormone has been reported.[3] Mental retardation is the rule and may be quite severe although it is masked by the personality of these children. They combine pleasant outgoing behavior with a flow of speech which is unusual. The questions they ask are often repetitive and trivial. The voice is high pitched and they may suffer from problems with pronunciation. All in all their friendliness, although charming, can be a little wearing. The children are frequently short statured and the bone age may be retarded. On rare occasions convulsions are noted.

Laboratory studies reveal little evidence of muscle abnormality. Serum muscle enzymes are usually normal. Electromyography reveals no abnormal-

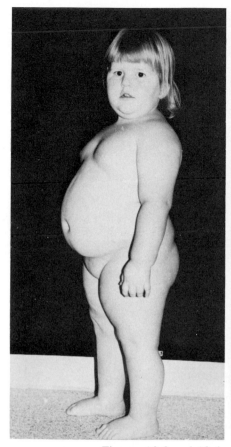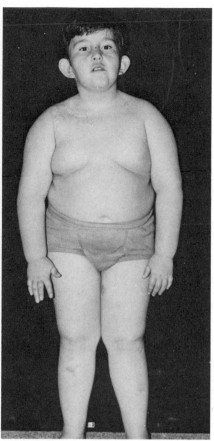

Figures 10.3 and 10.4. Prader-Willi syndrome.

ity and light microscopy shows normal muscle biopsy. Some changes have been described following electron microscopic studies[4] but are rather unconvincing.

There is no specific treatment for this disease. The obesity, complications of which present the major threat to the patient's life, responds poorly to dietary management. Although harsh restriction of diet may be of value, it is seldom attained.

CONGENITAL MUSCULAR DYSTROPHY

I reserve this diagnosis for children who are undoubtedly suffering from some malign muscle disease but whose diagnosis, in my ignorance, I am unable to ascertain. I suspect there are others who use the diagnosis in the same fashion. It is really not a diagnosis at all, and as investigations become increasingly sophisticated the category will probably disappear. One subcategory whose outlines are hazily glimpsed includes patients with weakness, wasting, and hypotonia of a progressive nature, presenting within the first year of life. The limb muscles are more involved than the bulbar muscles, which are often spared. Deep tendon reflexes are decreased and contractures of muscles seem to be quite common. We have not yet seen any familial cases

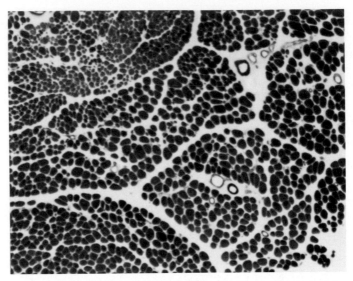

Figure 10.5. A biopsy from the biceps of a three year old girl with progressive weakness and contractures of muscle showed a total absence of Type 2 fibers. The diagnosis of congenital muscular dystrophy was based on the muscle biopsy, myopathic findings on the EMG examination, and elevated serum "muscle" enzymes (ATPase pH 9.4).

which may suggest that the term dystrophy is incorrect. The muscle biopsy shows a number of abnormal findings including a random variation in the size of fibers and increased fibrosis with some internal nuclei. The most striking finding is that there are no Type 2 fibers whatsoever (Figure 10.5). This total absence of Type 2 fibers in association with the other abnormalities mentioned implies a rather poor prognosis. Cardiorespiratory failure has been the cause of death in several patients. The serum muscle enzymes are always elevated but no other chemical abnormalities have been noted. Electromyographically, small, short, polyphasic potentials with an increased interference pattern have been seen.

CONGENITAL FIBER TYPE DISPROPORTION

Some children who are born with weakness and hypotonia have an unusual finding on the biopsy in which the size and number of the two principal muscle fiber types are abnormal. The Type 1 fibers are more numerous and smaller than the Type 2 fibers (Figure 10.6).[5-8] Because this type of biopsy was associated with a rather stereotyped clinical picture, it was suggested that it constituted a clinical syndrome and this was named congenital fiber type disproportion. The children were floppy at birth and had varying degrees of weakness. On occasion the disease was so severe that respiratory compromise and recurrent respiratory infections were seen in the first year of life. In over half of the cases, contractures of various muscles were noticed at birth. The muscle involved varied from the sternocleidomastoid to the muscles of the forearm and hand. Congenital hip dislocation was noted in a third of the patients, which may represent no more than the secondary effect of intrauterine weakness and hypotonia. The weakness seemed to be at its most severe during the first two years of life. After this, the disease either improved or became relatively stable. It should be emphasized that residual weakness is the rule in these patients. In only three out of the twelve original patients did muscle strength attain the normal. As the children grew older, their weight fell below the third percentile, and frequently the patients were also short. Other skeletal abnormalities included a high arched palate and kyphoscoliosis, which were seen in over half. Valgus or varus deformities of the feet were noted.

Investigation of other family members has shown that in some instances the disease is inherited. In two families it has occurred as an autosomal dominant. In some there are other members involved in different generations but the mode of inheritance is not clear. Both sexes seem to be involved. There is no disturbance of intellectual function. Clinical examination shows decreased to absent deep tendon reflexes with mild to moderate weakness of the arms and legs. The proximal muscles around the shoulders and hips are slightly more involved than the distal muscles. Mild facial weakness has been seen on occasions. Laboratory studies are not very helpful. The serum muscle enzyme may be slightly elevated. The EMG shows a combination of small, short potentials together with large amplitude potentials. Conduction velocities are normal. The muscle biopsy shows the disproportion in the number and size of the fiber types, sometimes with additional features such as scattered internal nuclei or occasional fibers with rods.

Some comment should be made with regard to the relationship between this illness and some of the other morphologically distinct myopathies. The illness closely resembles nemaline myopathy, in which the Type 1 fibers are also smaller than the Type 2 fibers, and there is frequently Type 1 fiber predominance. The profusion of rod-like structures in the muscles of patients

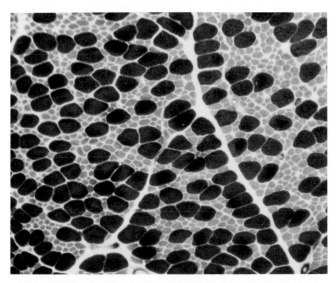

Figure 10.6. A biopsy from the biceps of a patient with congenital fiber type disproportion. Notice the discrepancy between the size of the Type 2 (dark) fibers and the Type 1 (light). In addition, there is a discrepancy in the numbers of fibers, the Type 1 fibers being far more numerous than usual (ATPase pH 9.4).

with nemaline myopathy not only has given the name to the disease but also has been considered a necessary part of the illness. The existence of rods in the muscle, however, is a nonspecific finding. Furthermore, patients with nemaline myopathy have been described in whom the rods are present in only one of several biopsies or in one part of the biopsy.

The question is unresolved. It seems illogical to make a diagnosis of nemaline myopathy without proof of the existence of rods in the muscle, and yet it may also be illogical to make such an important distinguishing point out of a structural alteration which may be nonspecific.

BIBLIOGRAPHY

1. Dubowitz, V. *The Floppy Infant.* Spastics International Medical Publications, 1969.
2. Zellweger, H., and Schneider, H. J. The syndrome of hypotonia, hypomentia, hypogonadism, obesity (HHHO) or Prader-Willi syndrome. Am. J. Dis. Child. *115:* 588, 1958.
3. Theodoridis, C. H., Brown, C. A., Chance, G. W., and Rudd, B. T. Plasma growth hormone levels in children with Prader-Willi syndrome. Aust. Paediatr. J. *7:* 24, 1971.
4. Afifi, A. K., and Zellweger, H. Pathology of muscular hypotonia in the Prader-Willi syndrome. Light and electron microscopic study. J. Neurol. *9:* 49–61, 1969.
5. Brooke, M. H. Congenital fiber type disproportion. In: *Clinical Studies in Myology,* edited by B. A. Kakulas. Excerpta Medica, Amsterdam, 1973.
6. Lenard, H. G., and Goebel, H. H. Congenital fiber type disproportion. Neuropaediatrie *6:* 220–231, 1975.
7. Kinoshita, M., Satoyoshi, E., and Kumagai, M. Familial Type 1 fiber atrophy. J. Neurol. Sci. *25:* 11–17, 1975.
8. Fardeau, M., Harpey, J. P., and Caille, B. Disproportion congénitale des différents types de fibre musculaire, avec petitesse relative des fibres de type I. Rev. Neurol. *131:* 745–766, 1975.

CENTRAL CORE DISEASE

In 1956 Shy and Magee observed a pathological change that was so striking that they embodied it in the name they gave the illness.[1] This was central core disease and it was the forerunner of a number of myopathies whose descriptive titles reflect the predominant change on the muscle biopsy. Some of these have stood the test of time. As in the original case report, the disease is often inherited as an autosomal dominant. However, sporadic instances have been described and it is possible that we should think not of central core disease but of central core diseases.

In most patients the onset is noted at or shortly after birth, when the patient is floppy and attains the motor milestones only slowly. In a number of patients congenital hip dislocation is noted. As the child grows older he finds that he cannot run as smoothly as other children and jumping is often impossible. Often the family expresses little concern over these symptoms since it is recognized in some of the other members as a mild abnormality and is regarded more as an annoyance than an illness. Only two of the twelve patients we have seen with central core disease came to the muscle clinic because of their complaint of weakness. Others arrived for reasons as various as needing a letter in order to be excused from military duty or, in the case of one patient, simply because he worked in the next laboratory to my own.

In adult life the patients are often slender and short statured, but without any focal muscle atrophy (Figure 10.7). The weakness may be diffuse although some reports have stressed a proximal distribution, particularly of the hips. Mild weakness of the face and neck muscles may also be seen. The deep

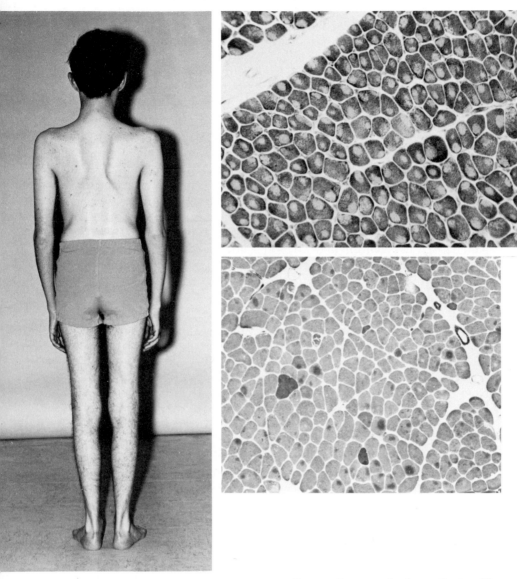

Figures 10.7 through 10.9. Central core disease. In general, the patients with central core disease have a rather diffuse weakness and are slender without any focal muscle wasting (10.7, *left*). With the NADH-tetrazolium reductase reaction there are unstained areas within each muscle fiber which give the disease its name (10.8, *upper right*). The ATPase reaction (pH 9.4) shows Type 1 fiber predominance (10.9, *lower right*). Only two or three Type 2 (dark) fibers are present in the entire biopsy.

tendon reflexes may be decreased but are often normal. Skeletal deformities are not uncommon, perhaps a reflection of the early onset of this illness. In addition to congenital hip dislocation, lordosis and kyphoscoliosis may be seen. Either high arched feet or flat feet are also relatively common findings. In some, only fragments of the disease are expressed and patients whose only complaint was pes cavus or tight heel cords have been recorded.[2]

Laboratory tests other than the muscle biopsy are usually unhelpful, serum enzymes are normal, and the EMG is rather nonspecific. The muscle biopsy is quite strikingly abnormal. Mild variability in the size of the fibers is seen. On occasions, extremely small atrophic fibers have been noted. There is often marked Type 1 fiber predominance (Figure 10.9), and there exists in the center of most of the fibers an area which is unreactive with the oxidative enzyme histochemistry (Figure 10.8). With the ATPase reaction the reactivity of the central areas is either decreased or on occasions increased. If the diagnosis is restricted to those patients demonstrating the changes shown above, then the clinical picture is always as described. It may even be that the presence of central cores is unnecessary for the diagnosis. In one family, although the patient's biopsy demonstrated such cores, the patient's children, both of whom had the illness, showed only the Type 1 predominance and slight variability in the size of fibers.[3] At the other end of the spectrum are patients whose biopsies demonstrate fairly good differentiation of the muscle fibers into two types with central cores only in the minority of fibers. These patients may not conform to the typical history and perhaps represent another disease. The question is further complicated by the resemblance of the changes in these patients to the target fiber, a change which indicates denervation and probably reinnervation.

In an attempt to clarify this situation (although in retrospect it may have compounded the confusion), the differentiation of cores into "structured" and "unstructured" was suggested.[4] In an earlier description of the pathological changes in central core disease, the myofibrillar cross striations were well preserved.[5] Indeed, this was one of the grounds for distinguishing the change from that of target fibers in which the cross striations are lost. In some patients, electron microscopy shows that the central core of altered myofibrillar material still retains perfect cross striations. Although the sarcomeres may be slightly contracted and the mitochondria are absent from the core region, the I and A band and even the Z line are undisturbed. This type of core ("structured") can be clearly distinguished from target fibers. In the unstructured core there is considerable disarray in the myofibrillar architecture with distortion of the cross banding pattern. We found it impossible to distinguish such changes from those of the target fiber, and indeed the name "core-targetoid" fiber has been coined to indicate this confusion.[6] If the patient's biopsy demonstrates only unstructured cores, if they are present in a minority of fibers, and if the associated Type 1 predominance is lacking, then the diagnosis should be accepted only with reservation.

Biochemical abnormalities have been described but may be nonspecific. Phosphorylase activity is reduced,[5, 7] a finding which might be expected in view of the paucity of Type 2 (glycolytic) fibers. The calcium dependent ATPase and the uptake of calcium by the sarcoplasmic reticulum is also reduced, which might correlate with the absence of this membrane from the core regions.

The treatment of central core disease is usually supportive. Genetic counseling should be given on the basis of an autosomal dominant disease unless the family history indicates clearly that this is a sporadic case. Most of the patients are so mildly handicapped that no specific treatment is necessary. The literature on central core disease has been reviewed by Telerman-Toppet et al.[2]

BIBLIOGRAPHY

1. Shy, G. and Magee, K. R. A new congenital nonprogressive myopathy. Brain *79:* 610–621, 1956.
2. Telerman-Toppet, N., Gerard, J. M., and Coers, C. Central core disease; a study of clinically unaffected muscle. J. Neurol. Sci. *19:* 207–223, 1973.
3. Morgan-Hughes, J. A., Brett, E. M., Lake, B. D., and Tome, F. M. S. Central core disease or not? Observations on a family with a nonprogressive myopathy. Brain *96:* 527–536, 1973.
4. Neville, H. E., and Brooke, M. H. Central core fibers; structured and unstructured. In: *Basic Research in Myology,* edited by B. A. Kakulas. Excerpta Medica, Amsterdam, 1973.
5. Engel, W. K., Foster, J. B., Hughes, B. P., Huxley, H. D., and Mahler, R. Central core disease; an investigation of a rare muscle cell abnormality. Brain *84:* 167–185, 1961.
6. Engel, W. K., Brooke, M. H., and Nelson, P. G. Histochemical studies of denervated or tenotomized cat muscle. Ann. N.Y. Acad. Sci. *138:* 160–185, 1966.
7. Isaacs, H., Heffron, J. J. A., and Badenhorst, M. Central core disease. J. Neurol. Neurosurg. Psychiatry *38:* 1177–1186, 1976.

NEMALINE MYOPATHY (ROD BODY DISEASE)

Nemaline myopathy is characterized by the presence of myriads of small, rod-like particles in the muscle (Figure 10.11).[1,2] The origin of these rod-like particles is still uncertain and they are not specific for this disease alone but have been found in many different situations. It is also possible, as will be discussed later, that they may not be an essential part of the illness. Nevertheless, the presence of an overwhelming number of rods in a muscle biopsy suggests the entity nemaline myopathy.

The disease has a genetic basis; in some families it is inherited as an autosomal dominant, whereas in others it occurs as an autosomal recessive with varying penetrance. Sporadic cases have also been reported. There are two clinical syndromes associated with nemaline myopathy. The most commonly recognized is of hypotonia and a rather diffuse weakness of the limbs and trunk beginning at a very early age. In addition to weakness of the arms and legs, some mild weakness of the face and other bulbar muscles has been noted.[3] These children are often dysmorphic with a long narrow face, high arched palate, and slender musculature. Often the patients are stronger than their muscle bulk would imply. High arched feet and kyphoscoliosis are not uncommon, particularly in the older patients. For the most part, the disease is not progressive and the patient learns to live with the moderate degree of weakness. Very rarely the illness may be severe, and death from respiratory complications has been seen.

Other patients present with a scapuloperoneal distribution of weakness, and a foot-drop is one of the earliest symptoms.[4-6] Sometimes this begins later in adolescence or even adult life. The hip muscles are involved in this type of illness, but this occurs later, and the most severe weakness is of the muscles of the anterior tibial compartment and of the shoulders. I have observed patients with kyphoscoliosis (Figure 10.10) and this may differentiate the illness from some of the other varieties of the scapuloperoneal syndrome.

The deep tendon reflexes are generally decreased and, as in many of the congenital myopathies, serum enzyme studies and EMG are really not helpful in making the diagnosis. There may be mild elevation of serum creatine phosphokinase and the EMG may show short polyphasic potentials. The muscle biopsy, however, is paramount in arriving at the diagnosis. Most

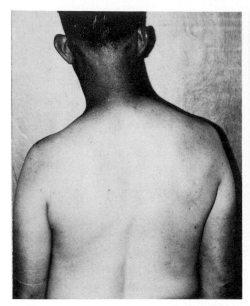

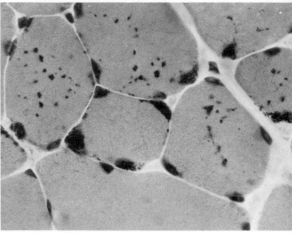

Figures 10.10 and 10.11. Nemaline myopathy. This patient presented to the hospital with a kyphoscoliosis. He was found to have scapular weakness and weakness of the anterior tibial muscles. The muscle biopsy from the biceps showed large numbers of rods scattered throughout the fibers. The small particles are seen at the corners of the muscle fibers and are also scattered throughout the centers of many of them.

patients show Type 1 fiber predominance which may at times comprise over 90 percent of the fibers in the biopsy. There is often Type 1 fiber atrophy, particularly in the diffuse childhood form of the disease.

The origin of the rods is uncertain. They are thought to be derived from the Z line, since they often seem to arise from this structure when muscle is examined under the electron microscope. Some similarities between the rod bodies and tropomyosin led to the suggestion that these structures actually represented storage of tropomyosin within the muscle. However, no increase in this substance was noted on biochemical analysis.[7] A recent study demonstrated no abnormality of tropomyosin and furthermore failed to demonstrate the relationship between the rods and adjacent Z lines, although most studies have shown such a relationship. These authors found evidence of an abnormal myosin characterized by an altered pattern of the light chain composition.[8] Experiments in which electron microscopic studies were combined with biochemical techniques suggested that a major component of the rod bodies was α-actinin.[9] This compound is a "structural" protein which holds the actin filaments to the Z line.

The problem of nemaline myopathy is further compounded by the undoubted presence of nemaline rods in other diseases which are far removed in their clinical appearance from nemaline myopathy. I have seen rods in patients with Parkinson's disease, rheumatoid arthritis, and polymyositis, and they have been recorded in equally unrelated conditions.[10–12] If, in fact, they are relatively nonspecific, perhaps the most significant change in nemaline myopathy is the Type 1 fiber atrophy and/or Type 1 fiber predominance, as has been suggested by Dahl and Klutzow.[13] If one disregards the rods then the entity becomes very similar to that described under congenital fiber type disproportion. Two of our patients with this entity had a few scattered rods, and another report records a similar family.[14]

BIBLIOGRAPHY

1. Shy, G. M., Engel, W. K., Somers, J. E., and Wanko, T. Nemaline myopathy; a new congenital myopathy. Brain 86: 793–810, 1963.
2. Conen, P. E., Murphy, G. E., and Donohue, W. L. Light and electron microscopic studies of "myogranules" in a child with hypotonia and muscle weakness. Can. Med. Assoc. J. 89: 983–986, 1963.
3. Kulakowski, S., Flament-Durand, J., Malaisse-Lagae, F., Chevallay, M., and Fardeau, M. Myopathie a batonnets. Arch. Franc. Pediatr. 30: 505–526, 1973.
4. Feigenbaum, J. A., and Munsat, T. L. A neuromuscular syndrome of scapuloperoneal distribution. Bull. Los Angeles Neurol. Soc. 35: 47–57, 1970.
5. Kuitunen, P., Rapola, J. Noponen, A.-L., and Donner, M. Nemaline myopathy. Acta Paediatr. Scand. 61: 353–361, 1972.
6. Kinoshita, M. and Satoyoshi, E. Type 1 fiber atrophy and nemaline bodies. Arch. Neurol. 31: 423–425, 1974.
7. Sugita, H., Masaki, T., Ebashi, S., and Pearson, C. M. Protein composition of rods in nemaline myopathy. In: Basic Research in Myology, edited by B. A. Kakulas. Excerpta Medica, Amsterdam, 1973.
8. Sreter, F. A., Astrom, K. E., Romanul, F. C. A., Young, R. R., and Royden-Jones, H. Characteristics of myosin in nemaline myopathy. J. Neurol. Sci. 27: 99–116, 1976.
9. Stromer, M. H., Tabatabai, L. B., Robson, R. M. Goll, D. E., and Zeece, M. G. Nemaline myopathy, an integrated study; selective extraction. Exp. Neurol. 50: 402–421, 1976.
10. Rewcastle, N. B., and Humphrey, J. G. Vacuolar myopathy; clinical, histochemical and microscopic study. Arch. Neurol. 12: 570–582, 1965.
11. Sato, T., Walker, D. L., Peters, H. A., Reese, H. H., and Chou, S. M. Chronic polymyositis and myxovirus-like inclusions. Arch. Neurol. 24: 409–418, 1971.
12. Meltzer, H. Y., McBride, E., and Poppei, R. W. Rod bodies in the skeletal muscle of an acute schizophrenic patient. Neurology 23: 769–780, 1973.
13. Dahl, D. S., and Klutzow, F. W. Congenital rod disease; further evidence of innervational abnormalities as the basis for the clinico-pathological features. J. Neurol. Sci. 23: 371–385, 1974.
14. Kinoshita, M. Satoyoshi, E., and Kumagai, M. Familial type 1 fiber atrophy. J. Neurol. Sci. 25: 11–17, 1975.

MYOTUBULAR MYOPATHY (CENTRONUCLEAR MYOPATHY)

In 1966 Spiro and others described an illness in which structures resembling fetal myotubes persisted into adult life. They christened this myotubular myopathy.[1] Others, noting that the resemblance may be superficial and that there are important differences between true myotubes and the changes seen in the disease, have suggested centronuclear myopathy.[2] However, the term "myotubular" has established its precedence and is picturesque enough to warrant retention until the basic cause of the disease is uncovered.

Since the disease has been characterized by the muscle biopsy, it is appropriate to describe this first. The most typical cases of myotubular myopathy have a combination of internal nuclei (Figure 10.12), a characteristic increase in the central staining of the muscle fibers with the oxidative enzyme reactions (Figure 10.13), and a central pale area with the ATPase reactions (Figure 10.14). The last two changes are far more frequent than the presence of internal nuclei, since the "myotube" represents rows of nuclei separated by

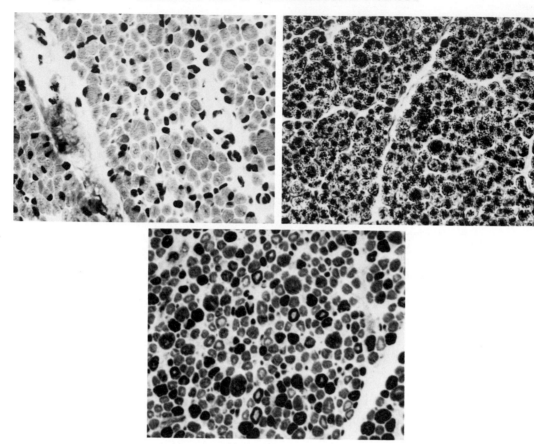

Figures 10.12 through 10.14. A three month old boy was born with severe weakness and floppiness and had considerable respiratory difficulty, dying from pulmonary complications at the age of three months. The H and E stain showed occasional fibers with large central nuclei (10.12, *upper left*). Oxidative enzyme reaction showed an alteration of the normal staining pattern. Instead of a diffuse stain of the intermyofibrillar network, there were increased areas of central staining in most of the fibers (10.13, *upper right*). Notice that many more of the fibers have this area of increased staining than demonstrate internal nuclei. The ATPase reaction (pH 9.4) shows these central areas to be nonreactive, giving the appearance of doughnuts. (10.14, *lower*).

spaces and the chances of a section cutting through a space are greater than of cutting through a nucleus. Most of the biopsies reveal Type 1 fiber predominance. The presence of Type 1 fiber atrophy has also been recorded, but this may not necessarily be a part of the picture.

A heterogeneous collection of clinical pictures is described under the title of myotubular or centronuclear myopathy. This is partly due to the inclusion of patients whose sole abnormality on the muscle biopsy is internal nuclei. If these patients are excluded, and only those whose biopsies include all the changes above are considered, then the clinical findings are not quite so variegated. Most of these patients are hypotonic at or shortly after birth. Ptosis and paralyses of the extraocular muscles occur early and facial weakness is often mentioned. Weakness of the axial musculature involves both the neck flexors and the limbs. In some cases the emphasis is on proximal weakness but in others more distal involvement is noted. On occasions, the degree of weakness may be alarming and death may occur in early childhood from cardiorespiratory failure. In one family all the affected members died within the neonatal period.[3] I have seen a similar patient dying in the neonatal period but without any family history of the illness. At other times the illness is milder and progresses only slowly or not at all.

Some reports[1, 2] indicate the presence of cerebral damage with an abnormal EEG and seizures, though whether this is part of the disease or due to some unrelated cause is not entirely clear. Most of the more recent reports have not shown evidence of such abnormal seizure activity.

The genetics of the illness vary. X-linked recessive inheritance has been described.[3, 4] In another family an autosomal dominant inheritance was found.[5] This family was slightly atypical clinically, and the muscle biopsy findings resembled Type 1 fiber hypotrophy with internal nuclei more than myotubular myopathy. An autosomal recessive pattern of inheritance has also been suggested. The occurrence of the illness in families provides an opportunity to study the muscle biopsy during the various stages of development of the illness, and a complex picture results. In families where the children have the very typical changes of myotubular myopathy, the adult members with the same disease may demonstrate only internal nuclei or the relatively infrequent occurrence of myotubes.[4] Similarly, asymptomatic carriers of the X-linked recessive variety have also shown abnormal changes with myotubes in the muscle. Two reviews of the literature on myotubular myopathy have been published and should be consulted.[6, 7]

TYPE 1 FIBER HYPOTROPHY WITH INTERNAL NUCLEI

This condition is often considered in the literature to be identical to myotubular myopathy, and it may indeed be related. It also has some features in common with congenital fiber type disproportion, differing pathologically in the presence of internal nuclei. It is not certain just how blurred the borderlines between these various illnesses will become. The original description of Type 1 fiber hypotrophy and internal nuclei stressed the association of internal nuclei with small Type 1 fibers in a boy who was born in respiratory distress with diffuse weakness and hypotonia.[8] The extraocular muscles and the facial muscle were not involved, and there was no ptosis. The child died at the age of eighteen months from respiratory complications. A second report documented a similar illness in the patient's brother, who died at the age of seven months.[9] The authors suggested that the pattern of inheritance was again that of an X-linked recessive disease. Karpati et al. reported a mother and daughter suffering from a very slowly progressive proximal weakness, probably beginning in childhood.[10] In another case in which the atrophy of Type 1 fibers was prominent, the patient, a girl, was floppy at birth, had delayed motor milestones, and had a predominantly distal distribution of weakness, particularly of the legs. She also developed a cardiomyopathy. Her brother had weakness of the anterior tibial and peroneal group of muscles, with bilateral pes cavus and diffuse areflexia.[11]

It is difficult to know what to make of these entities, if such they be. Perhaps there are various influences at work in the early stages of muscle development that may cause the central nuclei, myotube-like structures and abnormalities in the size and number of Type 1 fibers. We may be dealing with entirely separate diseases which are merely linked together because of the similar appearances of the muscle biopsy. Conversely it may be that the various illnesses at present described under different titles are artificially separated on the basis of essentially trivial differences in the muscle biopsy. Whatever the case, the common thread running through the fabric of so many of these congenital neuromuscular diseases seems to be Type 1 fiber predominance and atrophy.

BIBLIOGRAPHY

1. Spiro, A. J., Shy, G. M., and Gonatas, N. K. Myotubular myopathy. Arch. Neurol. *14:* 1–14, 1966.
2. Munsat, T. L., Thompson, L. R., and Coleman, R. F. Centronuclear (myotubular) myopathy. Arch. Neurol. *20:* 120–131, 1969.
3. Barth, P. G., Van Wijngaarden, G. K., and Bethlem, J. X-linked myotubular myopathy with fatal neonatal asphyxia. Neurology *25:* 531–536, 1975.
4. Van Wijngaarden, G. K., Fleury, T. Bethlem, J., and Meijer, A. E. F. H. Familial myotubular myopathy. Neurology *19:* 901–908, 1969.
5. McLeod, J. G., Baker, W. De C., Lethlean, A. K., and Shorey, C. D. Centronuclear myopathy with autosomal dominant inheritance. J. Neurol. Sci. *15:* 375–387, 1972.
6. Schochet, S. S., Zellweger, H., Ionasescu, V., and McCormick, W. F. Centronuclear myopathy; disease entity or syndrome. J. Neurol. Sci. *16:* 215–228, 1972.
7. Vital, C. Vallat, J.-M., Martin, F., Le Blanc, M., and Bergouignan, M. Étude clinique et ultrastructurale d'un cas de myopathie centronucléaire (myotubular myopathy) de l'adulte. Rev. Neurol. (Paris) *123:* 117–130, 1970.
8. Engel, W. K., Gold, G. N., and Karpati, G. Type 1 fiber hypotrophy and central nuclei. Arch. Neurol. *18:* 435–444, 1968.
9. Meyers, K. R., Gollomb, H. M., Hansen, J. L., and McKusick, V. A. Familial neuromuscular disease with "myotubes." Clin. Genet. *5:* 327–337, 1974.
10. Karpati, G., Carpenter, S., and Nelson, R. F. Type I muscle fiber atrophy and central nuclei; a rare familial neuromuscular disease. J. Neurol. Sci. *10:* 489–500, 1970.
11. Bethlem, J., Van Wijngaarden, G. K., Meijer, A. E. F. H., and Hulamann, W. C. Neuromuscular disease with Type 1 fiber atrophy; central nuclei and myotube-like structures. Neurology *19:* 705–710, 1969.

OTHER DISEASES

Some other neuromuscular diseases have been characterized by unusual changes within the muscles. This would include multicore disease, sarcotubular myopathy, reducing body myopathy, and myopathy with tubular aggregates. The number of case reports of these entities is so small that it is difficult to derive a general impression of the diseases. Furthermore, some of the changes which are used to characterize the illnesses may in fact be nonspecific.

Multicore Disease

Two cases of a benign, congenital and nonprogressive muscle disease were described by Engel et al.[1] Several muscle biopsies were obtained and revealed small focal areas of degeneration within the fibers. These bore some resemblance to the change seen in central core disease, but the abnormality extended over only a few sarcomeres rather than occupying large parts of the length of the fiber. As in central core disease, the abnormal areas showed a decrease in the number of mitochondria and some disorganization of sarcomere structure beginning in the Z disc.

The patients, who were unrelated, had a lifelong history of weakness and their early motor development was retarded. The weakness affected the limbs and trunk; in one patient it was diffuse, whereas in the other proximal muscles were more severely involved than distal and the shoulders were weaker than the legs. Deep tendon reflexes were decreased and the remainder of the laboratory results were not remarkable. In addition to the "multicores" the biopsy also demonstrated Type 1 fiber predominance, a common finding in congenital hypotonic patients.

Sarcotubular Myopathy

Another nonprogressive form of weakness was characterized by Jerusalem et al.[2] Two sons of consanguineous parents suffered from this illness. In both, the attainment of motor milestones was slightly delayed and, when the patients walked or ran, they were noted to be clumsy and awkward. Both demonstrated mild weakness of the neck flexors and of the proximal muscles of all the extremities. There was some weakness of the facial muscles in one patient, and the other was noted to have anterior tibial muscle weakness. Mental development was normal in both cases. The routine laboratory studies showed no specific abnormality; only the muscle biopsy was unusual. Abnormal spaces were found in the fibers. Ultrastructural studies including the use of markers for the membranes of the T system and of the sarcoplasmic reticulum showed that the spaces were probably derived from the membranes of the sarcotubular system (sarcoplasmic reticulum and T system). The limiting membranes of these spaces were reactive for the SR associated ATPase, and the peroxidase labeled T tubules were also closely associated with these spaces.

Fingerprint Myopathy

Another nonprogressive, congenital disease characterized by generalized weakness and hypotonia since infancy occurred in a 5 year old girl. The bulbar muscles and the extraocular muscles were spared, and there was no muscle wasting. Deep tendon reflexes were decreased and a static tremor of the arms was noticed. Intelligence was slightly below the normal level. Most of the laboratory tests were within normal limits. The muscle biopsy showed abnormal inclusions within the muscle fibers which were often subsarcolemmal. With electron microscopy, their structure appeared to be a series of concentric lamellae arranged in spiral fashion and bearing a remarkable resemblance to the pattern of a fingerprint.[3] The muscle biopsy also revealed small Type 1 fibers and hypertrophied Type 2 fibers, showing some similarity to congenital fiber type disproportion. Since this description, fingerprint bodies have also been found in myotonic dystrophy, dermatomyositis, and various other conditions.[4-6]

Reducing Body Myopathy

Two unrelated patients with a progressive and fatal disease were described whose muscle biopsies were characterized by the presence of numerous inclusion bodies within the fibers. These had a unique characteristic in that they could be demonstrated by histochemical reactions for sulfhydryl groups.[7] Both of these children showed hypotonia very early in life and the motor milestones were retarded. The weakness was progressive and involved both proximal and distal muscles. In one patient, ptosis and facial weakness were noted. Both children died from cardiorespiratory failure. Contracture of the muscles was a prominent feature of one case. A third case with onset at about the age of four years also showed a progressive course.[8] Other substances were also present within the reducing bodies (RNA and glycogen), but the presence of sulfhydryl groups was striking enough to make the histochemical reaction a useful screening technique (Figure 10.15). A few structures resembling reducing bodies were also seen in a boy of 14 with a benign congenital myopathy, although there were differences in the ultrastructure of these bodies compared to the ones described above.[9] Additionally, this latter case showed marked Type 1 fiber predominance and was quite similar to the congenital hypotonia with Type 1 predominance.

Myopathy with Tubular Aggregates

The tubular aggregate is a pathological change in which compact collections of tubules replace part of the muscle fiber. They are visible as tubules only under the electron microscope since they have a diameter of 500 to 600 Å. With the histochemical reaction at the light microscopic level they are easily recognized as intensely blue staining areas with some of the oxidative enzyme reactions (Figure 10.16). They have been seen in many different diseases, such as the periodic paralyses, and it has also been suggested that the change may be associated with toxins or medications.[10] Morgan-Hughes and associates described this change as the characteristic finding in a 60 year old man who experienced pain and stiffness in the muscles, particularly in the leg, after exercise. Over a six year period his exercise tolerance had decreased

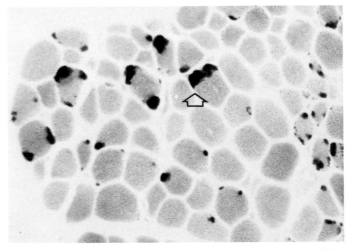

Figure 10.15. Reducing body myopathy. With this stain for reducing substances the abnormal structures are intensely staining (*arrow*) (direct nitro Blue Tetrazolium (NBT) stain).

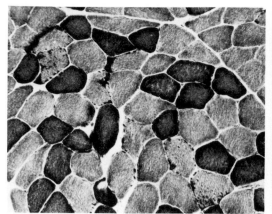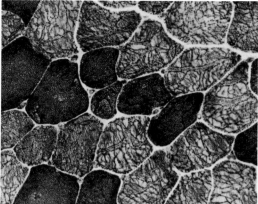

Figure 10.16 *(left)*. Myopathy with tubular aggregates. A forty-five year old man had a history of muscle pains for three years prior to the biopsy. He had taken aspirin to relieve his discomfort but had not been taking any other medications. The tubular aggregates can be seen as dark staining areas scattered throughout the muscle biopsy (NADH-tetrazolium reductase).

Figure 10.17 *(right)*. In a patient whose only complaint was "toe walking", the oxidative enzyme reaction revealed an abnormal "stranded" appearance to the muscle fibers particularly of the Type 2 fibers. The electron microscopy did not reveal any marked abnormality (NADH tetrazolium reductase).

until he was able to walk only half a mile on level ground or two to three minutes uphill. The pain and stiffness would then become severe and could persist for twenty-four hours or more following the exercise. He had been treated previously for depression and was taking diazepam and nialamide. There were no abnormal laboratory tests other than the muscle biopsy and the ischemic exercise test was normal.[11] Additional case reports, especially of patients who are not receiving any medication, will be needed before this entity can be defined more exactly. One patient with an identical history had the same findings of tubular aggregates in his muscle biopsy (Figure 10.16). He had been taking aspirin on an average of twice daily but had not taken any medication for 5 weeks prior to the biopsy.

"Toe Walkers"

A child who walks with the ball of the foot hitting the ground first rather than the heel may have some serious illness such as Duchenne's dystrophy, in which case the toe walking is no more than part of a spectrum of signs and symptoms. Occasionally children present with this as the only complaint. In the majority no diagnosis is ever made, passive stretching exercises are prescribed, and the child seems to recover, either because of or in spite of the physical therapy.

Sometimes the condition is familial as illustrated by the following example. A three year old girl was referred to the clinic because she was "stiff." Apart from a very slight hip waddle she usually walked in a normal fashion but on occasion, and particularly when excited, she would walk on her toes. She tired rather easily but she was able to run and keep up with the other children in a normal fashion. There was no other neuromuscular symptom in her history and her motor development had been quite normal. Eleven relatives in four generations had the same symptom including her father. The disease was inherited as an autosomal dominant. On examination, she had mild weakness of the hips so that she steppcd up onto a stool with transient unilateral hand support and used bilateral hand support to stand from a squatting position. The deep tendon reflexes were slightly decreased. The strength in the arms appeared normal. The heel cords were tight and dorsiflexion of the foot was possible only to 90°.

Her father was also examined at the age of thirty-one. His only complaint had been that he felt some stiffness of his joints, particularly of the knees and ankles. He also tired more easily than most people. When arising from a very low chair, he occasionally had to use his hands for support but he was able to take part in athletics at high school without any problem. On examination, there was no detectable weakness but the heel cords were tight and dorsiflexion of the foot was not possible beyond 90°. Deep tendon reflexes were normal. The laboratory studies were all normal with the exception of the muscle biopsy which is illustrated (Figure 10.17). Both father and daughter had identical changes. The oxidative enzyme reactions showed a lacy distortion of the intermyofibrillar network pattern which is, in my experience, unique. Electron microscopic examination of the tissue revealed no abnormality that we could detect, thereby compounding the mystery. The significance of these "lace fibers" remains in doubt.

BIBLIOGRAPHY

1. Engel, A. G., Gomez, M. R., and Groover, R. V. Multicore disease; a recently recognized congenital myopathy associated with multifocal degeneration of muscle fibers. Mayo Clin. Proc. *46:* 666–681, 1971.
2. Jerusalem, F., Engel, A. G., and Gomez, M. R. Sarcotubular myopathy. Neurology *23:* 897–906, 1973.
3. Engel, A. G., Angelini, C., and Gomez, M. R. Fingerprint body myopathy; a newly recognized congenital muscle disease. Mayo Clin. Proc. *47:* 377–388, 1972.
4. Tomé, F. H. S. and Fardeau, M. Fingerprint inclusions in muscle fibers in dystrophia myotonica. Acta Neuropathol. *24:* 62–67, 1973.
5. Carpenter, S., Karpati, G., Eisen, A, Andermann, F., and Watters, G. Childhood dermatomyositis and familial collagen disease. Neurology *22:* 425, 1972.
6. Sengel, A. and Stoebner, P. Une Inclusion Musculaire Atypique Rare: Les "Corps en Empreintes Digitales" ou "Fingerprint Bodies." Acta Neuropathol. *27:* 61–68, 1974.
7. Brooke, M. H. and Neville, H. E. Reducing body myopathy. Neurology *22:* 829–840, 1972.
8. Dubowitz, V. and Brooke, M. H. *Muscle Biopsy: A Modern Approach.* W. B. Saunders, London, 1973, p. 351.
9. Tomé, F. H. S. and Fardeau, M. Congenital myopathy with "reducing bodies" in muscle fibers. Acta Neuropathol. *31:* 207–217, 1975.
10. Engel, W. K., Bishop, D. W., and Cunningham, G. G. Tubular aggregates in Type II muscle fibers; ultrastructural and histochemical correlation. J. Ultrastruc. Res. *31:* 507–525, 1970.
11. Morgan-Hughes, J. A., Mair, W. G. P., and Lascelles, P. T. A disorder of skeletal muscle associated with tubular aggregates. Brain *93:* 873–880, 1970.

INDEX